McGraw-Hill's
EMT-Basic Exam Review

Third Edition

Peter A. DiPrima, Jr., CCEMT-P
EMS Instructor, Suffolk County
Paramedic/Firefighter
Lakeland Fire Department
Suffolk County, New York

McGraw Hill Education

New York   Chicago   San Francisco   Athens   London   Madrid   Mexico City
Milan   New Delhi   Singapore   Sydney   Toronto

McGraw-Hill's EMT-Basic Exam Review, Third Edition

1 2 3 4 5 6 7 8 9 0 RMN/RMN 20 19 18 17 16 15

ISBN 978-0-07-184719-3
MHID 0-07-184719-7

Notice

Medicine is an ever-changing science. As new research and clinical experience broaden our knowledge, changes in treatment and drug therapy are required. The authors and the publisher of this work have checked with sources believed to be reliable in their efforts to provide information that is complete and generally in accord with the standards accepted at the time of publication. However, in view of the possibility of human error or changes in medical sciences, neither the authors nor the publisher nor any other party who has been involved in the preparation or publication of this work warrants that the information contained herein is in every respect accurate or complete, and they disclaim all responsibility for any errors or omissions or for the results obtained from use of the information contained in this work. Readers are encouraged to confirm the information contained herein with other sources. For example and in particular, readers are advised to check the product information sheet included in the package of each drug they plan to administer to be certain that the information contained in this work is accurate and that changes have not been made in the recommended dose or in the contraindications for administration. This recommendation is of particular importance in connection with new or infrequently used drugs.

This book was set in Minion Pro by Cenveo® Publisher Services.
The editors were Andrew Moyer and Christina Thomas
The production supervisor was Richard Ruzycka.
Project management was provided by Anubhooti Saxena, Cenveo Publisher Services.
RR Donnelley/Menasha was printer and binder.

This book is printed on acid-free paper.

Library of Congress Cataloging-in-Publication Data

DiPrima, Peter A., Jr., author.
    [McGraw-Hill's EMT-basic]
  McGraw-Hill Education's EMT-basic exam review / Peter A. DiPrima Jr. — Third edition.
        p. ; cm.
    EMT-basic exam review
    Emergency medical technician-basic exam review
    Preceded by McGraw-Hill's EMT-basic / Peter A. DiPrima Jr., George P. Benedetto Jr. Second edition. 2011.
    Includes bibliographical references and index.
    ISBN 978-0-07-184719-3 (pbk. : alk. paper)
    ISBN 0-07-184719-7 (pbk.: alk. paper)   I. Title.   II. Title: EMT-basic exam review.
  III. Title: Emergency medical technician-basic exam review.
    [DNLM: 1. Examination Questions—United States.   2. Emergency Medical Services—United States.   3. Emergencies—United States. 4. Emergency Medical Technicians—United States.   5. Emergency Treatment—United States. WB 18.2]
    RC86.7
    616.02'5—dc23
                                                                                    2015007750

McGraw-Hill Education books are available at special quantity discounts to use as premiums and sales promotions, or for use in corporate training programs. To contact a representative please visit the Contact Us pages at www.mhprofessional.com.

To my wife, Sue, and our children, Gabrielle and Jack, thank you for being there, with love.

PAD

McGraw-Hill's
EMT-Basic Exam
Review

CONTENTS

Preface   ix
Exam Preparation Tips   xi

Section 1: Preparatory 1
Chapter 1:   Introduction to EMS Systems   3
Chapter 2:   Workforce Safety and Wellness   11
Chapter 3:   EMS Communication and Documentation   15
Chapter 4:   Medical, Legal, and Ethical Issues in EMS   26
Chapter 5:   The Human Body   35
Chapter 6:   Life Span Development   47

Section 2: Pharmacology 59
Chapter 7:   General Pharmacology   61

Section 3: Patient Assessment 73
Chapter 8:   Patient Assessment   75

Section 4: Airway 93
Chapter 9:   Airway Management, Ventilation, and Oxygen Therapy   95

Section 5: Medical Emergencies 113
Chapter 10: Respiratory Emergencies   115
Chapter 11: Cardiovascular and Hematological Emergencies   126
Chapter 12: Neurological Emergencies: Stroke, Seizures, and Syncope   141
Chapter 13: Immunological Emergencies   153
Chapter 14: Toxicological Emergencies   158
Chapter 15: Abdominal and Gastrointestinal Emergencies   169
Chapter 16: Infectious Diseases and Personal Protection   175
Chapter 17: Altered Mental Status and Diabetic Emergencies   181
Chapter 18: Psychiatric Emergencies   189
Chapter 19: Genitourinary and Renal Emergencies   197
Chapter 20: Gynecological Emergencies   207

Section 6: Shock 213
Chapter 21: Bleeding and Shock   215
Chapter 22: Mechanism of Injury, Kinematics of Trauma   226

Chapter 23: Soft Tissue Injuries　233

Chapter 24: Head, Face, Neck, and Spine Injuries　238

Chapter 25: Chest Trauma　254

Chapter 26: Abdominal and Genitourinary Trauma　259

Chapter 27: Orthopedic Trauma　263

Chapter 28: Environmental Emergencies　267

Section 7: Special Patient Populations..279

Chapter 29: Obstetric and Neonatal Emergencies　281

Chapter 30: Infants and Children　293

Chapter 31: Assessment of the Geriatric Patient　308

Chapter 32: Patients With Special Challenges　318

Section 8: EMS Operations...333

Chapter 33: Lifting and Moving Patients　335

Chapter 34: Ambulance Operations　341

Chapter 35: Gaining Access and Extrication　348

Chapter 36: Incident Management　350

Chapter 37: Response to Hazardous Materials and Terrorism　358

End of Book Crosswords...381

End of Chapter Answers...391

Index　399

PREFACE

The emergency medical technician (EMT) performs a very unique service at the scene of an emergency, which cannot be rendered by any other emergency services profession. The concept of the team approach is important in responding to emergencies in the pre-hospital environment. Each health-care professional must not only perform the duties of his or her own role, but must understand the roles of other professionals involved. Everyone must work together in a coordinated and efficient manner to achieve optimal results for patient survival.

This review book is a complete resource for EMT training, which contains reader-friendly step-by-step explanations with comprehensive, stimulating, and challenging material that prepares and equips users for real on-the-job situations. With its use of the case study model, and the inclusion of areas above and beyond the National Educational Standards, this new, third edition of *McGraw-Hill's EMT* prepares users for success. Topics covered include an excellent introductory section that contains an overview of the human body, baseline vital signs, history taking, and ethical and legal issues. Subsequent chapters cover the airway; patient assessment; medical, behavioral, and obstetrics/gynecology; trauma; infants and children; operations; and advanced airway management. In addition, we have added a robust practice examination at the end of the book, which will assist the new or seasoned EMT in studying for their local state or national registry examination.

A free practice examination is also available online to help you prepare for examination day. Visit www.mcgrawhillemt.com to take the test and assess your results.

The review book also provides the theory adapted by the American Heart Association, Guidelines for Cardiopulmonary Resuscitation and Emergency Cardiovascular Care, the National Education Standards, the National Incident Management System, and updated hazardous materials' information for the first responder.

I hope you enjoy utilizing this book as an adjunct learning tool. Be safe!

Peter A. DiPrima, Jr., EMT-P

Examination Preparation Tips

Start studying now! Give yourself ample time to prepare by arranging your notes and making sure you have covered all the required course material. Organize all information that was given to you during your course—this includes textbooks, lecture notes, handouts, and the like.

ANATOMY OF A MULTIPLE-CHOICE QUESTION

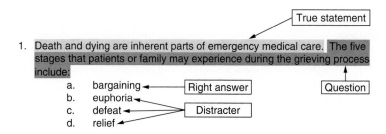

The Do's and Don'ts of Answering Multiple-Choice Questions

Do's

- If the question is "theoretical" carefully read and understand the stem of the question before looking at the alternatives. Circle or underline key words in the stem. Use your knowledge of headings to think about where in your text, lecture notes, etc that question is drawn from. Recall a few relevant points about the information. This does not have to take much time, but this recall is an essential step!

- Predict an answer, if possible.

- Uncover all of the alternatives and check the format of the question. Is one of the alternatives correct or can several or all of the alternatives be correct?

- Read each alternative carefully for understanding. Pay careful attention to qualifying words. Keeping the stem of the question in mind, respond to each alternative with a yes, no, or maybe/not sure.

- If you know the answer, carefully mark the correct answer on your answer sheet.

- If you do not know the answer, recheck the stem of the question. Narrow your choices, by eliminating any alternative that you know is incorrect. If two options still look equally tempting, compare each to the stem of the question, making sure that the one you eventually choose answers what is asked.

- If you are still not sure, make an educated guess.

- If you were unable to make a choice and need to spend more time with the question, or you answered the question but are not at all sure that you made the correct choice, put a big question mark beside that question, and move on to the next. Avoid getting bogged down on one question part of the way through the examination. It is much better to move on and finish all of those questions that you can answer and then to come back later to process the problematic questions. If necessary, when looking over the questions again, change an answer *only* if you can logically justify the change.

Don'ts

- Don't select an alternative just because you remember learning the information in the course; it may be a "true" statement in its own right, but you have to make sure that it is the "correct" answer to the question.
- Don't pick an answer just because it seems to make sense.
- Don't dismiss an alternative answer because it seems too obvious and simple.
- Don't be wowed by fancy terms in the question.
- Don't pick "c" every time you are unsure of the answer.
- Don't pick your answer based on a pattern of responses.

PHYSICAL PREPARATION

It is crucial to know the material to pass the examination, but it is equally important to be prepared physically as well. Physical preparation includes staying healthy, getting adequate sleep, eating balanced meals, and exercising regularly. Reward yourself after a successful study session.

Finally, keep anxiety in check! Stretch, breathe deeply, breathe often, take frequent short breaks, and stay positive.

McGraw-Hill's
EMT-Basic Exam
Review

Section 1

Preparatory

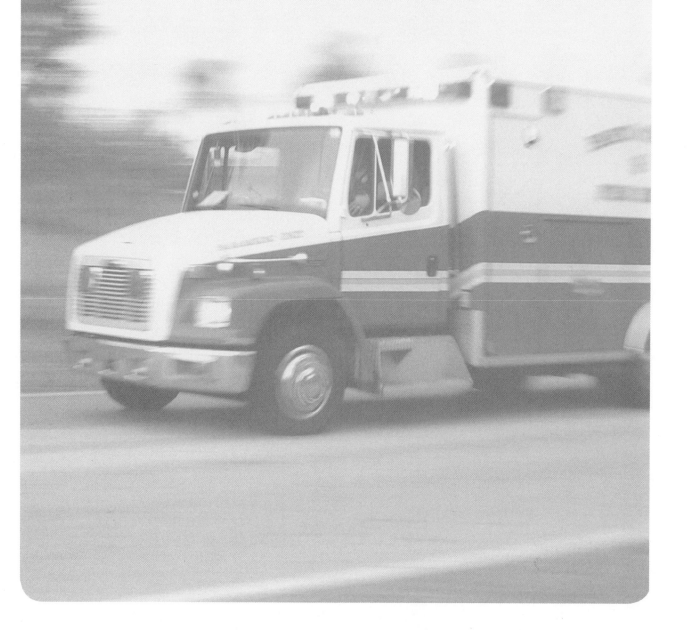

Chapter 1
Introduction to EMS Systems

It is 5 AM on an already hot summer morning. An elderly woman wakes up to start her day. She rolls over to attempt to wake her husband who is due to go out for some early golf with his friends. She attempts to wake him, with no response. She nervously begins to shake him and yell his name, no response. She notices his face is cyanotic (blue) and he is not breathing, she yells for help and runs across the room to find the bedroom phone. She dials 911 frantically and begins giving the 911 operator her address and phone number. The emergency medical services (EMS) operator ascertains the medical complaint and prioritizes the assignment. A first-responder unit and a basic and advanced life support unit are dispatched for a priority assignment, "Elderly Male Unconscious, Not Breathing." The elderly woman is asked to stay on the phone and begin resuscitation efforts through the direction of the emergency medical dispatcher.

EARLY HISTORY OF EMERGENCY MEDICAL SERVICES

Throughout the evolution of paramedicine, there has been an ongoing association with military conflict. One of the first indications of a formal process for managing injured people dates from the Imperial Legions of Rome, where aging Centurions, no longer able to fight, were tasked with organizing the removal of the wounded from the battlefield and providing some form of care. Such individuals, although not physicians, were probably among the world's earliest surgeons, suturing wounds and completing amputations, not through training, but by default. This trend would continue throughout the Crusades, with the Knights Hospitallers of the Order of St. John of Jerusalem, known throughout the Commonwealth of Nations today as St. John Ambulance, filling a similar function.

The first vehicle that was specifically designed as an ambulance was created during the Napoleonic War, and called the *ambulance volante*. Created by Napoleon's Chief Surgeon, Baron Dominique Jean Larrey, this new horse-drawn contrivance was intended to transport the wounded rapidly to surgeons waiting at the rear. Such vehicles were seen by the military as a general resource, and care of the wounded was not given much priority; it was not uncommon for such vehicles to be tasked with carrying fresh ammunition to the battlefront before they transported the wounded back. The basic design of such vehicles remained unchanged for nearly 100 years.

Early Civilian Ambulance Services

While communities had organized to deal with the care and transportation of the sick and dying as far back as the plague in London, England (1598, 1665), such arrangements were typically temporary. In time, however, such arrangements began to formalize and become permanent. During the American Civil War, Jonathan Letterman devised a system of forward first-aid stations at the regimental level, where principles of triage were first instituted. Letterman, with the rank of major, served as the medical director of the Army of the Potomac. The US Army had reeled from inefficient treatment of casualties, in part because of the adoption of new firearm technology such as breech-loading rifles and Minié ball systems. Letterman established mobile field hospitals to be located at division and corps headquarters. This was all connected by an efficient ambulance corps, established by him in August 1862, under the control of medical staff instead of the Quartermaster Department. He also arranged an efficient system for the distribution of medical supplies. His system was adopted by other Union armies and was eventually officially established as the medical procedure for the entirety of the United States' armies by an Act of Congress in March 1864.

Following the American Civil War, some veterans began to attempt to apply what they had seen on the battlefield to their own communities, through the creation of volunteer life-saving squads and ambulance corps. This translation to civilian use did not occur in the same way everywhere; in Britain, early civilian ambulances were often operated by the local hospital or police, while in some parts of Canada, it was common for the local undertaker (having the only transport in town in which one could lie down) to operate both the local furniture store (making coffins as a sideline) and the local ambulance service. In larger centers in various countries, such services might fall to the local Health Department, Police, Fire Department, or some combination of all of the above. Once again, the civilian model followed the lead of the military; although there were a handful of motorized ambulances just prior to the First World War (1914-1918), the concept of motorized ambulances was proven first on the battlefield, and spread rapidly to civilian systems immediately following the war.

There is some debate as to when the first formal training of "ambulance attendants" began. The generally accepted belief is that this occurred at Roanoke, Virginia, with the Roanoke Life Saving and First Aid Crew, under Julian Stanley Wise, in 1928. While this may have been true of the United States, Canadian records indicate the members of the Toronto Police Ambulance Service received a mandatory 5 days of training, conducted by St. John, as early as 1889, and well-developed printed manuals, clearly beyond the scope of simple first aid, were present in England even earlier. In terms of advanced skills, it is known that, once again, the military led the way. During the Second World War (1939-1945) and the Korean Conflict, battlefield "medics" were administering painkilling narcotics by injection, as emergency procedures, and "pharmacists'" mates on warships without physicians were permitted to do even more. Korea also marked the first widespread use of helicopters to evacuate the wounded from forward positions to medical units, coining the phrase "medevac." These innovations would not find their way into the civilian sphere for nearly 20 more years.

PRE-HOSPITAL MEDICINE

By the early 1960s, experiments in improving care had begun in some civilian centers. The first such experiment involved the provision of pre-hospital cardiac care by physicians in Belfast, Northern Ireland in 1966. This was repeated in Toronto, Canada in 1968, using a single ambulance called Cardiac One, staffed by a regular ambulance crew, plus a hospital intern, who was tasked with performing the advanced procedures. While both of these experiments had certain levels of success, technology had not yet reached the required level (the Toronto "portable" defibrillator/heart monitor was powered by lead-acid car batteries and weighed nearly 100 lb). The required telemetry and miniaturization technologies already existed in the military, and particularly in the space program, but it would take several more years before they found their way to civilian applications. In North America, physicians were judged to be too expensive to be used in the pre-hospital setting, although such initiatives were implemented, and in some cases still operate, in the United Kingdom, Europe, and Latin America.

Around 1966, in a published report entitled "Accidental Death and Disability: The Neglected Disease of Modern Society," (known in EMS trade as the "White Paper") medical researchers began to reveal, to their astonishment, that soldiers who were seriously wounded on the battlefields of Vietnam had a better survival rate than those individuals who were seriously injured in motor vehicle accidents on California freeways. Early research attributed these differences in outcome to a number of factors, including comprehensive trauma care, rapid transport to designated trauma facilities, and a new type of medical corpsman, one who was trained to perform certain critical advanced medical procedures such as fluid replacement and airway management, which allowed the victim to survive the journey to definitive care. As a result, a series of grand experiments began in the United States. Almost simultaneously, and completely independent from one another, experimental programs began in a handful of US centers: Miami, Florida, Seattle, Washington, Los Angeles, and California. The first of these to go from being an experiment to being a working unit was in Los Angeles. With the passage of the Wedsworth-Townsend Act, other states would soon push their own paramedic bills through, and soon, every fire department in every major city in the country had their own paramedic squads. Each was aimed at determining the effectiveness of using firefighters to perform many of these same advanced medical skills in the pre-hospital setting in the civilian world. Many in the senior administration of the fire departments were initially quite opposed to this concept of "firemen giving needles," and actively resisted and attempted to cancel pilot programs more than once.

THE PUBLIC DISCOVERS "EMS AND PARAMEDICINE"

In a curious example of life-imitating art, television producer Robert A. Cinader, working for producer Jack Webb of *Dragnet* and *Adam-12*, happened to be in Los Angeles' UCLA Harbor Medical Center, doing background research for a proposed new TV show about doctors, when he happened to encounter these "firemen who spoke like doctors and worked with them." This novel idea would eventually evolve into the *Emergency!* television series, which ran from 1972 to 1977, portraying the exploits of a new group called "paramedics." The show captured the imagination of emergency services personnel, the medical community, and the general public. When the show first aired in 1972, there were exactly six paramedic units operating in three pilot programs in the entire United States. No one had ever heard the term "paramedic"; it is reported that one of the show's actors was initially concerned that the "para" part of the term might involve jumping out of airplanes. By the time the program ended production in 1977, there were paramedics operating in every state. The show's technical advisor was a pioneer of paramedicine, James O. Page, then a Battalion Chief responsible for the paramedic program, but who would go on to help establish other paramedic programs in the United States, and to become the founding publisher of the *Journal of Emergency Medical Services* (JEMS).

Evolution and Growth

Throughout the 1970s and 1980s, the field continued to evolve, although in large measure on a local level. In the broader scheme of things, the term *ambulance service* was replaced by *emergency medical service* in order to reflect the change from a transportation system to a system which provided actual medical care. The training, knowledge base, and skill sets of both paramedics and emergency medical technicians (both competed for the job title, and "EMT-Paramedic" was a common compromise) were typically determined by what local medical directors were comfortable with, what it was felt that the community needed, and what could actually be afforded. There were also tremendous local differences in the amount and type of training required, and how it would be provided. This ranged from in-service training in local systems, through community colleges, and ultimately even to universities. In the United States, the community college training model remains the most common, although university-based paramedic education models continue to evolve. These variations in both educational approaches and standards led to tremendous differences from one location to another and, at its worst, created a situation in which a group of people with 120 hours of training, and another group (in another jurisdiction) with university degrees, were both calling themselves paramedics, there were some efforts made to resolve these discrepancies. The National Association of Emergency Medical Technicians (NAEMT) along with National Registry of Emergency Medical Technicians (NREMT) attempted to create a national standard by means of a common licensing examination, but to this day, this has never been universally accepted by all states, and issues of licensing reciprocity for paramedics continue. Nevertheless, if an EMT obtains certification through NREMT (NREMT-P, NREMT-I, NREMT-B), this is accepted by 40 of the 50 states in the United States. This confusion was further complicated by the introduction of complex systems of gradation of certification, reflecting levels of training and skill, but these too were for the most part purely local. The only truly common trend that would evolve was the relatively universal acceptance of the term Emergency Medical Technician being used to denote a lower level of training and skill than a Paramedic. In the United Kingdom, paramedics are being developed further, so a basic qualification of a paramedic is a foundation degree or diploma at university. Paramedics in the United Kingdom can now develop further into "Emergency Care Practitioner" and "Critical Care Practitioner," providing extra clinical skills to their patients.

During the evolution of paramedicine, a great deal of both curriculum and skill set was in a state of constant flux. Permissible skills evolved in many cases at the local level, and were based on the preferences of physician advisers and medical directors. Treatments would go in and out of fashion, and sometimes back in again. In some respects, the development seemed almost faddish. Technologies also evolved and changed, and as medical equipment manufacturers quickly learned, the pre-hospital environment was not the same as the hospital environment; equipment standards which worked fine in hospitals could not cope well with the less controlled pre-hospital environment. Physicians began to take more interest in paramedics from a research perspective as well. By about 1990, most of the trends in pre-hospital emergency care had begun to disappear, and was replaced by outcome-based research, the gold standard for the rest of medicine. This research began to drive the evolution of the practice of both paramedics and the emergency physicians who oversaw their work; changes to procedures and protocols began to occur only after significant outcome-based research demonstrated their need. Such changes affected everything from simple procedures, such as cardiopulmonary resuscitation (CPR), to changes in drug protocols. As the profession of paramedicine grew, some of its members actually went on to become not just research participants, but researchers in their own right, with their own projects and journal publications.

Changes in procedures also included the manner in which the work of paramedics was overseen and managed. In the earliest days of the field, medical control and oversight was direct and immediate, with paramedics calling into a local hospital and receiving orders for every individual procedure or drug. This still occurs in some jurisdictions, but is becoming very rare. As physicians began to build a bond of trust with paramedics, and experience in working with them, their confidence levels also rose. Increasingly, in many jurisdictions, day-to-day operations moved from direct and immediate medical control to pre-written protocols or "standing orders," with the paramedic typically only calling in for direction after the options in the standing orders had been exhausted. Medical oversight became driven more by chart review or rounds, than by step-by-step control during each call.

EMS SYSTEM

- EMS over the past 30 years has changed considerably.
- As an essential part of the EMS system, EMTs are usually one of the first medical professionals encountered by patients.

What Is an EMS System?

- EMS is a network of coordinated medical services that provide support and medical care to a given community.
- National Highway Traffic Safety Administration (NHTSA) Technical Assistance Program Standards for EMS include:
  1. Integration of health services
  2. EMS research
  3. Legislation and regulation
  4. System finance
  5. Human resources
  6. Medical direction
  7. Education systems
  8. Public education
  9. Prevention
  10. Public access
  11. Communication systems
  12. Clinical care
  13. Information systems
  14. Evaluation

Components of an EMS System

The "911" system emergency telephone number is utilized to gain access to emergency services such as fire, police, and EMS. Access to the EMS includes:

- Activation by citizens
- Dispatch of resources

- Out-of-hospital care (pre-hospital care)
- Transition of care (transfer of care between pre-hospital and in-hospital health-care providers)
- In-hospital care
- Rehabilitation

In some regions a non-emergent telephone number has been instituted, such as 311 in New York City.

There are four national recognized levels of pre-hospital care. They include:

1. First Responder (minimal training for emergencies)
2. EMT-Basic
3. EMT-Intermediate
4. EMT-Paramedic (highest level of pre-hospital care)

In various states other levels of training are available (ie, EMT-Cardiac Care).

Clinical Significance

Review local and/or state emergency and nonemergency access phone numbers.

KEY COMPONENTS OF A HEALTH-CARE SYSTEM

Emergency department (ED).
- Specialty facilities such as:
  - Trauma centers
  - Burn centers
  - Pediatric centers
  - Poison centers
  - Other specialty centers—locally dependent (ie, venomous bite center, hyperbaric center, cardiac centers, stroke centers, etc)
- Hospital personnel include:
  - Physicians
  - Nurses and other health professionals (physician assistant, respiratory therapist, nurse practitioners)

EMS personnel must be able to interact with other public safety workers, some examples include:

- Local law enforcement
- State and federal law enforcement
- Federal Emergency Management Agency (FEMA)—A division within the Department of Homeland Security
- Department of Homeland Security (DHS)

The roles and responsibilities of the EMT include:

- Personal safety (safety of crew, patient, and bystanders)
- Patient assessment
- Patient care based on assessment findings
- Lifting and moving patients safely
- Transport/transfer of care (transition of care)
- Record keeping/data collection
- Patient advocacy (protecting patient rights)

As an extension of the emergency department, EMTs are required to maintain professional attributes, such as:

- Neat and clean appearance
- A positive image
- Up-to-date knowledge and skills, which include continual medical education (CME), attending seminars, EMS regional updates
- Patient's needs prioritized without endangering self/crew
- Current knowledge of local, state, and national issues affecting EMS

Clinical Significance
EMS is an extension of the emergency department.

QUALITY IMPROVEMENT

Quality improvement (QI) is a system of internal/external reviews and audits of all aspects of an EMS system. QI is important to an EMS system to identify aspects needing improvement; this ensures that the public receives the highest quality of pre-hospital care. Our role as EMTs in quality improvement includes:

- Neat, legible, and accurate documentation
- Attending CME that includes run review and call audits
- Gathering feedback from patients and hospital staff
- Conducting preventive maintenance
- Maintaining mastery skills performance

Clinical Significance
The goal of quality improvement is to *improve* patient care, not to find fault.

ROLES OF THE SYSTEM MEDICAL DIRECTOR

The system medical director is a physician responsible for the clinical and patient care aspects of an EMS system or service.
- Every ambulance service/rescue squad must have physician medical direction. Types of medical direction include:
  - On-line (telephone, cell phone, satellite phone)
  - Radio (ultrahigh-frequency [UHF], very-high-frequency [VHF] radio)
  - Off-line (standing orders, protocols)
- The relationship of the EMT and the systems medical director:
  - An EMT is the designated agent of the physician.
  - Care rendered is considered an extension of the medical director's authority (varies by state law). The EMT should review specific statutes and regulations regarding EMS in their state regarding specific health laws.

The system medical director is directly responsible for reviewing quality improvement.

? CHAPTER QUESTIONS

1. One important responsibility of the EMT is *patient advocacy*. This means the emergency provider is responsible for:

   a. providing emergency medical care
   b. gaining access to the patient
   c. ensuring scene safety by wearing body substance isolation
   d. protecting the patient's rights

2. A physician who is legally responsible for the clinical and patient care rendered by an EMS system is known as the system's:

   a. system medical director
   b. clinical manager
   c. chief medical officer (CMO)
   d. none of the above

3. Quality improvement includes finding fault of an EMT who is producing illegible ambulance run reports.

   a. True
   b. False

Chapter 2
Workforce Safety and Wellness

In the previous chapter, you and your partner responded to an elderly man in cardiac arrest. Upon arrival at the scene you evaluate scene safety, and determine the scene is safe to operate. You and your partner enter the apartment to find an elderly woman hysterically crying, screaming, "why me!" She is frantically attempting to perform cardiopulmonary resuscitation (CPR). You evaluate the elderly patient and determine whether he meets the criteria for obvious death. The elderly woman, distraught and angry, starts yelling and screaming at you and your partner. What should your next step be?

The myth of saving lives . . .

Somewhere along the way, the myth of saving lives found its way into the EMS profession. There are indeed times when EMS saves lives, but even in large EMS systems, this is by no means a daily occurrence. The vast majority of EMS providers are called upon simply to take care of people in need. Sometimes those needs are met with a combination of advanced invasive procedures, sophisticated pharmacology, and technical expertise. Other times, what a patient may need is a caring attitude, a few kind words, or safe transportation to an extended-care facility. Between these two extremes lie many shades of gray. One measure of an outstanding EMS professional is the ability to perceive a patient's real needs and to meet them.[1]

EMOTIONAL ASPECTS OF EMERGENCY CARE

Emergency medical technicians (EMTs) encounter death more frequently than the average person. As health-care professionals, we have very little training in dealing with people's emotions when they have lost a friend or a family member. Dealing with a grieving family is quite difficult, and at times impossible. Therefore, understanding how to treat and react during these difficult times may allow us to better cope with survivors and their families.

The grieving process has five distinct or predictable stages. They are:

1. *Denial* ("Not me.")—Defense mechanism creating a buffer between shock of dying and dealing with the illness/injury.
2. *Anger* ("Why me?")—EMTs may be the target of the anger. Don't take anger or insults personally, be tolerant, and do not become defensive. Employ good listening and communication skills. Be empathetic.
3. *Bargaining* ("OK, but first let me . . .")—Agreement that, in the patient's mind, will postpone the death for a short time.
4. *Depression* ("OK, but I haven't . . .")—Characterized by sadness and despair. The patient is usually silent and retreats into his own world.

5. *Acceptance* ("OK, I am not afraid.")—Does not mean the patient will be happy about dying. The family will usually require more support during this stage than the patient.

Dealing with the needs of a dying patient and/or their family members includes performing the following:

- Show respect—Keep an open line of communication and allow the patient and family a means for privacy.
- Treat them with dignity by allowing them to feel in control.
- Family members may express rage, anger, and despair.
- Listen empathetically.
- Do not offer false reassurance.
- Use a gentle tone of voice.
- Let the patient know everything that can be done to help will be done.
- Use a reassuring touch, if appropriate.
- Comfort the family.
- Be respectful of religious beliefs and, when possible, honor requests of the family while adhering to regional or state protocols.

STRESS

In addition to responding to day-to-day assignments, EMTs encounter stressful situations while performing their duties. Examples of situations that may produce a stress response include:

- Mass casualty situations (ie, Oklahoma City bombing, September 11, Hurricane Katrina, Fort Hood Shooting, West Virginia mine explosion, etc)
- Infant and child trauma (ie, child struck by a car)
- Amputations
- Infant/child/elder/spouse abuse
- Death/injury of coworker or other public safety personnel

The EMT will experience personal stress as well as encounter patients and bystanders in severe distress. Therefore, understanding how to manage stress and stressful situations is paramount. Remember, what constitutes an emergency to others may not necessarily be an emergency to you; be respectful!

Stress Management

EMTs should recognize warning signs of stress:

- Irritability to coworkers, family, friends
- Inability to concentrate
- Difficulty sleeping/nightmares
- Anxiety
- Indecisiveness
- Guilt
- Loss of appetite
- Loss of interest in sexual activity
- Isolation
- Loss of interest in work

Keeping Stress Under Control

Reducing stress by making lifestyle changes is helpful for "burnout." Lifestyle changes include:

- Changing your diet
- Reducing sugar, caffeine, and alcohol intake
- Avoiding fatty foods
- Increasing carbohydrates
- Exercising regularly
- Practicing relaxation techniques, meditation, and visual imagery
- Balancing work, recreation, family, health, and the like

Work environment changes can reduce stress.

- Request work shifts allowing for more time to relax with family and friends.
- Request a rotation of duty assignment to a less busy area.
- Seek/refer professional help (employee assistance program [EAP]).

CRITICAL INCIDENT RESPONSE

Critical incident stress debriefing (CISD) or critical incident stress management (CISM) is a team of peer counselors and mental health professionals who help emergency care workers deal with critical incident stress.

A meeting is held within 24 to 72 hours of a major incident.

- Open discussion of feelings, fears, and reactions.
- Not an investigation or interrogation.
- All information is confidential.
- CISD leaders and mental health personnel evaluate the information and offer suggestions on overcoming the stress.

CISD/CISM is designed to accelerate the normal recovery process after experiencing a critical incident.

- Works well because feelings are vented quickly.
- Debriefing environment is nonthreatening.
- The EMT should review how to access their local CISD system.

Comprehensive critical incident stress management includes:

- Pre-incident stress education
- On-scene peer support
- One-on-one support
- Disaster support services
- Defusing
- CISD
- Follow-up services
- Spouse/family support
- Community outreach programs
- Other health and welfare programs such as EAP

? CHAPTER QUESTIONS

1. One of the five stages of death and dying is:

   a. relief
   b. bargaining
   c. elation
   d. overcoming

2. What stage of death or dying is characterized by sadness and despair? The patient is usually silent and retreats into his own world ("OK, but I haven't . . .").

   a. Depression
   b. Anger
   c. Despair
   d. Denial

Reference

1. American College of Emergency Physicians. In: Peter T, Pons MC, Cason D, eds. *Paramedic Field Care*. St. Louis, MO: Mosby-Year Book; 1997.

Chapter 3
EMS Communication and Documentation

Upon arriving at the scene of a patient in severe respiratory distress, you begin assessing the patient and determine the respiratory difficulty is secondary to being stung by a hornet. The patient is complaining of respiratory difficulty, urticaria, and angioedema, and the patient is describing a closing sensation of the throat. You and your partner decide the patient requires an intramuscular injection of epinephrine, and begin transport per local protocol. You contact medical control via cellular phone and give your presentation to the physician. The physician orders you to administer 0.3 mg of epinephrine IM using the Epipen. Your communication via cell phone for medication orders from the medical control physician are complete and the patient states the tightness feeling in the throat has subsided. This mode of communication is an example of what type of communication?

COMMUNICATION SYSTEM

System Components

- Base station—A radio which is located at a stationary site such as a hospital, mountaintop, or public safety agencies, tall building.
- Mobile two-way radios (transmitter/receivers).
  - Implies a vehicle-mounted device.
  - Mobile transmitters usually transmit at lower power than base stations (typically 20-50 W).
  - Typical transmission range is 10 to 15 mi over average terrain.
- Portable radios (transmitter/receivers).
  - Handheld device.
  - Typically has a power output of 1 to 5 W, limiting their range.
- Repeater/base station—Receives a transmission from a low-power portable or mobile radio on one frequency and retransmits at a higher power on another frequency.
- Digital radio equipment.
- Cellular telephones.

Radio Communications

- Radio frequencies are assigned and licensed by the Federal Communication Commission (FCC).

- Response to the scene.
  - The dispatcher needs to be notified that the call was received (acknowledgment of the assignment).
  - Dispatch needs to know that the unit is en route (response).
  - Other agencies, such as a local hospital, should be notified as appropriate.
  - Arrival at the scene—the dispatcher must be notified.

Communication With Medical Direction

- In some systems, medical direction is at the receiving facility, and in other systems, medical direction is at a separate site.
- In either case, the emergency medical technician (EMT) may need to contact medical direction for consultation, and to get orders for administration of medications. Radio transmissions need to be organized, concise, and pertinent.
- Since the physician will determine whether to order medications and procedures based on the information given by the EMT, information *must* be accurate.
- After receiving an order for a medication or procedure (or denial of such a request), repeat the order word for word.
- Orders that are unclear or appear to be inappropriate should be questioned.

Communication With Receiving Facilities

- EMTs provide information that allows hospitals to prepare for a patient's arrival by having the right room, equipment, and personnel prepared.

PATIENT REPORTING CONCEPTS

- When speaking on the radio, keep these principles in mind:
  - Radio is on and volume is properly adjusted.
  - Listen to the frequency and ensure it is clear before beginning a transmission.
  - Press the "press-to-talk" (PTT) button on the radio and wait for 1 second before speaking.
  - Speak with lips about 2 to 3 in from the microphone.
  - Address the unit being called, then give the name of the unit (and number if appropriate) where the transmission is originating from.
  - The unit being called will signal that the transmission should start by saying "go ahead" or some other term standard for that area. A response of "stand by" means wait until further notice.
  - Speak clearly and slowly, in a monotone voice.
  - Keep transmissions brief. If, on occasion, a transmission takes longer than 30 seconds, stop at that point and pause for a few seconds so that emergency traffic can use the frequency if necessary.
  - Use clear text.
  - Avoid codes.
  - Avoid meaningless phrases like "be advised."

- Courtesy is assumed, so there is no need to say "please," "thank you," and "you're welcome."
- When transmitting a number that might be confused (eg, a number in the teens), give the number, then give the individual digits.
- The airwaves are public and scanners are popular. Emergency medical services (EMS) transmissions may be overheard by more than just the EMS community. Do not give a patient's name over the air.
- For the same reason, be careful to remain objective and impartial in describing patients. An EMT may be sued for slander if he injures someone's reputation in this way.
- An EMT rarely acts alone—Use *we* instead of *I.*
- Do not use profanity on the air. The FCC takes a dim view of such language and may impose substantial fines.
- Avoid words that are difficult to hear like *yes* and *no.* Use *affirmative* and *negative.*
- Use the standard format for transmission of information.
- When the transmission is finished, indicate this by saying *over.* Get confirmation that the message was received.
- Avoid codes, especially those that are not standardized.
- Avoid offering a diagnosis of the patient's problem.
- Use EMS frequencies only for EMS communication.
- Reduce background noise as much as possible by closing the window.
- Notify the dispatcher when the unit leaves the scene.
- When communicating with medical direction or the receiving facility, a verbal report should be given. The essential elements of such a report, in the order they should be given, are:
    — Identify unit and level of provider (who and what)
    — Estimated time of arrival
    — Patient's age and sex
    — Chief complaint
    — Brief, pertinent history of the present illness
    — Major past illnesses
    — Mental status
    — Baseline vital signs
    — Pertinent findings of the physical examination
    — Emergency medical care given
    — Response to emergency medical care
- After giving this information, the EMT will continue to assess the patient. Additional vital signs may be taken and new information may become available, particularly on long transports. In some systems, this information should be relayed to the hospital (refer to local protocol). Information that must be transmitted includes deterioration in the patient's condition.
- Arrival at the hospital.
  - The dispatcher must be notified.
  - In some systems, the hospital should also be notified.
- Leaving the hospital for the station—The dispatcher should be notified.
- Arrival at the station—The dispatcher should be notified.

Verbal Communication (Transition of Care)

- After arrival at the hospital, give a verbal report to the staff.
- Introduce the patient by name (if known).
- Summarize the information given over the radio:
  - Chief complaint
  - History that was not given previously
  - Additional treatment given en route
  - Additional vital signs taken en route
  - Give additional information that was collected but not transmitted.

Interpersonal Communication

- Make and keep eye contact with the patient.
- When practical, position yourself at a level lower than the patient.
- Be honest with the patient.
- Use language the patient can understand.
- Be aware of your own body language.
- Speak clearly, slowly, and distinctly.
- Use the patient's proper name, either first or last, depending on the circumstances. Ask the patient what he wishes to be called.
- If a patient has difficulty hearing, speak clearly with lips visible.
- Allow the patient enough time to answer a question before asking the next one.
- Act and speak in a calm, confident manner.

Common Communication Issues With Elderly Patients

- Potential for visual deficit
- Potential for auditory deficit

Documentation

You and your partner have just completed an assignment involving a pedestrian auto accident. Your partner has begun the clean-up process in the ambulance, and you are going to begin documenting the assignment. You sit down in the crew room at the hospital and begin the difficult task of documenting all subjective and objective information. You include the patient's name, address, social security number, and date of birth. What are some of the necessary documentation requirements needed to complete a thorough pre-hospital care report (PCR)?

DOCUMENTATION

- Minimum documentation requirements that should be on every ambulance call report (Fig. 3-1):
  - Information gathered at time of the EMT's arrival at scene, at initial contact with patient, following all interventions, and on arrival at facility:
    — Chief complaint

MMDDYY RUN NO 5- 2 AGENCY VEH ID

COPY

AGENCY NAME
DISPATCH INFORMATION
CALL LOCATION

LOCATION CODE
CODE

MILEAGE
END
BEGIN
TOTAL

CALL REC'D
ENROUTE
AT SCENE
FROM SCENE
AT DESTINATION
IN SERVICE
IN QUARTERS

PATIENT INFORMATION

FIRST NAME LAST NAME
ADDRESS
APPT/UNIT NUMBER (PHO) NE -
CITY ST ZIP - +4
AGE D.O.B. MM / DD / YYYY F M SS# - -

O Residence
O Health
O Farm
O Industrial
O Other Work
O Residence
O Road
O Other

Call Received as
O EMERGENCY
O NON EMERGENCY
O STANDBY

Physician

CARE IN PROGRESS ON ARRIVAL: O None O Citizen O PD/FD/Other First Responder O Other EMS O PAD used

MECHANISM OF INJURY
O MVA (✓ seat belt used ➞) O Fall of ____ feet O GSW O Machinery
O Struck by vehicle O Unarmed assault O Knife O ____
O Extrication required ____ minutes
Seat belt used? O Yes O No O Unknown
Seat Belt Use Reported By O Crew O Patient O Police O Other

CHIEF COMPLAINT

SUBJECTIVE ASSESSMENT

PRESENTING PROBLEM
Fill in circle

O Airway Obstruction
O Respiratory Arrest
O Respiratory Distress
O Cardiac Related (Potential)
O Cardiac Arrest
O Allergic Reaction
O Syncope
O Stroke/CVA
O General Illness/Malaise
O Gastro-Intestinal Distress
O Diabetic Related (Potential)
O Pain ____
O Unconscious/Unresp.
O Seizure
O Behavioral Disorder
O Substance Abuse (Potential)
O Poisoning (Accidental)
O Shock
O Head Injury
O Spinal Injury
O Fracture/Dislocation
O Amputation
O Other ____
O Major Trauma
O Trauma-Blunt
O Trauma-Penetrating
O Soft Tissue Injury
O Bleeding/Hemorrhage
O OB/GYN
O Burns
Environmental
O Heat
O Cold
O Hazardous Materials
O Obvious Death

PAST MEDICAL HISTORY
O None
O Allergy to ____
O Hypertension O Stroke
O Seizures O Diabetes
O COPD O Cardiac
O Other (List) O Asthma

Current Medications (List)

VITAL SIGNS

TIME	RESP	PULSE	B.P.	LEVEL OF CONSCIOUSNESS	GCS	R PUPILS L	SKIN	STATUS
	Rate: O Regular O Shallow O Labored	Rate: O Regular O Irregular		O Alert O Voice O Pain O Unresp.		O Normal O / O Dilated O / O Constricted O / O Sluggish O / O No-Reaction O	O Unremarkable O Cool O Pale O Warm O Cyanotic O Moist O Flushed O Dry O Jaundiced	O C O U O P O S
	Rate: O Regular O Shallow O Labored	Rate: O Regular O Irregular		O Alert O Voice O Pain O Unresp.		O Normal O / O Dilated O / O Constricted O / O Sluggish O / O No-Reaction O	O Unremarkable O Cool O Pale O Warm O Cyanotic O Moist O Flushed O Dry O Jaundiced	O C O U O P O S
	Rate: O Regular O Shallow O Labored	Rate: O Regular O Irregular		O Alert O Voice O Pain O Unresp.		O Normal O / O Dilated O / O Constricted O / O Sluggish O / O No-Reaction O	O Unremarkable O Cool O Pale O Warm O Cyanotic O Moist O Flushed O Dry O Jaundiced	O C O U O P O S

OBJECTIVE PHYSICAL ASSESSMENT

COMMENTS

TREATMENT GIVEN *FILL IN CIRCLE*

O Moved to ambulance on stretcher/backboard
O Moved to ambulance on stair chair
O Walked to ambulance
O Airway Cleared
O Oral/Nasal Airway
O Esophageal Obturator Airway/Esophageal Gastric Tube Airway (EOA/EGTA)
O EndoTracheal Tube (E/T)
O Oxygen Administered @ ____ L.P.M., Method ____
O Suction Used
O Artificial Ventilation Method ____
O C.P.R. in progress on arrival by: O Citizen O PD/FD/Other First Responder O Other
O C.P.R. Started @ Time ____ Time from Arrest Until C.P.R. ____ Minutes
O EKG Monitored (Attach Tracing) [Rhythm(s) ____]
O Defibrillation/Cardioversion No. Times ____ O Manual O Semi-automatic
O Medication Administered (Use Continuation Form)
O IV Established Fluid ____ Cath. Gauge ____
O Mast Inflated @ Time ____)
O Bleeding/ Hemorrhage Controlled (Method Used: ____)
O Spinal Immobilization Neck and Back
O Limb Immobilized by O Fixation O Traction
O (Heat) or (Cold) Applied
O Vomiting Induced @ Time ____ Method ____
O Restraints Applied, Type ____
O Baby Delivered @ Time ____ In County ____
O Alive O Stillborn O Male O Female
O Transported in Trendelenburg position
O Transported in left lateral recumbent position
O Transported with head elevated
O Other ____

DISPOSITION (See list) DISP. CODE CONTINUATION FORM USED YES

CREW
IN CHARGE O EMT O AEMT #
DRIVER'S NAME O CFR O EMT O AEMT #
NAME O CFR O EMT O AEMT #
NAME O CFR O EMT O AEMT #

AGENCY COPY
EMS 100 (11/86) provided by NYS-EMS PROGRAM
DOH 3283 (7/02)

Figure 3-1 New York state PCR document.

- — Level of consciousness (AVPU [alert, verbal, painful, unresponsive])
- — Mental status
- — Systolic blood pressure for patients greater than 3 years old
- — Skin perfusion (capillary refill) for patients less than 6 years old
- — Skin color and temperature
- — Pulse rate and quality
- — Respiratory rate and effort
  - Administrative information.
    - — Time incident was reported.
    - — Time unit was notified.
    - — Time of arrival at patient side.
    - — Time unit left scene.
    - — Time of arrival at destination.
    - — Time transfer of care occurred.

THE PRE-HOSPITAL CARE REPORT (LEGAL MEDICAL DOCUMENT)

- Functions as
  - Continuity of care (a form that is not read immediately in the emergency department may very well be referred to later for important treatment rendered by EMTs).
  - Legal document—A good report has documentation of what emergency medical care was provided, the status of the patient on arrival at the scene, and any changes upon arrival at the receiving facility. Information should include objective and subjective information.
    - — All documentation should be clear, concise, and legible.
  - Educational—Used to demonstrate proper documentation and how to handle unusual or uncommon cases.
  - Administrative—Used for billing and service statistical analysis for research.
  - Evaluation and continuous quality improvement.

Types of Ambulance Call Reports

- Traditional reports are written forms with check boxes and a section for a narrative.
- Computerized versions are filled in by means of an electronic clipboard or a similar device.
- Sections include date, times, service, unit, names of crew, patient data (patient's name, address, date of birth, insurance information, sex, age, nature of call, mechanism of injury, location of patient, treatment administered prior to arrival of EMT, signs and symptoms, care administered, baseline vital signs, SAMPLE [signs/symptoms, allergies, medications, past medical problems, last oral intake, events] history, and changes in condition).
- Check boxes should be filled in completely.
  - Avoid stray marks.
- Narrative section (if applicable):
  - Describe, don't conclude.

- Include pertinent negative/positive findings (**Pertinent negative:** absence of a sign or symptom that helps substantiate or identify a patient's condition).
- Record important observations about the scene, that is, suicide note, weapon, and the like.
- Avoid radio codes.
- Use abbreviations only if they are standard medical abbreviations.
- When information of a sensitive nature is documented, note the source of that information, for example, communicable diseases.
- State reporting requirements such as child abuse, animal bites, and the like.
- Be sure to spell words correctly, especially medical words. If you do not know how to spell it, find out or use another word.
- For every reassessment, record time and findings.
- Confidentiality—The ambulance call report and the information on the form are considered confidential. Be familiar with state laws.
- Distribution—Local/state protocols will determine where the different copies of the form should be distributed.
- Falsification issues.
  - When an error of omission or commission occurs, the EMT should not try to cover it up. Instead, document what did or did not happen and what steps were taken (if any) to correct the situation.
  - Falsification of information on the Pre-Hospital Care Report may lead not only to suspension or revocation of the EMT's certification/license, but also to poor patient care because other health-care providers have a false impression of which assessment findings were discovered or what treatment was given.
- Difficult documentation issues.
  - Vital signs—Document only the vital signs that were actually taken.
  - Treatment—If a treatment like oxygen was overlooked, do not chart that the patient was given oxygen.

DOCUMENTATION OF PATIENT REFUSAL

- Competent adult patients have the *right to refuse* treatment.
- Before the EMT leaves the scene, he/she should:
  - Try again to persuade the patient to go to a hospital.
  - Ensure the patient is able to make a rational, informed decision.
  - Inform the patient why he/she should go and what may happen to him if he does not.
  - Consult medical direction as directed by local protocol.
  - If the patient still refuses, document any assessment findings and emergency medical care given, and then have the patient sign a refusal form.
  - Have a family member, police officer, or bystander sign the form as a witness. If the patient refuses to sign the refusal form, have a family member, police officer, or bystander sign the form verifying that the patient refused to sign.
  - Complete the PCR for a patient refusal.
    — Complete patient assessment.

— Care EMT wished to provide for the patient.
— Statement that the EMT explained to the patient, the possible consequences of failure to accept care, including potential death.
— Offer alternative methods of gaining care.
— State willingness to return even if patient refuses treatment and transport.

SPECIAL SITUATIONS/REPORTS/INCIDENT REPORTING

Correction of Errors

- Draw a single horizontal line through the error, initial it, and write the correct information beside it.
- Do not try to obliterate the error—This may be interpreted as an attempt to cover up a mistake.

Errors Discovered After the Report Form Is Submitted

- Preferably in a different color ink, draw a single line through the error, initial, and date it and add a note with the correct information.
- If information was omitted, add a note with the correct information, the date, and the EMT's initials.

Documentation at Multiple Casualty Incidents

- When there is not enough time to complete the form before the next call, the EMT will need to fill out the report later.
- The local multiple casualty incident's (MCI) plan should have some means of recording important medical information temporarily, that is, triage tag that can be used later to complete the form.
- The standard for completing the form in an MCI is not the same as for a typical call. Your local plan should have guidelines.

Special Situation Reports

- Used to document events that should be reported to local authorities, or to amplify and supplement primary report (Fig. 3-2).
- Should be submitted in timely manner.
- Should be accurate and objective.
- The EMT should keep a copy for his/her own records.
- The report, and copies, if appropriate, should be submitted to the authority described by local protocol.
- Exposure.
- Injury.

CONTINUOUS QUALITY IMPROVEMENT

- Information gathered from the Pre-Hospital Care Report can be used to analyze various aspects of the EMS system.
- This information can then be used to improve different components of the system and prevent problems from occurring in the future.

Emergency Medical Services Agency
Unusual Occurrence Report
EMS-903

(Refer to The Back of This Form For Directions)

1. Incident Date/Time	2. Provider Agency Name	3. Event #	4. Reporting Date
5. Address or Location of Incident			
6. Person Reporting Incident			

7. Preferred Method of Contact	
Email:	Address:
Phone:	Fax:

8. Affiliation	9. Unit

10. Type of Incident

11. Incident Description: Be as specific as possible. Include names, addresses, times, dates, etc. Use separate sheets of paper if necessary.

12. Attachments YES/NO # of pages or documents_____

FOR EMS AGENCY USE	EMSA Incident #
Final Disposition:	Date received:
Reviewed By:	Date closed:

Figure 3-2   Emergency Medical Services Agency Unusual Occurrence Report (EMS-903). (*Reproduced with permission from http://www.sccgov.org/portal/site/ems/.*)

? CHAPTER QUESTIONS

1. In the emergency pre-hospital care communications system, a mobile transmitter/receiver:

   a. is a portable, hand-carried radio useful when working at a distance from your vehicle

   b. is a device that receives transmissions and rebroadcasts them at a higher power

   c. serves as a dispatch and coordination area

   d. is a vehicle-based radio which comes in a variety of power ranges

2. Components of an emergency communications system may include:

   a. cellular phones
   b. a base station
   c. digital equipment
   d. all of the above

3. As an EMT you will be expected to communicate with partners, dispatch, medical direction, and hospitals. The progression of radio transmissions includes:

   a. notifying dispatch of your arrival at the hospital
   b. contacting law enforcement with medical information about the patient
   c. contacting the patient's personal physician while en route to the hospital
   d. notifying dispatch when you are 5 minutes from the scene

4. The ground rules for radio communication include:

   a. using EMS frequencies for all radio traffic, including personal messages
   b. pressing your lips against the microphone for clarity while speaking
   c. pushing the press-to-talk button and waiting for 1 second before speaking
   d. giving the receiving hospital what you feel the patient's diagnosis is

5. When receiving orders from medical direction, the EMT should do all of the following *except*:

   a. repeat the order(s) word for word
   b. give the patient's name over the radio
   c. ask for clarification of an order you did not understand or feel is inappropriate
   d. avoid phrases such as *please, thank you,* and *you're welcome*

6. When communicating with medical direction, you should provide the following information:

   a. the patient's chief complaint
   b. the patient's marital status
   c. the patient's ethnic origin
   d. the patient's name

7. Once you arrive at the hospital with your patient, it is important to give the emergency room (ER) staff an oral report. This report should include:

   a. personal information about the patient not pertinent to medical care
   b. only new information, it is not necessary to repeat your broadcast (radio) report
   c. treatment given to the patient en route and his response to it
   d. the patient's billing and insurance information

8. Documentation you assemble as an EMT has a variety of functions. These include:

   a. helping to ensure the continuity of care for the patient
   b. providing data for researchers and scientists
   c. submitting records to insurance companies
   d. all of the above

9. The medical documentation you prepare has legal and administrative functions. Which of the following is true regarding these uses of your documentation?

    a. Since the documentation is not considered a legal document, you will not be able to refer to it when testifying in court.

    b. Since the EMT is the only person who will read the documentation, legibility and use of abbreviations are not of importance.

    c. The EMTs documentation is generally not used when preparing bills.

    d. The medical documentation you provide typically becomes a part of the patient's permanent hospital record.

10. An important division of a PCR is the patient's vital signs. Which of the following is true regarding this division of the PCR?

    a. Once the baseline vital signs are assessed, the second set of vital signs can be estimated.

    b. At least two complete sets of vital signs should be taken and recorded.

    c. The exact time the patient's vital signs were taken is not critical.

    d. All of the above.

11. Information that is measurable or verifiable in some way is called:

    a. pertinent negatives

    b. objective information

    c. subjective information

    d. pertinent information

Suggested Reading

US Department of Transportation, National Highway Traffic Safety Administration. *EMT-Basic National Standard Curriculum.* Washington, DC: US Department of Transportation, National Highway Traffic Safety Administration; 1994.

Chapter 4
Medical, Legal, and Ethical Issues in EMS

You respond to an unconscious patient at an adult community within your response area. Upon arrival, the patient's wife meets you at the door and briefs you on the patient's extensive cancer medical history and provides you and your partner with a valid out-of-hospital do not resuscitate (DNR) order. You assess the patient and determine he meets the criteria for death. A few moments later, the patient's children show up and begin questioning why resuscitative efforts have not started. Your partner explains to the family the patient's wishes, and they begin to get very upset about the decision not to resuscitate. What should you and your partner do?

MEDICAL ETHICS

Eth-ics\'e-thiks\ n: the principles of conduct governing an individual or a group. In 1978, the National Association of Emergency Medical Technicians (NAEMTs) adopted the EMT Code of Ethics. Professional status as an emergency medical technician (EMT) and EMT-Paramedic is maintained and enriched by the willingness of the individual practitioner to accept and fulfill obligations to society, other medical professionals, and the profession of EMT. As an EMT-Paramedic, I solemnly pledge myself to the following code of professional ethics: A fundamental responsibility of the EMT is to conserve life, to alleviate suffering, to promote health, to do no harm, and to encourage the quality and equal availability of emergency medical care.

The emergency medical technician provides services based on human need, respect for human dignity, and is unrestricted by consideration of nationality, race, creed, color, or status. The emergency medical technician does not use professional knowledge and skills in any enterprise detrimental to the public well-being.

LEGAL DUTIES TO THE PATIENT, MEDICAL DIRECTOR, AND PUBLIC

- Providing for the well-being of the patient by rendering necessary interventions outlined in the scope of practice.
- Legal duties are defined by state legislation and are enhanced by medical direction through the use of protocols and standing orders.
- Legal right to function as an EMT may be contingent upon the following:
  - Medical direction
  - Telephone/radio communications

○ Approved standing orders/protocols
○ Responsibility to medical direction

MEDICAL ETHICS AND ETHICAL RESPONSIBILITIES

- Always make the physical/emotional needs of the patient a priority.
- Practice/maintain skills to the point of mastery.
- Attend continuing education/refresher programs.
- Critically review performances, seeking ways to improve response time, patient outcome, and communication.
- Honesty in reporting.

ADVANCE DIRECTIVES

Honoring patient preferences is a critical element in providing quality end-of-life care. To enable physicians and other health-care providers to discuss and convey a patient's wishes regarding cardiopulmonary resuscitation (CPR) and life-sustaining treatment.

Out-of-hospital DNR orders (Fig. 4-1) are:

- Patient has the right to refuse resuscitative efforts.
- Requires written order from a physician.
- The EMT should review state and local legislation/protocols relative to DNR orders and advance directives.
- When in doubt or when written orders are not present, the EMT should begin resuscitation efforts.

State of New York
Department of Health

Nonhospital Order Not to Resuscitate
(DNR Order)

Person's name _____
Date of Birth __/__/__

Do not resuscitate the person named above.

Physician's Signature _____
Print Name _____
License Number _____
Date __/__/__

It is the responsibility of the physician to determine, at least every 90 days, whether this order continues to be appropriate, and to indicate this by a note in the person's medical chart. The issuance of a new form is NOT required, and under the law this order should be considered valid unless it is known that it has been revoked. This order remains valid and must be followed, even if it has not been reviewed within the 90-days period.

Figure 4-1   DNR order. *(Reproduced with permission from http://www.health.state .ny.us/publications/ 4182/index.htm)*

- In New York State the Medical Orders for Life-Sustaining Treatment (MOLST) form was created by the Community-wide End-of-Life Palliative Care Initiative to provide a single document that would function as an actionable medical order and could transition with a patient through all health-care settings. It is intended that the form will be transported with the patient between different health-care settings, in order that their wishes for life-sustaining treatment and CPR will be clearly indicated.

If the EMT is unsure about the next course of action, the EMT should begin resuscitation and contact medical control for definitive direction.

FORMS OF CONSENT

Expressed Consent

- Patient must be of legal age and able to make a rational decision.
- Patient must be informed of the steps of the procedures and all related risks.
- Consent must be obtained from every conscious, mentally competent adult before rendering any treatment.

Implied Consent

- Consent assumed from the unconscious patient requiring emergency intervention.
- Based on the assumption that the unconscious patient would consent to life-saving interventions.

Children and Mentally Incompetent Adults

- Consent for treatment must be obtained from the parent or legal guardian.
- When life-threatening situations exist and the parent or legal guardian is not available for consent, emergency treatment should be rendered based on implied consent.

Emancipation Issues

A patient legally underage but is recognized by the state as having the legal capacity to consent. Criteria for being emancipated vary among states.

ASSAULT/BATTERY

- An EMT can be charged with assault/battery when proper consent is not elicited. This includes the following instances:
    - Unlawfully touching a patient without his/her consent.
    - Providing emergency care when the patient does not consent to the treatment.

Refusals of Treatment and/or Transport

- The patient has the right to refuse treatment.
- The patient may withdraw from treatment at any time. Example: an unconscious patient regains consciousness and refuses transport to the hospital.
- Refusals must be made by mentally competent adults following the rules of expressed consent.

> **REFUSAL OF MEDICAL ASSISTANCE**
>
> You have been advised that you require medical assistance and that this pre-hospital care provider is prepared to render pre-hospital care and to transport you to a hospital. You have further been advised that your refusal to accept such medical assistance may imperil your health, or result in death.
>
> You have nonetheless refused to accept pre-hospital care and/or transportation to a hospital, as documented on Page 2 of the pre-hospital Care Report. You have agreed to assume all risks, consequences and costs of your decision not to accept pre-hospital care and/or transportation to a hospital, and you release the provider of pre-hospital care service, and its employees, agents and independent contractors, from any liability arising from your decision.

Figure 4-2   Patient privacy practices from the electronic patient care reporting (ePCR). HealthEMS ePCR form.

- The patient must be informed of, and fully understand, all the risks and consequences associated with refusal of treatment/transport, and must sign a "release from liability" form (Fig. 4-2).
- When in doubt, err in favor of providing care.
- Documentation is a key factor in protecting the EMT legally during, and after a patient refuses treatment and transportation.

    ○ Competent adult patients have the right to refuse treatment.
    ○ Before the EMT leaves the scene, he/she should:
        — Try again to persuade the patient to go to a hospital.
        — Ensure the patient is able to make a rational, informed decision, that is, ensure the patient is not under the influence of alcohol or drugs, or illness/injury affecting rational decision making.
        — Inform the patient why he should go and what may happen to him if he does not.
        — Consult medical direction as directed by local protocol.
        — Consider assistance of law enforcement.
        — Document any assessment findings and emergency medical care given, and if the patient still refuses, then have the patient sign a refusal form.
        — The EMT should never make an independent decision not to transport.

ABANDONMENT

Termination of care without assuring the continuation of care at the same level or higher.

NEGLIGENCE

Deviation from the accepted standard of care resulting in further injury to the patient. Components needed to prove negligence include:

- Duty to act
- Breach of the duty
- Injury/damages were inflicted (physical/psychological)
- The actions of the EMT that caused the injury/damage

DUTY TO ACT

A contractual or legal obligation must exist.

- *Implied*
  - Patient calls for an ambulance and the dispatcher confirms that an ambulance will be sent.
  - Treatment has begun.
- *Formal*
  - Ambulance service has a written contract with a municipality. Specific clauses within the contract should indicate when service can be refused to a patient.
- Legal duty to act may not exist, may be a moral/ethical consideration.
- In some states, while off duty, if the EMT comes upon an accident while driving, they must stop and help.
- When driving the ambulance not in the company's service area and EMT observes an accident.
  - Moral/ethical duty to act
  - Risk management
  - Documentation
- "- - - how a reasonably prudent person with similar training & experience would act under similar circumstances, with similar equipment, and in the same place."

PATIENT CONFIDENTIALITY/CONFIDENTIAL INFORMATION

- Patient history gained through interview
- Assessment findings
- Treatment rendered

HEALTH INSURANCE PORTABILITY AND ACCOUNTABILITY ACT

These are the requirements that are most relevant to ambulance service providers. For more detail, see the HHS Fact Sheet or the complete Privacy Rule.

- A covered provider must provide patients with notice of their privacy rights and its privacy practices, but need not obtain prior consent that would inhibit patient access to health care.
- Patients must grant permission in advance for each type of nonroutine use or disclosure, but providers may use one form for all of them.
- A covered entity must obtain prior written authorization to use protected health information for marketing purposes.
- Only the minimum necessary protected health information may be disclosed without authorization.
- A covered entity must account for disclosures of protected health information in the 6 years prior to the individual's request, with some exceptions, such as individual authorization.
- An individual may request restriction of use and disclosure of protected health information.

- Administratively, a covered entity must implement administrative, technical, and physical safeguards:
  - It must implement policies and procedures to comply with HIPAA, document all policies and procedures, written communications, required actions, and personnel designations, and maintain them for 6 years.
  - It must train its workforce, provide a complaint process, apply workforce sanctions for violations, mitigate harmful effects of improper use and disclosure, not retaliate, not require rights waived, designate a privacy official and contact person, and establish permitted uses and disclosures for its business associates.
- Releasing confidential information:
  - Requires a written release form signed by the patient. Do not release on request, written or verbal, unless legal guardianship has been established.
  - When a release is not required, other health-care providers need to know information to continue care. State law requires reporting incidents such as rape, abuse, or gunshot wounds.

SPECIAL SITUATIONS
Donor/Organ Harvesting

Donor/organ harvesting requires a signed legal permission document. The EMT's role in organ harvesting includes:

- Identifying the patient as a potential organ donor
- Establishing communication with medical direction
- Providing care to maintain viable organs

Medical Identification Insignia (Medical Alert Tag)

- Bracelet, necklace, card (Fig. 4-3)
- Indicates a serious medical condition of the patient, such as:
  - Allergies to food, medication, and the like
  - Serious medical conditions (epilepsy, diabetes, stroke, etc)
  - Others (DNR bracelet)

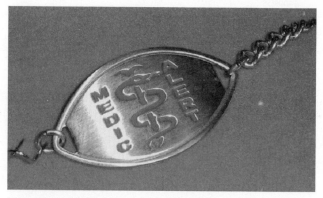

Figure 4-3 Medical alert tag. *(Reproduced with permission from http://dhfs.wisconsin.gov/ ems/ images/MedAlert_front.jpg)*

LDSS-2221A (Rev. 9/2007) FRONT

NEW YORK STATE
OFFICE OF CHILDREN AND FAMILY SERVICES
REPORT OF SUSPECTED
CHILD ABUSE OR MALTREATMENT

Report Date	Case ID	Call ID
Time : ☐ AM ☐ PM	Local Case #	Local Dist/Agency

SUBJECTS OF REPORT

List all children in household, adults responsible and alleged subjects.

Line #	Last Name	First Name	Aliases	Sex (M, F, Unk)	Birthday or Age Mo/Day/Yr	Race Code	Ethnicity (Ck Only If Hispanic/Latino)	Relation Code	Role Code	Lang. Code
1.							☐			
2.							☐			
3.							☐			
4.							☐			
5.							☐			
6.							☐			
7.							☐			

☐ MORE

List Addresses and Telephone Numbers (Using Line Numbers From Above) — (Area Code) Telephone No.

BASIS OF SUSPICIONS

Alleged suspicions of abuse or maltreatment. Give child(ren)'s line number(s). If all children, write **"ALL"**

_____ DOA/Fatality
_____ Fractures
_____ Internal Injuries (e.g., Subdural Hematoma)
_____ Lacerations/Bruises/Welts
_____ Burns/Scalding
_____ Excessive Corporal Punishment
_____ Inappropriate Isolation/Restraint (Institutional Abuse Only)
_____ Inappropriate Custodial Conduct (Institutional Abuse Only)

_____ Child's Drug/Alcohol Use Poisoning/Noxious Substances
_____ Choking/Twisting/Shaking
_____ Lack of Medical Care
_____ Malnutrition/Failure to Thrive
_____ Sexual Abuse
_____ Inadequate Guardianship
_____ Other (specify)

_____ Swelling/Dislocation/Sprains _____
_____ Educational Neglect _____
_____ Emotional Neglect _____
_____ Inadequate Food/Clothing/Shelter _____
_____ Lack of Supervision _____
_____ Abandonment _____
_____ Parent's Drug/Alcohol Misuse _____

State reasons for suspicion, including the nature and extent of each child's injuries, abuse or maltreatment, past and present, and any evidence or suspicions of "Parental" behavior contributing to the problem.

(If know, give time/date of alleged incident)
MO
DAY
YR
Time : ☐ AM ☐ PM

☐ Additional sheet attached with more explanation.   **The Mandated Reporter Requests Finding of Investigation** ☐ YES ☐ NO

CONFIDENTIAL	SOURCE(S) OF REPORT	*CONFIDENTIAL*
NAME	(Area Code) TELEPHONE / NAME	(Area Code) TELEPHONE
ADDRESS	ADDRESS	
AGENCY/INSTITUTION	AGENCY/INSTITUTION	

RELATIONSHIP

____ Med. Exam/Coroner   ____ Physician   ____ Hosp. Staff   ____ Law Enforcement   ____ Neighbor   ____ Relative   ____ Instit. Staff

____ Social Services   ____ Public Health   ____ Mental Health   ____ School Staff   ____ Other (Specify)

For Use By Physicians Only	Medical Diagnosis on Child	Signature of Physician who examined/treated child X	(Area Code) Telephone No.
	Hospitalization Required: ☐ None ☐ Under 1 week ☐ 1–2 weeks ☐ Over 2 weeks		
Actions Taken Or About To Be Taken	☐ Medical Exam ☐ X-Ray ☐ Removal/Keeping ☐ Not. Med Exam/Coroner ☐ Photographs ☐ Hospitalization ☐ Returning Home ☐ Notified DA		

Signature of Person Making This Report: X | Title | Date Submitted Mo. Day Yr.

Figure 4-4 Report of suspected child abuse. *(Reproduced with permission from http://www.health.state.ny.us/publications/4182/index.htm)*

Potential Crime Scene/Evidence Preservation

- Dispatch should notify police personnel.
- Responsibilities of the EMT:
  - Emergency care of the patient is the EMT's *first* priority.
  - Every attempt should be made *not* to disturb any item at the scene unless emergency care requires it. Observe and document anything unusual at the scene using an Unusual Occurrence document.
  - Documentation on the Pre-Hospital Care Report should include patient assessment and treatment only. Any other documentation related to the incident or assignment should be included on a report of Unusual Occurrence document.

SPECIAL REPORTING SITUATIONS

These situations are established by state legislation and may vary from state to state. Common reporting situations for EMS providers include instances of abuse, such as:

- Child abuse (Fig. 4-4)
- Elderly abuse
- Spousal abuse

Incidents Involving a Crime

- Wounds obtained by violent crime, sexual assault, or animal bites
- Infectious disease exposure
- Patient restraint laws (forcing someone to be transported against their will)
- Mental incompetence (ie, intoxication with injuries)

? CHAPTER QUESTIONS

1. Refusals must be made by a mentally competent adult following the rules of expressed consent.

   a. True

   b. False

2. All of the following are components of establishing negligence, except when:

   a. the EMT's action or lack of action incurs injury to the patient

   b. the EMT has violated the standard of care

   c. there was a duty to act

   d. the EMT was being paid at the time of the incident

3. When a patient is unable to make a rational decision regarding consent to emergency care, the EMT will care for the patient based on what form of consent?

   a. Expressed
   b. Minor
   c. Informed
   d. Implied

4. An EMT performed his primary assessment on a patient who was experiencing chest pain and shortness of breath. After initiating care, the EMT transported the patient to the hospital and did not provide a proper transition of care between the hospital staff and the EMS crew. In addition, the EMT did not wait to get a proper signature from the receiving hospital nurse or physician. This EMT could be legally liable for:

   a. negligence
   b. gross negligence
   c. abandonment
   d. violating the standard of care

5. By law, the EMT is authorized to release confidential information without the patient's permission in all of the following situations except when:

   a. information is requested by a member of the press
   b. another health-care provider needs information for the continuity of care
   c. the EMT is legally subpoenaed
   d. the third-party billing form requires the information

Chapter 5
The Human Body

You arrive on-scene and ensure the scene is safe to operate. In the apartment you find an 89-year-old woman semi-Fowler on a couch. She is complaining of crushing substernal chest pain radiating to her midscapular region, left shoulder, and mandible. She also complains of associated shortness of breath, nausea, and vomiting. You begin performing the initial assessment and determine any life threats. You and your partner form a general impression of the patient. You then move on to assessing mental status and note the patient is alert to person, place, and time. As you determine if the patient's airway is patent, you ask the patient to open her mouth and inspect her oropharynx. As you move on in the assessment, you establish the patient is breathing at a rate of 20, shallow and labored. Upon auscultation, you listen to the right and left midaxillary line and note equal lung sounds bilateral, equal chest rise, and no signs of trauma. Oxygen is administered via nonrebreather at 15 L/min. Circulation is assessed by taking a radial pulse located on the distal end of the arm just proximal to the thumb in the ridge located where the radius bone meets the hand. You establish that her heart rate is 88 and irregular. The patient is kept in a position of comfort and your assessment continues.

ANATOMIC TERMINOLOGY

Normal *anatomical position* is defined as a person standing, facing forward, palms facing forward (Fig. 5-1).

- An anatomical plane is a surface in which if any two points are taken, a straight line that is drawn to join these two points lies wholly within that plane or surface.
- Midline—Imaginary line drawn vertically through the middle of the body: nose through the umbilicus (belly button).
  - Divides the body into right and left halves.
- Midaxillary—Imaginary line drawn vertically from the middle of the armpit to the ankle.
  - Divides the body into anterior and posterior.

Descriptive Anatomical Terms/Definitions

- *Torso*—Trunk of the body
- *Medial*—Toward the middle
- *Lateral*—A point that is more distant from the midsagittal or median plane

Clinical Significance

Anatomical terms are used in medicine to describe location, comparison, or position. These terms are vital in proper communication/documentation.

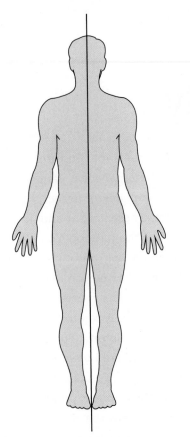

Figure 5-1   Anatomical position.

- *Proximal*—Closer to any point of reference
- *Distal*—Farther from any point
- *Superior*—Toward the head
- *Inferior*—Toward the feet
- *Anterior*—Toward the front
- *Posterior*—Toward the back
- *Right and left*—Toward the right or left
- *Midclavicular*—Imaginary line in the center of the clavicle
- *Bilateral*—Both sides
- *Dorsal*—Toward the back
- *Ventral*—Toward the front
- *Plantar*—Pertaining to the sole of the foot
- *Palmar*—Pertaining to the palm
- *Prone*—Face down
- *Supine*—Face up
- *Fowler*—Sitting in a 90-degree angle
- *Trendelenburg*—Supine, lower body elevated above head
- *Shock position*—Body supine, legs elevated 8 to 12 in

COMPONENTS OF THE SKELETAL SYSTEM

The function of the skeletal system is to provide the body shape, protect vital internal organs, and assist in body movement. The skeletal system consists of 206 bones (Fig. 5-2).

Skull

It houses and protects the brain.

Facial Bones

- Orbit
- Nasal bone
- Maxilla
- Mandible (jaw)
- Zygomatic bones (cheeks)

Spinal Column

- Cervical (neck)—7 vertebrae
- Thoracic—12 vertebrae
- Lumbar—5 vertebrae
- Sacral (sacrum)—5 vertebrae
- Coccyx—4 vertebrae

Thorax

Ribs

- 12 pairs
- Attached posterior to the thoracic vertebrae
- Pairs 1 to 10 attached anterior to the sternum
- Pairs 11 and 12 floating

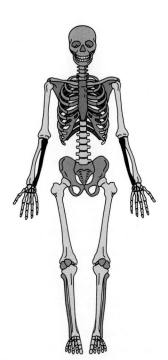

Figure 5-2   Skeletal system.

Sternum (Breastbone)

- Manubrium (superior portion of sternum)
- Body (middle)
- Xiphoid process (inferior portion of sternum)

Pelvis

- Iliac crest (wings of pelvis)
- Pubis (anterior portion of pelvis)
- Ischium (inferior portion of pelvis)

Lower Extremities

- Greater trochanter (ball) and acetabulum (socket of the hip bone)
- Femur
- Patella (knee cap)
- Tibia
- Fibula
- Medial and lateral malleolus
- Tarsals and metatarsals
- Calcaneus
- Phalanges

Upper Extremities

- Clavicle
- Scapula
- Acromion (tip of shoulder)
- Humerous
- Olecranon (elbow)
- Radius
- Ulna
- Carpals
- Metacarpals
- Phalanges

Joints—Where Bones Connect to Other Bones

Types of joints include:

- Ball and socket (eg, hip and shoulder)
- Hinge (eg, elbow and knee)

RESPIRATORY SYSTEM

Brings oxygen into the body and eliminates carbon dioxide (CO_2) from the body.

- Nose and mouth
- Pharynx
- Oropharynx
- Nasopharynx

- Epiglottis—A leaf-shaped structure that prevents food and liquid from entering the trachea during swallowing
- Trachea (windpipe)
- Cricoid cartilage—Firm cartilage ring forming the lower portion of the larynx
- Larynx (voice box)
- Bronchi—Two major branches of the trachea to the lungs (bronchus subdivides into smaller air passages ending at the alveoli)
- Lungs
- Diaphragm

Inhalation (Active)

- Diaphragm and intercostal muscles contract, increasing the size of the thoracic cavity.
- Diaphragm moves slightly downward, flares lower portion of rib cage.
- Ribs move upward/outward.
- Air flows into the lungs.

Exhalation (Passive)

- Diaphragm and intercostal muscles relax, decreasing the size of the thoracic cavity.
- Diaphragm moves upward.
- Ribs move downward/inward.
- Air flows out of the lungs.

Respiratory Physiology

How does the respiratory system work?

Alveolar/Capillary Exchange

- Oxygen-rich air enters the alveoli during each inspiration.
- Oxygen-poor blood in the capillaries passes into the alveoli.
- Oxygen enters the capillaries as carbon dioxide enters the alveoli.

Capillary/Cellular Exchange

- Cells give up carbon dioxide to the capillaries.
- Capillaries give up oxygen to the cells.

Adequate Breathing—Normal Rate/Ranges

- Adult—12 to 20/min
- Child—15 to 30/min
- Infant—25 to 50/min

Respiratory Assessment

Rhythm

- Regular/irregular

Clinical Significance

Sellick maneuver—The application of digital pressure to the cricoid cartilage to reduce gastric distention.

Clinical Significance

Primary Assessment
- *Airway*
  - Suction the oropharynx/nasopharynx as needed.
  - Insert an oropharyngeal or nasopharyngeal airway; if the patient gags, remove the airway and prepare for suction.
- *Breathing*
  - *Inspect* the chest.
  - *Palpate* the chest for symmetry, paradoxical movement, and crepitus.
  - *Auscultate* lung sounds.
  - *Seal/stabilize* any punctures or flail segments.
  - *Administer oxygen* non-rebreather mask, bag-valve-mask with reservoir, or nasal cannula.

Quality

- Breath sounds—Present and equal
- Chest expansion—Adequate and equal
- Effort of breathing—Use of accessory muscles predominantly in infants and children

Depth (Tidal Volume)

- Adequate/inadequate breathing.
- Rate—Outside of normal ranges.
- Rhythm—Regular/irregular.
- Quality.
  - Breath sounds—Diminished or absent
  - Chest expansion—Unequal or inadequate
  - Increased effort of breathing—Use of accessory muscles, predominantly in infants and children
- Inadequate/shallow.
- The skin may be pale or cyanotic (blue) and cool and clammy. **Hypoxia** is a pathological condition in which the body as a whole (**generalized hypoxia**) or a region of the body (**tissue hypoxia**) is deprived of adequate oxygen supply.
- There may be retractions above the clavicles, between the ribs, and below the rib cage, especially in children.
- Nasal flaring may be present, especially in children.
- In infants, there may be "see-saw" breathing where the abdomen and chest move in opposite directions.
- Agonal respirations (occasional gasping breaths) may be seen just before death.

PEDIATRIC ANATOMY CONSIDERATIONS

- Mouth and nose—All structures are smaller and more easily obstructed than in adults.
- Pharynx—Infants' and children's tongues take up proportionally more space in the mouth than adults.
- Trachea (windpipe).
  - Infants and children have narrower tracheas that are obstructed more easily by swelling.
  - The trachea is softer and more flexible in infants and children.
- Cricoid cartilage—Like other cartilage in the infant and child, the cricoid cartilage is less developed and less rigid.
- Diaphragm—The chest wall is softer, so infants and children tend to depend more heavily on the diaphragm for breathing.

CIRCULATORY (CARDIOVASCULAR) SYSTEM

Heart (Size, Shape, and Position)

- Muscular pump
- Size of the patient's fist
- Weighs 10 oz

Clinical Significance

Although these ranges are considered normal for the adult, child, and infant, it is important to remember that abnormal findings, such as perioral cyanosis, tripoding, tachypnea, and altered mental status, in conjunction with these ranges, are clinical findings of respiratory distress/failure.

Clinical Significance

Signs of accessory muscle use in infants and children include intercostal/supraclavicular retractions.

Clinical Significance

A swollen throat from the streptococcus infection (strep throat) can cause significant narrowing of the pediatric airway.

- Located in *mediastinum*, area between the lungs
- *Base*—Broad superior portion of heart
- *Apex*—Inferior end, tilts to the left, tapers to point

Heart Muscle

- Epicardium (visceral pericardium)
  - Serous membrane that covers the heart
- Myocardium
  - Thick muscular layer
  - Fibrous skeleton—Network of collagenous and elastic fibers
    — Provides structural support
    — Attachment for cardiac muscle
    — Nonconductor important in coordinating contractile activity
- Endocardium
  - Smooth inner lining

Heart Chambers

- Four chambers (two atria, two ventricles)
- Right and left atria
  - Two superior chambers.
  - Receive blood returning to heart from veins; veins carry blood back to the heart.
- Right and left ventricles
  - Two inferior chambers.
  - Pump blood into arteries; arteries carry blood away from the heart.

Atrium

- Right atrium—Receives blood from the veins of the body; pumps oxygen-poor blood to the right ventricle.
- Left atrium—Receives oxygenated blood from the pulmonary veins (lungs); pumps oxygen-rich blood to the left ventricle.

Ventricle

- Right ventricle—Pumps oxygen-poor blood to the lungs.
- Left ventricle—Pumps oxygen-rich blood to the body.

▶Note:

Valves prevent backflow of blood.

Follow a Drop of Blood Through the Heart

Deoxygenated blood enters the right atrium through the superior and inferior vena cava, and the coronary sinus. Deoxygenated blood is then pumped from the right atrium to the right ventricle through the tricuspid valve. Once deoxygenated blood fills the right ventricle, it is then pumped through the pulmonic semilunar valve into the pulmonary artery (still deoxygenated blood). Blood flows through the pulmonary artery to the lungs for gas exchange through the alveolar/capillary membrane. Once gas exchange occurs (oxygen/carbon dioxide), blood flows into the left atrium through the pulmonary vein (oxygenated blood). As it fills the left atrium, oxygenated blood is then pumped to the left ventricle passing through the mitral valve. Once the left ventricle is filled, oxygenated blood is pumped through the aortic semilunar valve into the aorta to the entire body (Fig. 5-3).

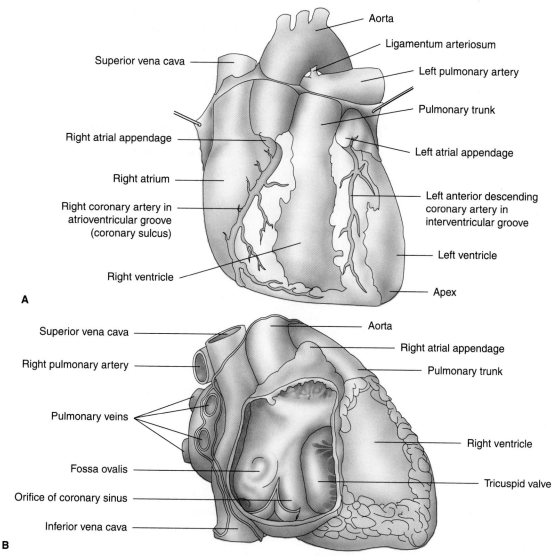

Figure 5-3 Anatomy of the heart. A. Anterior view of the heart. B. View of the heart with the right atrial wall reflected to show the right atrium. *(Reproduced with permission from Cheitlin MD, Sokolow M, McIllroy MB. Clinical Cardiology. 6th ed. New York: McGrawHill Companies, Inc; 1993)*

CARDIAC CONDUCTIVE SYSTEM

- The heart is more than just a muscle.
- The heart has specialized contractile and conductive tissue.

  ○ *Automaticity*—Ability to generate an electrical impulse without stimulation from another source
  ○ *Excitability*—Ability to respond to an electrical stimulus (This is a property of all myocardial cells.)
  ○ *Conductivity*—Ability to propagate an impulse from cell to cell

Electrical Impulses

- *Sinoatrial (SA) node*—Primary pacemaker, initiates heartbeat, sets heart rate
- *Fibrous skeleton insulates atria from ventricles*

- *Atrioventricular (AV) node*—Electrical gateway to ventricles
- *AV bundle*—Pathway for signals from AV node
- *Right and left bundle branches*—Divisions of AV bundle that enter inter-ventricular septum and descend to apex
- *Purkinje fibers*—Upward from apex spread throughout ventricular myocardium

Sinoatrial Node (Dominant Pacemaker of the Heart)
- Located in the right atrium near the entrance of the superior vena cava.
- Intrinsic rate is *60 to 100* beats/min.

Atrioventricular Node
- Responsible for creating a slight delay in conduction before sending the impulse to the ventricles.
- Impulse travel time is 0.08 to 0.16 second.
- No pace-making properties are found in the node itself.
- AV junction tissue has intrinsic rate of *40 to 60* beats/min.

Bundle of His
- Bundle of fibers coming from the AV node, located at the top of the interventricular septum.
- Considered as part of the AV junction.
- Makes the electrical connection between the atria and ventricles.

Bundle Branches
- Created by the bifurcation of the bundle of His into left and right bundle branches.
- Carry electrical impulse at high velocity to the interventricular septum and each ventricle simultaneously.
- Has a rate of *20 to 40* beats/min.

Purkinje Fibers
- Terminal ends of the bundle branches.
- Network of fibers helping to spread the impulse throughout the ventricular walls.
- Rapid impulse is 0.08 to 0.09 second
- Has a rate of *20 to 40* beats/min

Blood Vessels

Arteries—Carry blood away from the heart to the rest of the body.

Major Arteries of the Body
- Coronary arteries—Vessels that supply the heart with oxygen-rich blood.
- Aorta (oxygen-rich blood)—Major artery originating from the heart, lying in front of the spine in the thoracic and abdominal cavities.
  - Divides at the level of the navel into the iliac arteries.
- Pulmonary (oxygen-poor blood) artery—Originating at the right ventricle, carries oxygen-poor blood to the lungs.

- Carotid (oxygen-rich blood)—Major arteries of the neck.
  - Supplies the head with blood.
  - Pulsations can be palpated on either side of the neck.
- Femoral (oxygen-rich blood)—Major artery of the thigh.
  - Supplies the lower extremities with blood.
  - Pulsations can be palpated in the groin area (the crease between the abdomen and thigh).
- Radial (oxygen-rich blood)—Major artery of the lower arm.
  - Pulsations can be palpated at the wrist thumb side.
- Brachial (oxygen-rich blood)—An artery of the upper arm.
  - Pulsations can be palpated on the inside of the arm between the elbow and the shoulder.
  - Used when determining blood pressure (BP) using a BP cuff (sphygmomanometer) and a stethoscope.
- Posterior tibial—Pulsations can be palpated on the posterior surface of the medial malleolus.
- Dorsalis pedis—An artery in the foot.
  - Pulsations can be palpated on the anterior surface of the foot.
- Arteriole—The smallest branch of an artery leading to the capillaries.
- Capillaries—Tiny blood vessels that connect arterioles to venules.

  - Found in all parts of the body.
  - Allow for the exchange of nutrients and waste at the cellular level.

Major Veins

- Venule—The smallest branch of a vein leading to the capillaries.
- Veins—Vessels that carry blood back to the heart.
- Pulmonary vein (only vein that carries oxygen-rich blood in the adult body)—Carries *oxygen-rich* blood from the lungs to the left atrium.
- Venae cavae—Carries oxygen-poor blood back to the right atrium.
- Superior vena cava.
- Inferior vena cava.

Blood Composition

- Red blood cells
  - Carry oxygen to organs utilizing hemoglobin found in the cytoplasm.
  - Carries carbon dioxide away from organs.
  - Hemoglobin is what gives the blood its distinctive red color.
- White blood cells—Part of the body's defense against infections.
- Plasma—Fluid that carries the blood cells and nutrients.
- Platelets—Essential for the formation of blood clots.

Cardiovascular Physiology

How is a pulse generated?
- Left ventricle contracts sending a wave of blood through the arteries. Can be palpated anywhere an artery simultaneously passes near the skin surface and over a bone.

Clinical Significance

In the initial assessment it is important to assess circulation. While assessing the "C" in ABC (airway, breathing, circulation), we will:
- Correct any life-threatening bleeding.
- Assess skin color, temperature, and moisture.
- Assess pulse rate and quality.

Peripheral Circulation

- Radial
- Brachial
- Posterior tibial
- Dorsalis pedis

Where are these pulses palpated?

Central Circulation

- Carotid artery
- Femoral artery

Where are these pulses palpated?

Blood Pressure

- Systolic—The pressure exerted against the walls of the artery when the left ventricle contracts
- Diastolic—The pressure exerted against the walls of the artery when the left ventricle is at rest

MUSCULOSKELETAL SYSTEM

Functions of the musculoskeletal system:

- Gives the body shape.
- Protects internal organs.
- Provides for movement.

Types of Muscle

Voluntary (Skeletal)

- Attached to the bones.
- Form the major muscle mass of the body.
- Controlled by the nervous system and brain; voluntary muscles can be contracted and relaxed by the will of the individual.
- Responsible for movement.

Involuntary (Smooth)

- Found in the walls of the tubular structures of the gastrointestinal tract and urinary system, as well as the blood vessels and bronchi.
- Control the flow through these structures.
- Carry out the automatic muscular functions of the body.
- Individuals have no direct control over these muscles.
- Respond to stimuli such as stretching, heat, and cold.

Cardiac

- Found only in the heart.
- Involuntary muscle—Has its own supply of blood through the coronary artery system.
- Can tolerate interruption of blood supply for only very short periods.
- Automaticity—The ability of the muscle to contract on its own.

NERVOUS SYSTEM

Function—Controls the voluntary and involuntary activity of the body.

- Central nervous system (consists of the brain and spinal cord)
  ○ Brain—Located within the cranium
  ○ Spinal cord—Located within the spinal column from the brain through the lumbar vertebrae
- Peripheral nervous system
  ○ Sensory—Carry information from the body to the brain and spinal cord
  ○ Motor—Carry information from the brain and spinal cord to the body

INTEGUMENTARY SYSTEM

Functions of the skin

- Protects the body from the environment, bacteria, and other organisms.
- Helps regulate the temperature of the body.
- Senses heat, cold, touch, pressure, and pain; transmits this information to the brain and spinal cord via the sensory portion of the peripheral nervous system.

Layers of the Skin

(Fig. 5-4)

- Epidermis—Outermost layer of skin
- Dermis—Deeper layer of skin containing sweat and sebaceous glands, hair follicles, blood vessels, and nerve endings
- Subcutaneous layer—Fatty tissue

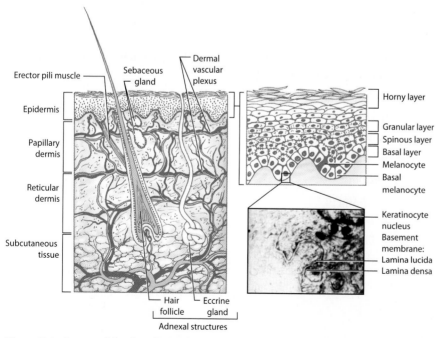

Figure 5-4 Layers of the skin. *(Reproduced with permission from Brunicardi FC, Andersen DK, Billiar TR, et al (eds). Schwartz's Principles of Surgery, 8th ed. New York: McGrawHill; 2005)*

ENDOCRINE SYSTEM

- Function—Secretes chemicals, such as insulin and adrenalin, responsible for regulating body activities and functions. The endocrine system is a vital system that aids in maintaining homeostasis in the body.
- Homeostasis—The ability or tendency of an organism or a cell to maintain internal equilibrium by adjusting its physiological processes.

? CHAPTER QUESTIONS

1. The functions of the body are called its:

   a. physiology
   b. kinesiology
   c. pathology
   d. microbiology

2. The term that refers to a position closer to the midline is:

   a. medial
   b. lateral
   c. posterior
   d. anterior

3. The structure that carries air downward from the larynx to the lungs is the:

   a. bronchus
   b. pharynx
   c. epiglottis
   d. trachea

4. The chamber that pumps oxygen-rich blood out of the heart for distribution to the rest of the body is the:

   a. right atrium
   b. right ventricle
   c. left atrium
   d. left ventricle

5. The pulse that is located in the foot is the:

   a. carotid
   b. femoral
   c. brachial
   d. dorsalis pedis

Chapter 6
Life Span Development

PHYSIOLOGICAL

Table 6-1 shows the ranges of normal vital signs for all age groups in the life span.

INFANCY (BIRTH TO 1 YEAR)
Weight

- Normally 3.0 to 3.5 kg at birth.
- Normally drops 5% to 10% in the first week of life due to excretion of extracellular fluid.
- Exceeds birth weight by second week.
- Grows at approximately 30 g/d during the first month.
- Should double weight by 4 to 6 months.
- Should triple weight at 9 to 12 months.
- Infant's head equal to 25% of the total body weight.

Cardiovascular System

- Circulation changes soon after birth include:
  - Closing of the ductus arteriosus
  - Closing of the ductus venosus
  - Closing of the foramen ovale
  - Immediate increase in systemic vascular resistance
  - Decrease in pulmonary vascular resistance
- Left ventricle strengthens throughout the first year.

Pulmonary System
- Airways are shorter, narrower, less stable, and more easily obstructed.
- Infants are primarily nose breathers until 4 weeks.
- Lung tissue is fragile and prone to barotrauma.
- Fewer alveoli with decreased collateral ventilation.
- Accessory muscles immature, susceptible to early fatigue.
- Chest wall is less rigid.
- Ribs positioned horizontally, causing diaphragmatic breathing.
- Higher metabolic and oxygen consumption rates than adults.
- Rapid respiratory rates lead to rapid heat and fluid loss.

TABLE 6-1: **Normal Vital Sign Ranges for All Age Groups**

Age	Heart Rate	Respiratory Rate/Tidal Volume	Systolic Blood Pressure	Temperature
Infancy (birth to 1 year)	• First 30 minutes the heart rate is 100-160 bpm • Averaging out around 120 bpm	• Initially 40-60 • Dropping to 30-40 after the first few minutes of life • Slowing to 20-30 by 1 year of life • 6-8 mL/kg initially • Increasing to 10-15 mL/kg by 1 year	Systolic blood pressure increases from 70 mm Hg at birth to 90 mm Hg at 1 year	98-100°F
Toddler (12-36 months) Preschool (3-5 years old)	• Toddlers: 80-130 bpm • Preschoolers: 80-120 bpm	• Toddlers: 20-30 bpm • Preschoolers: 20-30 bpm	• Toddlers: 70-100 mm Hg • Preschoolers: 80-110 mm Hg	96.8-99.6°F
School age (6-12 years old)	70-110 bpm	20-30 bpm	80-120 mm Hg	98.6°F
Adolescence (13-18 years old)	55-105 bpm	12-20 bpm	100-120 mm Hg	98.6°F
Early adulthood (20-40 years old)	70 bpm	16-20 bpm	120 mm Hg	98.6°F
Middle adulthood (40-60 years old)	70 bpm	16-20 bpm	120 mm Hg	98.6°F
Late adulthood (61 years and older)	Depends on health status	Depends on health status	Depends on health status	98.6°F

Renal System

- Kidneys are unable to concentrate urine.
- Specific gravity rarely exceeds 1.020.

Immune System

- Passive immunity is retained through the first 6 months of life.
- Based on maternal antibodies.

Nervous System

- Movements
  - Strong, coordinated suck and gag
  - Well-flexed extremities
  - Extremities move equally when infant is stimulated
- Reflexes
  - Moro reflex
  - Palmar grasp
  - Sucking reflex
  - Rooting reflex
- Fontanelles
  - Posterior fontanelle closes at 3 months.
  - Anterior fontanelle closes between 9 and 18 months.
  - Fontanelles may provide an indirect estimate of hydration.

- Sleep
  - Initially sleeps 16 to 18 hours per day with sleep and wakefulness evenly distributed over 24 hours.
  - Gradually decreases to 14 to 16 hours per day with 9 to 10 hours concentration at night.
  - Sleeps through the night at 2 to 4 months.
  - Normal infant is easily arousable.

Musculoskeletal System

- Bone growth
  - Epiphyseal plate—length.
  - Growth in thickness occurs by deposition of new bone on existing bone.
  - Is influenced by:
    — Growth hormone
    — Genetic factors
    — Thyroid hormone
    — General health
- Muscle weight is about 25% in infants.

Dental System

- Teeth begin to erupt at 5 to 7 months.

Growth and Development

Rapid changes occur over the first year of life.

- 2 months
  - Tracks objects with eyes.
  - Recognizes familiar faces.
- 3 months
  - Moves objects to mouth with hands.
  - Displays primary emotions with distinct facial expressions.
- 4 months
  - Drools without swallowing.
  - Reaches out to people.
- 5 months
  - Sleeps throughout night without food.
  - discriminates between family and strangers.
- 6 months
  - Sits upright in a high chair.
  - Makes one-syllable sounds, that is, ma, mu, da, di.
- 7 months
  - Fear of strangers.
  - Quickly changes from crying to laughing.
- 8 months
  - Responds to "no."
  - Sits alone.
  - Plays "peek-a-boo."

- 9 months
  - Responds to adult anger.
  - Pulls self to standing position.
  - Explores objects by mouthing, sucking, chewing, and biting.
- 10 months
  - Pays attention to own name.
  - Crawls well.
- 11 months
  - Attempts to walk without assistance.
  - Shows frustration to restrictions.
- 12 months
  - Walks with help.
  - Knows own name.

Psychosocial Development

- Family processes—Reciprocal socialization
  - Scaffolding
  - Attachment
  - Trust versus mistrust
  - Secure attachment
- Temperament—Infants may be:
  - Easy child
  - Difficult child
  - Slow to warm-up child
- Crying
  - Basic cry
  - Anger cry
  - Pain cry
- Trust—Based on consistent parental care
- Situational crisis—Parental separation reactions
  - Protest
  - Despair
  - Withdrawal
- Growth charts
  - Good for comparing physical development to norm

TODDLER (12-36 MONTHS)

Weight

- Rate of gain slows dramatically.
- Average child gains 2 kg/y.

Cardiovascular System

- Capillary beds are better developed to assist in thermoregulation.
- Hemoglobin levels approach normal adult levels.

Pulmonary System

- Terminal airways continue to branch.
- Alveoli increase in number.

Renal System

- Kidneys are well developed in toddler years.
- Specific gravity and other urine findings are similar to adults.

Immune System

- Passive immunity is lost, more susceptible to minor respiratory and gastrointestinal infections.
- Develops immunity to common pathogens as exposure occurs.

Nervous System

- Brain weighs 90% of what the adult brain weighs.
- Myelination increases cognitive development.
- Development allows effortless walking and other basic motor skills.
- Development of fine motor skills.

Musculoskeletal System

- Muscle mass increases.
- Bone density increases.

Dental System

- All primary teeth have erupted by 36 months.

Elimination Patterns

- Toilet training
- Physiologically capable by 12 to 15 months
- Psychologically ready between 18 and 30 months
- Average age for completion—28 months

Sensory

- Visual acuity—20/30 during the toddler years
- Hearing—Essential maturity at 3 to 4 years

Psychosocial

Cognitive

- Basics of language mastered by approximately 36 months, with continued refinement throughout childhood.
- Understands cause and effect between 18 and 24 months.
- Develops separation anxiety—approximately 18 months.
- Develops magical thinking—between 24 and 36 months.

Play

- Exploratory behavior accelerates.
- Able to play simple games and follow basic rules.
- Begins to display competitiveness.
- Observation of play may uncover frustrations otherwise unexpressed.

Sibling Relationships

- Sibling rivalry.
- First-born children.
- Usually maintain special relationship with parents.
- Expected to exercise self-control and show responsibility in interacting with younger siblings.

Peer Group Functions

- Children about the same age and maturity levels.
- Provide a source of information about the outside world and other families.
- Become more important to the child throughout childhood.

Parenting Styles and Its Effect on Children

- Authoritarian parenting
- Authoritative parenting
- Permissive-indifferent parenting
- Permissive-indulgent parenting

Divorce Effects on Child Development

- Age
- Cognitive and social competencies
- Amount of dependency on parents
- Type of day care
- Parents' ability to respond to the child's needs

Television

- May be a cause in aggression at this age.
- Careful screening of television exposure may be effective.

Modeling

- Children begin to recognize the differences of sex.
- Begin to model themselves based on sex.

SCHOOL-AGE CHILDREN (6-12 YEARS OLD)

Growth Rate

- Average child gains 3 kg/y and 6 cm/y.

Bodily Functions

- Most reach adult levels during this period.
- Lymph tissues proportionately larger than adult.
- Brain function increases in both hemispheres.
- Loss of primary teeth and replacement with permanent teeth begins.

Psychosocial

Families

- Children allowed more self-regulation.
- Parents still provide general supervision.
- Parents spend less time with children in this age group.

Develop Self-Concept

- More interaction with adults and children.
- Begin comparing themselves with others.
- Develop self-esteem.
- Tends to be higher during early years of school than later years.
- Often based on external characteristics.
- Effected by peer popularity, rejection, emotional support, and neglect.
- Negative self-esteem can be damaging to further development.

Moral Development

- Preconventional reasoning.
- Punishment and obedience.
- Individualism and purpose.
- Conventional reasoning.
- Interpersonal norms.
- Social system morality.
- Postconventional reasoning.
- Community rights versus individual rights.
- Universal ethical principles.
- Individuals move through development throughout school age and young adulthood at different paces.

ADOLESCENCE (13-18 YEARS OLD)

Growth Rate

- Most experience a rapid 2 to 3 year growth spurt.
- Begins distally with enlargement of feet and hands.
- Enlargement of the arms and legs follows.
- Chest and trunk enlarge in final stage.
- Girls are mostly done growing by age 16; boys are mostly done growing by age 18.
- Secondary sexual development occurs.
- Noticeable development of the external sexual organs.
- Pubic and axillary hair develops.
- Vocal quality changes occur (mostly in males).
- Menstruation initiates (in females).

Endocrine Changes

- Female
  - Follicle-stimulating hormone (FSH) and luteinizing hormone (LH) release.
  - Gonadotropin promotes estrogen and progesterone production.
  - Other biological changes.

- Male
  - Gonadotropins promote testosterone production.
  - Reproductive maturity.
  - Muscle mass and bone growth nearly complete.
  - Body fat decreases early in adolescence, and begins to increase later.
- Females require 18% to 20% body fat percentage for menarche to occur.
- Blood chemistry nearly equals to adult levels.
- Skin toughens through sebaceous gland activity.

Psychosocial

Family

- Conflicts arise.
- Adolescents strive for autonomy.
- Biological changes associated with puberty.
- Increased idealism.
- Independence and identity changes.

Develop Identity

- Self-consciousness increases.
- Peer pressure increases.
- Interest in the opposite sex increases.
- Want to be treated like adults.
- Progress through various stages based on how they handle crises, etc.
- Antisocial behavior peaks around eighth or ninth grade.
- Minority adolescents tend to have more identity crises than nonminority.
- Body image of great concern.
- Continual comparison among peers.
- Eating disorders are common.
- Self-destructive behaviors begin.
- Tobacco.
- Alcohol.
- Illicit drugs.
- Depression and suicide are more common than any other age group.

Ethical Development

- Develop capability for logical, analytical, and abstract thinking.
- Develop a personal code of ethics.

EARLY ADULTHOOD (20-40 YEARS)

- Peak physical conditioning between 19 and 26 years of age.
- Adults develop lifelong habits and routines during this time.
- All body systems at optimal performance.
- Accidents are a leading cause of death in this age group.

Psychosocial

- Experience highest levels of job stress during this time.
- Love develops.

- ◦ Romantic love
- ◦ Affectionate love
- Childbirth is most common in this age group.
- New families provide new challenges and stress.
- This period is less associated with psychological problems related to well-being.

MIDDLE ADULTHOOD (41-60 YEARS)

- Body still functions at high level with varying degrees of degradation.
- Vision changes.
- Hearing less effective.
- Cardiovascular health becomes a concern.
- Cardiac output decreases throughout this period.
- Cholesterol levels increase.
- Cancer strikes in this age group often.
- Weight control more difficult.
- Menopause in women in late 40s to early 50s.

Psychosocial

Adults in this group are more concerned with "social clock."

- Task oriented.
- Pressed for time to accomplish lifelong goals.
- Approach problems more as challenges than threats.
- Empty-nest syndrome.
- Often burdened by financial commitments for elderly parents as well as young adult children.

LATE ADULTHOOD (61 YEARS AND OLDER)

- Life span—Maximum approximately 120 years
- Life expectancy—Average length based on year of birth

Cardiovascular Function Changes

Blood Vessels

- Thickening.
- Increased peripheral vascular resistance.
- Reduced blood flow to organs.
- Decreased baroreceptor sensitivity.
- By 80 years of age, there is approximately 50% decrease in vessel elasticity.

Heart

- Increased workload causes include:
    - ◦ Cardiomegaly
    - ◦ Mitral and aortic valve changes
    - ◦ Decreased myocardial elasticity
- Myocardium is less able to respond to exercise.

- Fibrous tissues in sinoatrial (SA) node.
- Pacemaker cells diminish, resulting in arrhythmia.
- Tachycardia not well tolerated.
- Blood cells.
    - Decrease in functional blood volume
    - Decrease in platelet count
    - Diminished red blood cells (RBCs)
    - Poor iron levels

Respiratory System

- Changes in mouth, nose, and lungs.
- Metabolic changes lead to decreased lung function.
- Muscular changes.
- Diaphragm elasticity diminished.
- Chest wall weakens.
- Diffusion through alveoli diminished.
- Lifelong exposure to pollutants, etc:
    - Diminished lung capacity
    - Ineffective coughing
    - Weakened chest wall
    - Weakened bone structure

Endocrine System Changes

- Decreased glucose metabolism.
- Decreased insulin production.
- Thyroid shows some diminished T_3 production.
- Cortisol diminished by 25%.
- Pituitary gland 20% less effective.
- Reproductive organs' atrophy in women.

Gastrointestinal System

- Mouth, teeth, and saliva changes.
- Peristalsis decreased.
- Esophageal sphincter less effective.
- Gastrointestinal (GI) secretions decreased.
- Vitamin and mineral deficiencies.
- Internal intestinal sphincters lose tone.

Renal System

- Fifty percent nephrons are lost.
- Abnormal glomeruli more common.
- Decreased elimination.

Sensory Changes

- Loss of taste buds.
- Olfactory diminished.

- Diminished pain perception.
- Diminished kinesthetic sense.
- Visual acuity diminished.
- Reaction time diminished.
- Presbycusis is defined as problems with hearing.

Nervous System

- Neuron loss.
- Neurotransmitters diminish.
- Sleep-wake cycle disrupted.

Psychosocial

Terminal Drop Hypothesis

- Death preceded by a decrease in cognitive functioning over a 5-year period prior to death.
- Wisdom attributed to age in some cultures.
- Ninety-five percent of older adults live in communities.
- Challenges.
- Self-worth
- Declining well-being.
- Financial burdens.
- Death or dying of companions.

? CHAPTER QUESTIONS

1. A "toddler" is defined as:

    a. 12 to 36 months of age
    b. 36 to 48 months of age
    c. 1 to 12 months of age
    d. none of the above

2. Gonadotropins promote testosterone production in females.

    a. True
    b. False

Suggested Readings

Birren J. *The Psychology of Aging.* Englewood Cliffs, NJ: Prentice Hall; 1964.

US Department of Transportation, National Highway Traffic Safety Administration. *EMT-Paramedic: National Standard Curriculum.* Washington, DC: US Department of Transportation, National Highway Traffic Safety Administration; 1998.

Section 2
Pharmacology

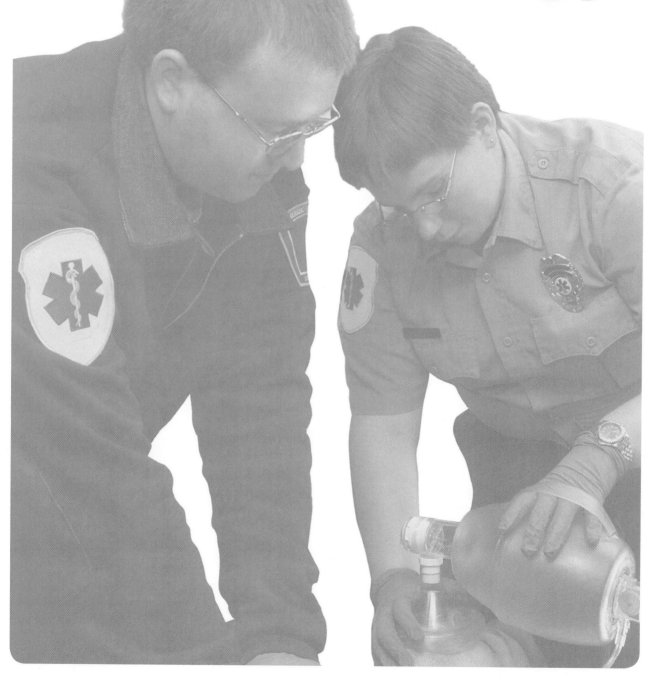

Chapter 7
General Pharmacology

Your emergency medical services (EMS) unit is dispatched to the staging area of a mass casualty incident (MCI). Upon arrival at the staging area, the staging officer orders you and your partner to wear the appropriate personal protective equipment and report to the treatment sector "cold zone." The report of a possible terrorist attack was confirmed when the first arriving units surveyed the scene and determined there were multiple casualties in a shopping mall which described an explosion and a device that disseminated a gas that has patients experiencing signs and symptoms of SLUDGEM (*s*alivation, *l*acrimation, *u*rination, *d*efecation, *G*I upset—nausea/vomiting/cramps/diarrhea, *e*mesis, *m*uscle twitching).

Report given by the incident commander reveals "a device was disseminated, and a chemical released of what was determined by the HAZMAT team to be a nerve agent." You and your partner don the appropriate gear and grab your HAZMAT response bag that contains the Mark-I auto-injectors needed to begin treatment. How would you begin treatment using the Mark-I auto-injectors?

As an emergency medical technician (EMT), it is important to understand what medications are used and the dangers associated with their administration.

- Medications typically carried on an EMS unit:
  - Activated charcoal (Fig. 7-1)
  - Oral glucose
  - Oxygen
  - Nebulized medication (ie, albuterol sulfate)
  - Epipen and Epipen Jr (Figs. 7-2, 7-3)
  - Mark-I auto-injector (Fig. 7-4)
  - Aspirin (Fig. 7-5)
  - Nitroglycerin (Fig. 7-6)
- Medication names.
  - Generic—The name listed in the *US Pharmacopeia*, a governmental publication listing all drugs in the United States, and is assigned to the drug before it becomes officially listed. Usually a simple form of the chemical name.
  - Trade (brand)—The name a manufacturer uses in marketing the drug.
- *Indications*—The indication for a drug's use includes the most common uses of the drug in treating a specific illness.

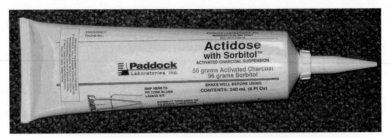

Figure 7-1   Activated charcoal. *(Used with permission of Peter DiPrima.)*

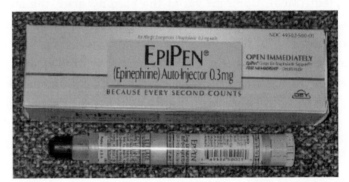

Figure 7-2   Epipen auto-injector. *(Used with permission of Peter DiPrima.)*

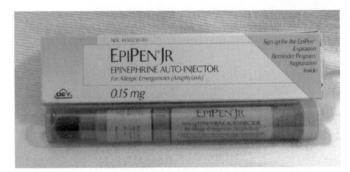

Figure 7-3   Epipen Jr auto-injector. *(Used with permission of Peter DiPrima.)*

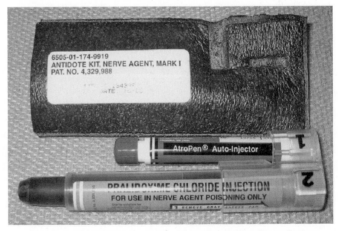

Figure 7-4   Mark-I auto-injector. *(Used with permission of Peter DiPrima.)*

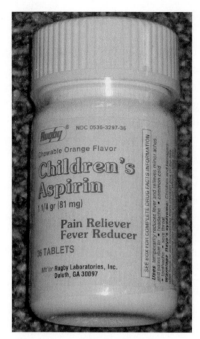

Figure 7-5 Children's chewable aspirin. *(Used with permission of Peter DiPrima.)*

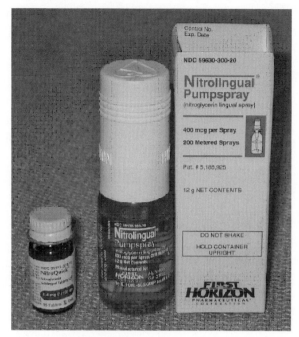

Figure 7-6 Nitrolingual spray and nitroglycerin tablets. *(Used with permission of Peter DiPrima.)*

- *Contraindications*—Situations in which a drug should not be used because it may cause harm to the patient or offer no effect in improving the patient's condition or illness.
- *Expiration date*—Date that indicates that the medication is expired and should not be used.

FORMS OF MEDICATIONS

- Compressed powders or tablets—Nitroglycerin.
- Liquids for injection—Epinephrine.
- Gels—Instaglucose (Fig. 7-7).
- Suspensions—Activated charcoal.
- Fine powder for inhalation—Prescribed inhaler.
- Gases—Oxygen.
- Sublingual (SL) spray—Nitroglycerin.
- Liquid/vaporized fixed-dose nebulizer.
- Dose—State how much of the drug should be given.
- Administration—State route by which the medication is administered, such as oral, sublingual (under the tongue), injectable, or intramuscular.

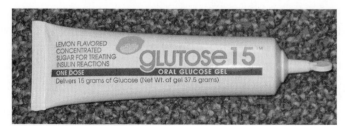

Figure 7-7 Instaglucose gel. *(Used with permission of Peter DiPrima.)*

- Actions—State desired effects a drug has on the patient and/or his body systems.
- Side effects—State any actions of a drug other than those desired. Some side effects may be predictable.
- Reassessment strategies after the administration of a medication include:
  - Repeat baseline vital signs
  - Part of the ongoing patient assessment
  - Documentation of response to intervention

PRE-HOSPITAL MEDICATIONS USED BY EMTS

Oral Glucose

▶Note:

Each drug is in a specific medication form to allow properly controlled concentrations of the drug to enter into the bloodstream where it has an effect on the target body system.

Class: Caloric

Actions: Needed for adequate utilization of amino acids

Indications: Hypoglycemia

Contraindications: Hyperglycemia

Precautions: Renal and hepatic disease

Side Effects: Confusion and dizziness

Dosage: One tube (15 g)

Routes: By mouth (PO)

Oxygen

Class: Gas.

Actions: Necessary for cellular metabolism.

Indications: Hypoxia.

Contraindications: None.

Precautions: Use cautiously in patients with chronic obstructive pulmonary disease (COPD), humidify when providing high-flow rates.

Side Effects: Drying of mucous membranes.

Dosage: Cardiac arrest: 100%. Other critical patients: 100%.

Routes: Inhalation.

Pediatric Dosage: 24% to 100% as required.

Albuterol Sulfate (Proventil, Ventolin)

Class: Relatively selective beta-2 adrenergic bronchodilator.

Description: Albuterol is a sympathomimetic that is selective for beta-2 adrenergic receptors. It relaxes smooth muscles of the bronchial tree and peripheral vasculature by stimulating adrenergic receptors of the sympathetic nervous system.

Onset and Duration: Onset: 5 to 15 minutes after inhalation; 30 minutes PO.

Duration: 3 to 4 hours after inhalation; 4 to 6 hours PO.

Indications: Relief of bronchospasm in patients with reversible obstructive airway disease. Prevention of exercise-induced bronchospasm.

Contraindications: Prior hypersensitivity reaction to albuterol cardiac dysrhythmias associated with tachycardia. Tachycardia caused by digitalis intoxication.

Adverse Reactions: Tachycardia, restlessness, apprehension, headache, dizziness, nausea, palpitations, increase in blood pressure, dysrhythmias, hypokalemia.

Drug Interactions: Sympathomimetics may exacerbate adverse cardiovascular effects. Antidepressants may potentiate the effects on the vasculature. Beta blockers may antagonize albuterol.

How Supplied:

MDI: 90 μg/metered spray (17-g canister with 200 inhalations)

Solution for aerosolization: 0.5% (5 mg/mL)

Prediluted nebulized solution: 2.5 mg in 3-mL normal saline (NS) (0.083%)

Dosage and Administration for Bronchial Asthma

Adult: Albuterol sulfate solution 0.083% (one unit dose bottle of 3.0 mL), by nebulizer, at a flow rate that will deliver the solution over 5 to 15 minutes. May be repeated twice (total of three doses).

Pediatric: Albuterol sulfate 0.083% (one unit dose bottle of 3.0 mL), by nebulizer, at a flow rate that will deliver the solution over 5 to 15 minutes. May be repeated twice during transport (total of three doses).

Special Considerations

Pregnancy Safety: Category C.

May precipitate angina pectoris and dysrhythmias. Should be used with caution in patients with diabetes mellitus, hyperthyroidism, prostatic hypertrophy, or seizure disorder.

Epinephrine

Class: Sympathomimetic.

Description: Epinephrine stimulates alpha, beta-1, and beta-2 adrenergic receptors in dose-related fashion. It is the initial drug of choice for treating bronchoconstriction and hypotension resulting from anaphylaxis.

Indications: Acute allergic reaction.

Contraindications: Hypersensitivity.

Adverse Reactions: Headache, nausea, restlessness, weakness, dysrhythmias, hypertension, precipitation of angina pectoris.

Drug Interactions: Monoamine oxidase (MAO) inhibitors and bretylium may potentiate the effect of epinephrine. Beta-adrenergic antagonists may blunt inotropic response.

How Supplied: Auto-injector (Epipen) 0.5 mg/mL (1:2000).

Dosage and Administration—Anaphylactic Reaction

Adult: 0.3 mg

Pediatric: 0.15 mg

Special Considerations

Pregnancy Safety: Category C

May increase myocardial oxygen demand.

Mark-I Auto-Injector

The Mark-I kit contains two separate auto-injectors with the following medications:

AtroPen—*atropine sulfate*, 2 mg in 0.7 mL

ComboPen—*pralidoxime chloride* (2-PAM), 600 mg in 2 mL

Each auto-injector is a disposable, spring-loaded, pressure-activated system prefilled with medication. The Mark-I kit consists of one atropine and one pralidoxime auto-injector linked together with a plastic clip. The atropine is administered first followed by the pralidoxime.

Pralidoxime (2-PAM)

Class: Antidote to cholinesterase inhibitors, organophosphate chemicals, organophosphate pesticides.

Mechanism of Action: Pralidoxime (pra-li-DOX-eem) is used together with another medicine called atropine to treat poisoning caused by organic phosphorus pesticides (ie, diazinon, malathion, mevinphos, parathion, and sarin) and by organophosphate chemicals ("nerve gases") used in chemical warfare. Poisoning with these chemicals causes your muscles, including the muscles that help you breathe, to become weak. Pralidoxime is used to help you get back strength in your muscles. Pralidoxime is to be given only by, or under the direct supervision of, a doctor or trained military personnel.

Effects: Along with its needed effects, this medicine may cause some unwanted effects. Although not all of these side effects may occur, if they do occur they may need medical attention. Check with your doctor as soon as possible if any of the following side effects occur:

Blurred or double vision, difficulty in focusing your eyes, difficulty in speaking, difficult or rapid breathing, dizziness, fast heartbeat, muscle stiffness or weakness, pain at the place of injection (after injection into a muscle).

Pregnancy

Studies on effects in pregnancy have not been done in either humans or animals.

Children

Although there is no specific information comparing use of pralidoxime in children with use in other age groups, this medicine is not expected to cause different side effects or problems in children than it does in adults.

Common Emergency Indications

When an emergency arises, you will need to know how to inject the pralidoxime auto-injector. It is important that you do not remove the safety cap on the auto-injector until you are ready to use it. This prevents spillage of the medicine from the device during storage and handling.

To Use the Pralidoxime Auto-Injector

1. Remove the gray safety cap.
2. Place the black tip of the device on the thigh, with the injector pointed straight at the thigh.
3. Press hard into the thigh until the auto-injector functions. Hold in place for several seconds.
4. Remove the auto-injector and dispose it of as directed.
5. Massage the injected area for 10 seconds.

Treatment of Organic Phosphorus Chemical Poisoning

Adults

The usual dose is 600 mg injected into a muscle. The dose may be repeated 15 minutes after the first dose and again 15 minutes after the second dose, if needed.

Children

Dose must be determined by your doctor.

Treatment of Overdose of Medicines Used to Treat Myasthenia Gravis in Adults and Teenagers

At first, the dose is 1 to 2 g injected into a vein. Then, the dose is 250 mg injected into a vein every 5 minutes.

Children

Dose must be determined by your medical director.

Precautions While Using This Medicine

This medicine will add to the effects of central nervous system (CNS) depressants (medicines that may make you drowsy or less alert). Some examples of CNS depressants are antihistamines or medicine for hay fever, other allergies, or colds; sedatives, tranquilizers, or sleeping medicine; prescription pain medicine or narcotics; barbiturates; medicine for seizures; muscle relaxants or anesthetics, including some dental anesthetics. Check with your doctor before taking any of the above while you are using this medicine.

Atropine

Class: Antimuscarinic, parasympathetic blocker, anticholinergic. It is better to refer to atropine as an antimuscarinic rather than an anticholinergic. The word cholinergic refers to the neurotransmitter acetylcholine (ACh) and therefore, anticholinergic implies antagonism of ACh everywhere. Atropine does not block ACh everywhere. For example, voluntary muscle contraction occurs when ACh (liberated from motor nerves) stimulates nicotinic receptors located in the membranes of skeletal muscle. If atropine was truly anticholinergic, then it would paralyze people, which, of course, it does not. Atropine is antimuscarinic, meaning that it blocks ACh primarily at muscarinic receptor sites. Muscarinic receptors are found predominantly in the heart, lungs, gastrointestinal tract (GIT), genitourinary tract, and glands.

Mechanism of Action: Competitively blocks ACh at muscarinic receptor sites by competing for the muscarinic receptors.

Effects: An easy way to learn the effects of atropine is to remember that its effects are opposite to that of parasympathetic nervous system stimulation. As mentioned, this is because it blocks the action of the ACh liberated from the parasympathetic nerve endings.

Heart: Accelerates heart rate (HR), conduction velocity, and force of contraction (slightly). The major parasympathetic nerve to the head is the vagus nerve (tenth cranial). When the vagus nerve is stimulated, ACh is liberated and upon combining with the muscarinic receptors of the brain, decreases the HR, conduction velocity, and force of contraction (slightly). Thus, atropine causes the opposite to occur.

Lungs: Inhibits glandular secretion in the respiratory tract. Relaxes smooth muscle in the bronchial tree resulting in bronchodilation. Liberation of ACh from parasympathetic nerves adjacent to respiratory tract structures (nose, mouth, pharynx, and bronchi) results in increased respiratory tract secretions and bronchial smooth muscle contraction. Atropine causes the opposite. The drying of respiratory secretions and the prevention of anesthesia-induced bradycardia are the basis of using atropine preoperatively.

Gastrointestinal Tract: Inhibits gastrointestinal secretions. Decreases gastrointestinal motility. Parasympathetic stimulation of the gastrointestinal tract via ACh combining with muscarinic receptors results in increased gastrointestinal secretions and an increase in gastrointestinal motility. By blocking muscarinic receptors, atropine decreases gastrointestinal secretions and decreases motility. Atropine all but stops the secretion of saliva, which is why it causes a dry mouth with difficulty in swallowing.

Pupils: Pupillary dilation. ACh liberated upon stimulation of parasympathetic nerves adjacent to the sphincter muscle of the iris combines with muscarinic receptors and constricts the pupil. Atropine does the opposite. Atropine is a far more effective mydriatic when instilled directly into the eye rather than when given intravenously. Actually, 0.5 mg of atropine given intravenously has little ocular effects, and atropine administration during cardiac arrest does not cause fixed and dilated pupils.

Genitourinary Tract: Decreases normal bladder tone and intensity of bladder contractions. The effect of ACh on muscarinic receptors of the bladder is to increase bladder tone and the intensity of bladder contractions. In other words, it facilitates urination. Atropine blocks the effects of ACh on muscarinic receptors and thus inhibits bladder motility. This is why atropine-containing drugs can cause urinary retention— especially in elderly males with prostate problems.

Cholinergic Poisonings

Organophosphate poisoning and certain types of mushroom poisonings. The symptoms of cholinergic poisoning result from excessive muscarinic stimulation by acetylcholine, or by acetylcholine-like drugs. Atropine is the drug of choice for cholinergic poisoning because it blocks the muscarinic receptor sites and therefore protects the individual from the effects of muscarinic overstimulation. The symptoms of cholinergic poisonings are salivation, lacrimation, urination, abdominal cramps, diarrhea, vomiting, bradycardia, dyspnea (secondary to bronchoconstriction and excessive bronchial secretions), seizures, and death. Atropine may be life-saving in this situation.

Treatment of Organic Phosphorus Chemical Poisoning

For significant organophosphate poisonings, start with 1 to 2 mg IV, may repeat as necessary. Severe organophosphate poisonings may require very little amounts of atropine. Best guide for atropinization is cessation of secretions.

Children

Dose: 0.02 mg/kg IV—may repeat every 3 to 5 minutes. Maximum single IV dose in child is 0.5 mg, minimum single IV dose in child is 0.1 mg. May be administered intratracheally at a dose of 0.05 mg.

Class: Antimuscarinic, parasympathetic blocker, anticholinergic.

Mechanism of Action: Competitively blocks ACh at muscarinic sites.

Effects: Heart—Accelerates HR, conduction velocity, and force of contraction (slightly). Lungs—Inhibits glandular secretion in the respiratory tract, relaxes smooth muscle in the bronchial tree resulting in bronchodilation.

Gastrointestinal tract: Inhibits gastrointestinal secretions, decreases gastrointestinal motility.

Pupils: Pupillary dilation.

Genitourinary tract: Decreases normal bladder tone and intensity of bladder contractions.

Common Emergency Indications: Symptomatic bradyarrhythmias, cholinergic poisonings, asystole, refractory bronchospasms. Symptomatic bradyarrhythmias—0.5 to 1 mg IV, may repeat every 3 to 5 minutes, 0.4 mg/kg total dose. Asystole—1 mg IV; may repeat in 3 to 5 minutes to a total dose of 3 mg.

Organophosphate Poisonings: 1 to 2 mg IV prn (best guide is cessation of secretions). Refractory bronchospasm—1 mg combined with a beta-2 agonist via nebulizer.

PEDS: 0.02 mg/kg IV may repeat every 5 minutes to a total dose of 0.04 mg/kg. Maximum single dose in child is 0.5 mg, minimum is 0.1 mg.

Side effects: Tachyarrhythmias, exacerbation of glaucoma, precipitation of myocardial ischemia.

Aspirin

Class: Platelet inhibitor/anti-inflammatory

Actions: Blocks platelet aggregation

Contraindications: Patients with history of hypersensitivity to the drug

Precautions: GI bleeding, and upset

Side Effects: Heartburn, nausea, vomiting, wheezing

Dosage: 162 to 325 mg PO or chewed

Routes: PO

Pediatric Dosage: Not recommended

Nitroglycerin

Nitroglycerin Spray (Nitrolingual Spray)

Class: Antianginal/vasodilator.

Actions: Smooth muscle relaxant, decreases cardiac work, dilates coronary arteries, dilates systemic arteries.

Indications: Angina pectoris, chest pain associated with myocardial infarction.

Contraindications: Hypotension.

Precautions: Constantly monitor vital signs. Syncope can occur.

Side Effects: Dizziness, hypotension, headache.

Dosage: One spray administered under the tongue; may be repeated in 10 to 15 minutes; no more than three sprays in a 15-minute period; spray should not be inhaled.

Routes: Sprayed under tongue on mucous membrane.

Pediatric Dosage: Not indicated.

Nitroglycerin (Nitrostat and Others)

Class: Antianginal/vasodilator.

Description: It was originally believed that nitrates and nitrites dilated coronary blood vessels, thereby increasing blood flow to the heart. It is now believed that atherosclerosis limits coronary dilation and that the benefits of nitrates and nitrites result from dilation of arterioles and veins in the periphery. The resulting reduction in preload, and to a lesser extent in afterload, decreases the workload of the heart and lowers myocardial oxygen demand. Nitroglycerin is a very lipid soluble and is thought to enter the body from the Gl tract through the lymphatics rather than the portal blood.

Onset and Duration: Onset: 1 to 3 minutes; duration: 20 to 30 minutes.

Indications: Ischemic chest pain, hypertension, congestive heart failure.

Contraindications: Hypersensitivity.

Adverse Reactions: Transient headache, postural syncope, reflex tachycardia, hypotension, nausea and vomiting, allergic reaction, muscle twitching, diaphoresis.

Drug Interactions: Other vasodilators may have additive hypotensive effects.

How Supplied:

Tablets (sublingual): 0.15 mg (1/400 g), 0.3 mg (1/200 g), 0.4 mg (1/150 g), 0.6 (1/100 g)

Aerosol (translingual): 0.4-mg metered dose

Parenteral: 0.5 mg/mL, 0.8 mg/mL, and 5.0 mg/mL

Tablets (sustained release): 2.6 mg, 6.5 mg, and 9 mg

Capsules (sustained release): 6.5 mg, 9 mg

Topical: 2% ointment

Dosage and Administration: 1/150 g or spray 0.4 mg, sublingually, every 5 minutes, for a total of three doses.

Special Considerations:

Pregnancy Safety: Category C.

Susceptibility to hypotension in older adults increases.

Nitroglycerin decomposes when exposed to light or heat.

Must be kept in airtight containers. Active ingredient of nitroglycerin "stings" when administered SL.

? CHAPTER QUESTIONS

1. An EMT is permitted, with medical direction, to administer, or assist the patient in administering, all of the following *except*:

   a. nitroglycerin

   b. oxygen

   c. penicillin

   d. oral glucose

2. Medications administered sublingually are:

   a. swallowed

   b. inhaled

   c. dissolved under the tongue

   d. injected under the skin

3. Which of the following is true regarding medication routes of administration?

   a. Most medications administered by the EMT are administered by injection.

   b. All medications are administered by the oral route.

   c. The route that is chosen controls how quickly the medication is absorbed by the body.

   d. Drugs administered by the sublingual route have a relatively slow rate of absorption.

4. A drug administered by an EMT, and used for a wide range of medical and traumatic emergencies, is:

   a. Tylenol

   b. glucose

   c. nitroglycerin

   d. oxygen

5. The EMT may administer which of the following medications to treat a severe allergic reaction?

   a. Glutose

   b. Adrenalin

   c. Liqui-Char

   d. Alupent

6. A 26-year-old female patient has breathing difficulty, and has been pre-scribed a bronchodilator. Having met all the requirements to administer the medication, the steps include:

   a. placing the patient on a nasal cannula for convenience

   b. leaving the oxygen off the patient until you can assess if the medica-tion worked

   c. having the patient inhale fully, then place her lips around the mouthpiece

   d. having the patient hold her breath as long as is comfortable after inhal-ing the medication

7. When administering a metered-dose inhaler, tips for the procedure include:

   a. depressing the canister just before the patient begins inhaling

   b. coaching the patient to hold his breath as long as possible

   c. having the patient breathe in and out quickly

   d. being careful not to shake the canister

Suggested Readings

Halperin HR, Tsitlik JE, Gelfand M, et al. A preliminary study of cardiopulmonary resuscitation by circumferential compression of the chest with use of a pneumatic vest. *N Engl J Med.* 1993;329:762-768.

Paradis NA, Martin GB, Rivers EP, et al. Coronary perfusion pressure and the return of spontaneous circulation in human cardiopulmonary resuscitation. *JAMA.* 1990;263:1106-1113.

2007 Physicians' Desk Reference. 61st ed PDR. The Thomson Corporation.

US Department of Transportation, National Highway Traffic Safety Administration. *EMT-Basic National Standard Curriculum.* Washington, DC: US Department of Transportation, National Highway Traffic Safety Administration; 1994.

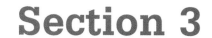

Section 3
Patient Assessment

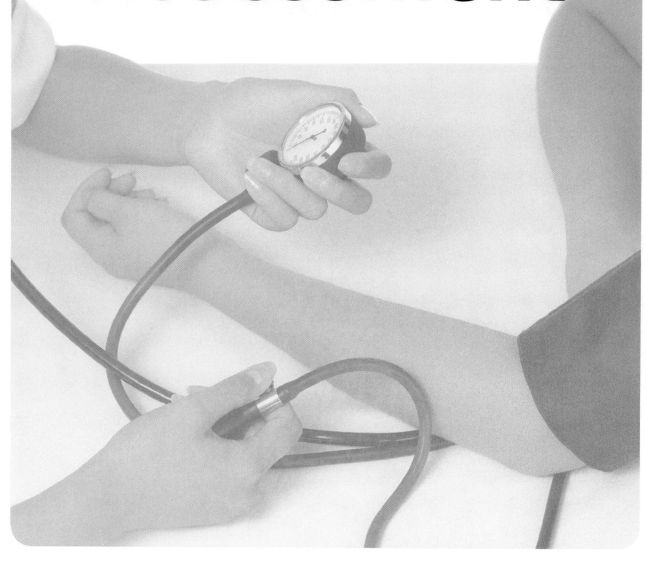

Chapter 8
Patient Assessment

Scenario 1:

You arrive on-scene of an overturned vehicle collision (Fig. 8-1), you establish scene safety and begin evaluating a 21-year-old man still in the vehicle, who was the unrestrained driver of a truck that ran into a cement barrier at approximately 50 mph, causing it to overturn. You notice the steering wheel is bent and observe "starring" on the windshield with no skid marks present. The patient has a small amount of blood in his oropharynx. His breathing is labored and tachypneic at 32 breaths/min. His pulse is thready at 154. What do you do next?

Scenario 2:

The emergency medical dispatcher sends you to the scene of a motor vehicle collision at Avenue Z and Ocean Parkway. The emergency involves a single car that has struck a large boulder. When you arrive at the scene, you do a quick scene size-up. The vehicle has major damage, and no electrical lines are down. First responders from the fire department have secured the scene, and have initiated cardiopulmonary resuscitation (CPR) on a male patient. You notice no obvious signs of trauma on the patient, except a 1-in laceration on the forehead. A police officer on-scene states, "The patient's driver's license indicates he is 24 years old. When we arrived, he was breathing agonally. He then went into cardiac arrest. We extricated him from the vehicle while providing c-spine stabilization and began CPR."

SCENE SIZE-UP

The first step in the entire process actually begins before your involvement, with a properly trained dispatcher. The dispatcher, who takes the initial call for help, should collect as much pertinent information as possible. Knowing where you are going, a familiarity with the location, and an understanding of the problem, are all "pieces" of information that will help you make a proper "preassessment." While responding to the scene, "armed" with the information supplied by the dispatcher and associating that information with your available equipment, your knowledge of the area, and your ability to deal with the upcoming anticipated problems, will better prepare you (mentally and emotionally) to deal with this patient. That preparation will also serve to present an "organized" group of rescuers to onlookers, family members, and the patient, when your ambulance arrives at the scene, adding to the degree of professionalism perceived by the public.

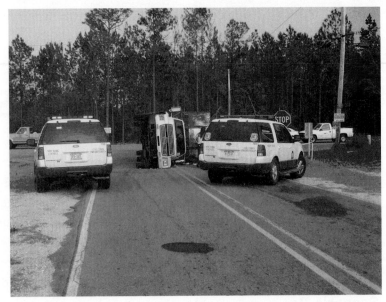

Figure 8-1   Overturned vehicle collision. New York-Presbyterian EMS First Responders. *(Used with permission of Peter DiPrima.)*

Body Substance Isolation

Body substance isolation (BSI)—Assumes all body fluids present a possible risk for infection. Protective equipment includes:

- Latex or vinyl gloves should always be worn.
- Eye protection.
- Respiratory protection such as filtering face piece respirators, full-face air-purifying respirators (APRs), powered air-purifying respirators (PAPRs), to name a few.
- Gown.
- Turnout gear.

Scene safety is an assessment to assure the safety and well-being of the emergency medical treatment (EMT).

- Personal protection—The EMT should ask, "Is it safe to approach the patient?"
  - Crash/rescue scenes.
  - Toxic substances—Low-oxygen areas.
  - Crime scenes—Potential for violence.
  - Unstable surfaces—Slope, ice, water, and the like.
  - Protection of the patient—Environmental considerations.
  - Protection of bystanders—If appropriate, prevent bystanders from becoming patients.
  - If the scene is unsafe, make it safe. Otherwise, do not enter.

Scene size-up is an assessment of the scene and surroundings that will provide valuable information to the EMT.

Mechanism of Injury/Nature of Illness

- Medical (nature of illness [NOI])
  - Nature of illness—Determine from the patient, family, or bystanders why emergency medical services (EMS) was activated.

Clinical Significance

The most important way to prevent infection is to wash your hands after every assignment.

- Determine the total number of patients. If there are more patients than the responding unit can effectively handle, request additional help (Medical Council of India [MCI] Plan).
- Obtain additional help prior to contact with patients—Law enforcement, fire, rescue, advanced life support (ALS), and utilities. EMT is less likely to call for help if involved in patient care.
- Begin triage.
- Trauma (mechanism of injury [MOI])
  - Mechanism of injury—Determine from the patient, family, or bystanders, and from inspection of the scene what the mechanism of injury is.
  - Determine the total number of patients.
    — If there are more patients than the responding unit(s) can effectively handle, initiate a mass casualty plan.
    — Obtain additional help prior to contact with patients.
    — Begin triage utilizing simple triage and rapid treatment (START).
    — If the responding crew can manage the situation, consider spinal precautions and continue care.

PATIENT ASSESSMENT (MEDICAL) AND PATIENT ASSESSMENT (TRAUMA)

Primary Assessment

- The general impression is formed to determine priority of care and is based on the EMT's immediate assessment of the environment and the patient's chief complaint (Table 8-1).
  - Determine if ill or injured (trauma).
  - If injured, identify mechanism of injury.

TABLE 8-1: **Patient Assessment**

Scene Size-Up
Take the appropriate body substance isolation (BSI) precautions, is the scene safe?
Determine mechanism of injury (MOI) or nature of illness (NOI) and the number of patients. Requests additional help if necessary. Consider stabilization of cervical spine.

Primary Assessment		
General impression of the patient: What is the patient's chief complaint? Are they a medical or trauma patient? What is the patient's age, gender, and are there any obvious life-threatening problems?		
Level of consciousness: AVPU (Alert, Verbal, Painful stimulus, Unresponsive)		
Airway and breathing assessment: Responsive patient: Is the patient breathing adequately?		
Unresponsive patient: Is the airway open? Suction as needed, insert an oropharyngeal or nasopharyngeal airway as needed.		
Responsive patient: If breathing adequately, administer high-concentration oxygen via non-rebreather mask. Unresponsive patient: If breathing adequately, administer high-concentration oxygen via non-rebreather mask. If inadequate, assist ventilations with a bag-valve-mask with reservoir and high-concentration oxygen. Inspect and palpate the chest, seal and stabilize any flail segments, and auscultate two lung fields.		
Circulatory assessment: Perform a rapid pulse check, is there any bleeding? Assess the skin; color, temperature, and moisture. In children less than 6 y of age assess capillary refill (<2 s is normal).		
Identify priority patients; perform transport decision and the need for advanced life support (ALS)		
Poor general impression	Difficulty breathing	Chest pain
Unresponsive patient	Hypoperfusion	Uncontrolled bleeding
Altered mental status	Complicated birth	Severe pain

- Age.
- Gender.
- Race.
- Assess patient and determine if the patient has a life-threatening condition.
  - If a life-threatening condition is found, treat immediately.
- Assess patient's mental status. Maintain spinal immobilization if needed.
  - Begin by speaking to the patient. Introduce yourself, tell the patient that you are an emergency medical technician, and explain that you are there to help.
  - Assess mental status using AVPU.
    — Alert—Alert to person, place, and time
    — Responds to verbal stimuli
    — Responds to painful stimuli
    — Unresponsive—No gag or cough
- Assess the patient's airway status.
  - Responsive patient—Is the patient able to speak?
    — If yes, assess for adequacy of breathing.
    — If no, open airway. (Remember, jaw-thrust maneuver for trauma patients.)
  - Unresponsive patient—Is the airway open?
    — Open the airway.
    — For medical patients, perform the head-tilt-chin-lift.
    — Suction as necessary.
  - For trauma patients or those with an unknown nature of illness, the cervical spine should be stabilized/immobilized and the jaw-thrust maneuver performed.
    — Suction as necessary.
- Assess the patient's breathing.
  - If breathing is adequate and the patient is responsive, administer appropriate oxygen therapy.
  - If the patient is unresponsive and the breathing is adequate, open and maintain the airway, and provide high-concentration oxygen via non-rebreather.
  - If the breathing is inadequate, open and maintain the airway, assist the patient's breathing, and utilize ventilatory adjuncts. In all cases, high-concentration oxygen should be used.
  - If the patient is not breathing, open and maintain the airway and ventilate using ventilatory adjuncts. In all cases oxygen should be used and rescue breathing should be performed by giving one breath every 5 to 6 seconds.
- Assess the patient's circulation.
  - Assess the patient's pulse.
  - Circulation is assessed by feeling for a radial pulse on a conscious patient.
    — In a patient 1-year old or less, palpate a brachial pulse.
    — If no radial pulse is felt, palpate carotid pulse.
    — If no radial pulse is present, following the appropriate AHA Basic Cardiac life Support Guideline pertaining to cardiac arrest.
  - Assess if major bleeding is present. If bleeding is present, control bleeding.

- Assess the patient's perfusion by evaluating skin color, temperature, and moisture.
  - The patient's skin color is assessed by looking at the nail beds, lips, and eyes.
    — Normal—Pink
    — Abnormal conditions
      Pale
      Cyanotic or blue-gray
      Flushed or red
      Jaundice or yellow
- Assess the patient's skin temperature by feeling the skin.
  - Normal—Warm
  - Abnormal skin temperatures
    — Hot
    — Cool
    — Cold
    — Clammy—Cool and moist (Diaphoresis is profuse sweating.)
- Assess the patient's skin condition. This is an assessment of the amount of moisture on the skin.
  - Normal—Dry
  - Abnormal—Moist or wet
- Assess capillary refill in pediatric patients.
  - Normal capillary refill is (<) 2 seconds.
  - Abnormal capillary refill is (>) 2 seconds.

IDENTIFY PRIORITY PATIENTS

- Consider the following:
  - Poor general impression
  - Unresponsive patients—No gag reflex or inability to cough
  - Responsive, but not following commands
  - Difficulty breathing
  - Shock (hypoperfusion)
  - Complicated childbirth
  - Chest pain with BP less than 100 systolic
  - Uncontrolled bleeding
  - Severe pain anywhere
- Expedite transport of the patient. Consider *ALS backup* as outlined in local/state protocol.
- Proceed to the appropriate history and secondary assessment.

HISTORY AND SECONDARY ASSESSMENT, "TRAUMA"

(Tables 8-2 and 8-3)

- Reconsider mechanism of injury.
- Look for injuries that have possibly been overlooked and injuries consistent with a significant mechanism of injury, such as (as outlined in the CDC, 2011 Guidelines for the Field Triage of the Injured Patient):

TABLE 8-2: **History and Secondary Assessment**

Mechanism of Injury—Trauma	Nature of Illness—Medical
All Patients: • Ejection from a vehicle • Death of a passenger from the same vehicle • Fall >20 ft • Rollover of vehicle • High-speed crash • Vehicle versus pedestrian • Motorcycle crash • Unresponsive or AMS • Penetrations of the head, neck, chest, abdomen • Hidden injuries (seat belt/air bag) **Infants and Children:** • Falls >10 ft • Medium-speed vehicle crash • Bicycle crash	Assess complaint, signs and symptoms: (OPQRSTI): O = Onset—When or how did the symptoms start? P = Provocation—What caused or makes the symptoms change or worsen? Q = Quality—Describe symptoms/sensations/pain. R = Radiation—Does sensation move to other body areas? S = Severity—How severe is the discomfort? Scale of 1-10. T = Time—How long have the symptoms lasted? I = Interventions—Any interventions performed prior to EMS arrival? • If the patient is unresponsive or they are a priority NOI • Reassess airway and protect the airway • Perform rapid assessment

TABLE 8-3: **Important Considerations for Priority Patients**

Respiratory	Cardiac	AMS	Allergic Reaction	Poisoning/ OD	Environmental	Obstetrics	Behavioral
Onset? Provocation? Quality? Radiation? Severity? Time? Interventions?	Onset? Provocation? Quality? Radiation? Severity? Time? Interventions?	Description of episode. Onset? Duration? Associated symptoms? Evidence of trauma? Interventions? Seizures? Fever?	History? What were they exposed to? How? Effects? Progression? Interventions?	Substance? When did they get exposed or ingest substance? How much? Over what period? Interventions? Patients' esti- mated weight?	Source? Environment? Duration? Loss of consciousness? Effects local or general?	Are you pregnant? How long have you been pregnant? Pain or contractions? Bleeding or discharge? Has your water broken? Do you feel the urge to push? Last menstrual cycle?	How do you feel? Determine sui- cidal tendencies? Is the patient a threat to them- selves or others? Is there an underlying medi- cal problem? Interventions?

Falls

  ○ Adults: greater than 20 ft (one story is equal to 10 ft)

  ○ Children: greater than 10 ft, or two or three times the height of the child

High-risk auto crash

  ○ Intrusion, including roof: greater than 12 in occupant site

  ○ Greater than 18 in any site

  ○ Ejection (partial or complete) from automobile

  ○ Death in same passenger compartment

  ○ Vehicle telemetry data consistent with a high risk of injury

  ○ Auto versus pedestrian/bicyclist thrown, run over, or with

  ○ Significant (>20 mph) impact

  ○ Motorcycle crash greater than 20 mph

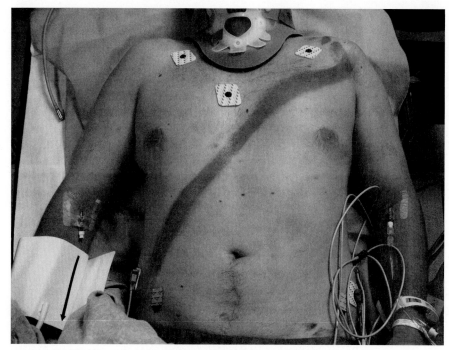

Figure 8-2 Chest and Abdominal Injury *(Reproduced with permission from Knoop KJ, Stack LB, Storrow AB, (eds): The Atlas of Emergency Medicine, 3rd edition. New York: McGraw-Hill; 2014. Photo contributor Brad Russell, MD)*

- ○ Unresponsive or altered mental status
- ○ Penetrations of the head, chest, or abdomen
- ○ Look for hidden injuries from:
  — Seat belts
    - If buckled, may have produced injuries (Fig. 8-2).
    - If patient had seat belt on, it does not mean they do not have injuries.
  — Air bags
    - May not be effective without seat belt.
    - Patient can hit wheel after deflation.
    - Lift the deployed air bag and look at the steering wheel for deformation.
    - "Lift and look" under the bag after the patient has been removed.
    - Any visible deformation of the steering wheel should be regarded as an indicator of potentially serious internal injury, and appropriate action should be taken.

High-Risk Trauma Patients

Older Adults

- ○ Risk of injury/death increases after the age of 55.
- ○ Systolic blood pressure (SBP) less than 110 may represent shock after age 65.
- ○ Low-impact mechanisms (eg, ground level falls) may result in severe injury.

Children

- ○ Should be triaged preferentially to pediatric capable trauma centers.

○ Anticoagulants and bleeding disorders.

○ Patients with head injury are at high risk for rapid deterioration.

Burns

○ Without other trauma mechanism: triage/transport to a burn facility

○ With trauma mechanism: triage/transport to a trauma center

Pregnancy More Than 20 Weeks

- Specific MOI involving pediatric patients:
  ○ Falls greater than 10 ft
  ○ Bicycle collision
  ○ Vehicle in medium-speed collision, restrained, or unrestrained
    — Perform rapid trauma assessment on patients with significant mechanism of injury to determine life-threatening injuries. In the responsive patient, symptoms should be sought before and during the trauma assessment.
    — Consider spinal stabilization.
    — Consider ALS request, but *do not delay* transport awaiting arrival of ALS.
    — Reconsider transport decision (transport to the appropriate 911 receiving hospital such as a trauma center).
    — Assess mental status.
    — As you inspect and palpate, look and feel for the following examples of injuries or signs of injury (Table 8-4):
- Assess the *head*, inspect and palpate for injuries or signs of injury.
- Assess the *neck*, inspect and palpate for injuries or signs of injury.
- Apply cervical spinal immobilization collar (CSIC).
- Assess the *chest*, inspect and palpate for injuries or signs of injury:
  ○ Paradoxical motion
  ○ Crepitation

TABLE 8-4: **Guidelines for Assessment of Trauma Patients**

If unresponsive or priority MOI or NOI. Reassess mental status, perform spinal immobilization as required, and complete a head-to-toe examination. **Remember to roll the patient and assess the posterior body.**

Assess baseline vital signs

Breathing: rate, rhythm, depth

Pulse: rate/quality (strong/weak/regular/irregular)

Pupils: size, reactivity to light and are they equal?

Blood pressure (systolic/diastolic)

Capillary refill: children <6 y of age

Assess SAMPLE history

S = Signs and symptoms

A = Allergies (medications, food, bee stings, etc)

M = Medications (prescribed or over the counter), are they compliant with taking their medications as prescribed?

P = Past pertinent medical history

L = Last oral intake

E = Events leading to history of present illness (HPI)

- Breath sounds in the apices, midclavicular line, bilaterally, bases, midaxillary line, and are they:
  - Present?
  - Absent?
  - Equal?
- Assess the *abdomen*, inspect and palpate for injuries or signs of injury.
  - Firm
  - Soft
  - Distended
- Assess the *pelvis*, inspect and palpate for injuries or signs of injury.
  - If no pain is noted, gently compress the pelvis to determine tenderness or motion.
- Assess *all four extremities*, inspect and palpate for injuries or signs of injury.
  - Distal pulse
  - Sensation
  - Motor function
- Roll patient with spinal precautions and assess posterior body, inspect and palpate, examining for injuries or signs of injury.
- Assess *baseline* vital signs.
- Assess *SAMPLE* history.
- For patients with no significant mechanism of injury:
  - Perform a history and physical examination of injuries.
  - Assess baseline vital signs.
  - Assess *SAMPLE* history.

HISTORY AND SECONDARY ASSESSMENT, "MEDICAL"

- Assess history of present illness. Obtaining an accurate history is the critical first step in determining the etiology of a patient's problem. A large percentage of the time, you will actually be able to make a diagnosis based on the history alone. The value of the history, of course, will depend on your ability to elicit relevant information. Your sense of what constitutes important data will grow exponentially in the coming years as you gain a greater understanding of the pathophysiology of disease through increased exposure to patients and illness.
- Assess patient complaint. Signs are what the EMT can physically see. Symptoms are what the patient describes to the EMT (such as complaining of nausea, headache, and so on).
- OPQRST.
  - *Onset*—What were you doing when the problem began?
  - *Provocation*—What makes the problem better or worse?
  - *Quality*—How would you describe the problem or pain?
  - *Radiation*—Does the pain radiate, or are there associated problems?
  - *Severity*—How intense is the pain on a scale from 1 to 10?
  - *Time*—How long ago did the problem begin?
- Assess *SAMPLE* history.
  - *Signs/symptoms?*

- ○ *Allergies*—Are you allergic to any medications?
- ○ *Medications*—Are you taking any prescribed or over-the-counter medications? When did you take them last? Are you compliant with taking your medications?
- ○ *Past medical problems*—Have you had any past or recent surgeries? Are you under the care of a physician?
- ○ *Last oral intake*—What have you had to eat or drink in the past 24 hours?
- ○ *Events* leading to the emergency—What happened, and what were you doing before the incident?

- Perform a physical assessment.
  - ○ Assess the head as needed.
  - ○ Assess the neck as needed.
  - ○ Assess the chest as needed.
  - ○ Assess the abdomen as needed.
  - ○ Assess the pelvis as needed.
  - ○ Assess the extremities as needed.
  - ○ Assess the posterior body as needed.
- Assess *baseline* vital signs.
- Provide emergency medical care based on signs and symptoms in consultation with medical direction.

Clinical Significance

S—Signs and symptoms; A—Allergies; M—Medications; P—Past history; L—Last oral intake; E—Events leading up to the present illness or injury. The goal during this phase of the medical patient assessment is to *focus* on the problem.

UNRESPONSIVE MEDICAL PATIENTS

- Position patient to protect airway.
- Perform rapid assessment.
  - ○ Assess the head.
  - ○ Assess the neck.
  - ○ Assess the chest.
  - ○ Assess the abdomen.
  - ○ Assess the pelvis.
  - ○ Assess the extremities.
  - ○ Assess the posterior aspect of the body.
- Assess baseline vital signs.
- Obtain *SAMPLE* history from bystanders, family, and friends prior to leaving.

PHYSICAL EXAMINATION

(Table 8-5)

- Patient and injury specific, that is, minor cut finger would not require a detailed examination.
- Perform a physical examination on the patient to gather additional information.
  - ○ As you inspect and palpate, look and/or feel for the following examples of injuries or signs of injury.
  - ○ Assess the head, inspect and palpate for injuries or signs of injury.
  - ○ Assess the face, inspect and palpate for injuries or signs of injury.
  - ○ Assess the ears, inspect and palpate for injuries or signs of injury plus drainage.

TABLE 8-5: Detailed Assessment

Complete head-to-toe assessment: Perform a full body assessment of areas not previously examined. The purpose is to identify previously unknown wounds and injuries and manage secondary problems.

Assess the head

Assess the neck: jugular vein distention and crepitation

Assess the chest: paradoxical movement, crepitation, and lung sounds

Assess the abdomen: swelling (firm/soft)

Assess the pelvis: if there is no pain present—compress

Assess the extremities: (pulse, motor, sensory)

Assess the posterior body

Performance is patient and injury specific. The detailed assessment is utilized to gather detailed patient information in addition to initial and focused assessments. Patient illness/injury will guide the EMT as to whether to perform this assessment or not.

○ Assess the eyes, inspect for injuries or signs of injury plus discoloration, unequal pupils, foreign bodies, and blood in the anterior chamber.

○ Assess the nose, inspect and palpate for injuries or signs of injury plus drainage and bleeding.

○ Assess the mouth, inspect for injuries or signs of injury plus teeth, obstructions, swollen or lacerated tongue, odors, and discoloration.

○ Assess the neck, inspect and palpate for injuries or signs of injury plus jugular vein distention and crepitus.

○ Assess the chest, inspect and palpate for injuries or signs of injury plus crepitus and paradoxical motion.

○ Breath sounds in the apices, midclavicular line, bilaterally, and at the bases, midaxillary line, bilaterally.

— Check for presence, absence, and whether they are equal.

○ Assess the abdomen, inspect and palpate for injuries or signs of injury plus check for a firm, soft, or distended abdomen.

○ Assess the pelvis, inspect and palpate for injuries or signs of injury. If the patient does not complain of pain or is unresponsive, gently flex and compress the pelvis to determine stability.

○ Assess all four extremities, inspect and palpate for injuries or signs of injury plus distal pulses, sensation, and motor function.

○ Roll with spinal precautions and assess posterior aspect of body, inspect and palpate for injuries or signs of injury.

ASSESS BASELINE VITAL SIGNS

See Table 8-6.

TABLE 8-6: Reassessment

Repeat the primary assessment; Reassess mental status; monitor airway, breathing, and circulatory status; and adjust priorities as needed. Reassess vital signs; repeat focused examination regarding complaint or injuries (HPI). Reassess interventions. *Stable patients repeat every 15 min; unstable patients repeat every 5 min.*

Baseline Vital Signs and History Taking

You respond to an adult female having difficulty breathing. Upon arrival you find a 23-year-old woman in obvious respiratory distress secondary to asthma. You perform a primary assessment and begin treatment with an albuterol nebulizer at 6 L/min. As treatment is being rendered, your partner begins eliciting the past medical history. What questions should you ask?

GENERAL INFORMATION

- Chief complaint—Why emergency medical services (EMS) was notified (ie, "My chest hurts.")
- Age—Years, months, days
- Gender—Male or female
- Race
- Estimated weight of patient

BASELINE VITAL SIGNS

Breathing

- Assessed by observing the patient's chest rise and fall.
- Rate is determined by counting the number of breaths in a 30-second period and multiplying by 2. Care should be taken not to inform the patient, to avoid influencing the rate.
- Quality of breathing can be determined while assessing the rate. Quality can be placed in one of the following categories:
  - Normal—average chest wall motion, not using accessory muscles
  - Shallow—slight chest or abdominal wall motion
  - Labored
    - An increase in the effort of breathing
    - Grunting and stridor
    - Use of accessory muscles
    - Nasal flaring, supraclavicular, and intercostal retractions in infants and children
    - Sometimes gasping
    - Noisy—an increase in the audible sound of breathing, may include snoring, wheezing, gurgling, crowing

Pulse

- Initially a radial pulse should be assessed in all patients who are 1 year or older. In patients less than 1 year of age, a brachial pulse should be assessed.
- If the pulse is present, assess rate and quality.
- Rate is the number of beats felt in 30 seconds multiplied by 2.

- Quality of the pulse can be characterized as:
  - Strong/Weak
  - Regular/Irregular
  - Absent (If absent, begin cardiopulmonary resuscitation [CPR] at a compression to ventilation rate of 30:2.)
- If peripheral pulse is not palpable, assess carotid pulse.
- Use caution. Avoid excess pressure on geriatrics. Never attempt to assess carotid pulse on both sides at one time.

Skin

Assess skin to determine perfusion.

- The patient's color should be assessed in the nail beds, oral mucosa, and conjunctiva.
- In infants and children, palms of hands and soles of feet should be assessed.
- Normal skin appearance—Pink.
- Abnormal skin colors:
  - Pale—Indicating poor perfusion (impaired blood flow)
  - Cyanotic (blue-gray)—Indicating inadequate oxygenation or hypoperfusion
  - Flushed (red)—Indicating exposure to heat or carbon monoxide poisoning (late sign)
  - Jaundice (yellow)—Indicating liver abnormalities such as hepatitis, liver failure, liver cancer
- The patient's temperature should be assessed by placing the back of your hand on the patient's skin.

  - Normal—Warm
  - Abnormal skin temperatures:
    — Hot—Indicating fever or an exposure to heat
    — Cool—Indicating poor perfusion or exposure to cold
    — Cold—Indicating extreme exposure to cold
- Assess the condition of the patient's skin.
  - Normal—Dry.
  - Abnormal—Skin is wet (diaphoretic), moist, or dry.
- Assess capillary refill in infants and children less than 6 years of age.
  - Capillary refill in infants and children is assessed by pressing on the patient's skin or nail beds and determining the time for return to initial color.
  - Normal capillary refill in infants and children is less than 2 seconds.
  - Abnormal capillary refill in infants and children is greater than 2 seconds.

> **Clinical Significance**
> Skin temperature is best assessed by using a thermometer (ie, tympanic thermometer or oral thermometer).

Pupils

Pupils are assessed by briefly shining a light into the patient's eyes, and determining size and reactivity.

- Dilated (very big), normal, or constricted (small)
- Equal or unequal

- Reactivity—Whether or not the pupils change in response to the light
  - Reactive—Change when exposed to light
  - Nonreactive—Do not change when exposed to light
  - Equally or unequally reactive

Blood Pressure

- Assess systolic and diastolic pressures.
- Systolic blood pressure is the first distinct sound of blood flowing through the artery as the pressure in the blood pressure cuff is released. This is a measurement of the pressure exerted against the walls of the arteries during contraction of the heart.
- Diastolic blood pressure is the point during deflation of the blood pressure cuff at which sounds of the pulse beat disappear. It represents the pressure exerted against the walls of the arteries while the left ventricle is at rest.
- There are two methods of obtaining blood pressure:
  - Auscultation—The EMT will listen for the systolic and diastolic sounds.
  - Palpation—In certain situations, the systolic blood pressure may be measured by feeling for return of pulse with deflation of the cuff.
- Blood pressure should be measured in all patients older than 3 years of age.
- The general assessment of the infant or child patient, such as appearing sick, in respiratory distress, or unresponsive, is more valuable than vital sign numbers.
- Reassessment of vital signs:
  - Vital signs should be assessed and recorded every 15 minutes at a minimum in a stable patient.
  - Vital signs should be assessed and recorded every 5 minutes in an unstable patient.
  - Vital signs should be assessed following all medical interventions.

OBTAIN A SAMPLE HISTORY

Use the mnemonic *SAMPLE*:

Signs/Symptoms

- Sign—Any medical or trauma condition displayed by the patient and identifiable by the EMT, that is, hearing = respiratory distress, seeing = bleeding, feeling = skin temperature
- Symptom—Any condition described by the patient, that is, shortness of breath, nausea, chest pain

Allergies

- Medications
- Food
- Environmental allergies
- Consider medical identification tag

Medications (Prescription)

- Nonprescription
- Current
- Recent
- Consider medical identification tag

Pertinent Past History

- Medical (prior intubations in an asthmatic)
- Surgical (recent surgery)
- Trauma
- Consider medical identification tag

Last Oral Intake—Solid or Liquid

- Time
- Quantity

Events

Leading to the injury or illness (ie, chest pain with exertion, or chest pain while at rest)

- Repeat primary assessment. For a stable patient, repeat and record every 15 minutes. For an unstable patient, repeat and record at a minimum every 5 minutes.
  - Reassess mental status.
  - Maintain open airway.
  - Monitor breathing for rate and quality.
  - Reassess pulse for rate and quality.
  - Monitor skin color and temperature.
  - Reestablish patient priorities.
- Reassess and record vital signs.
- Repeat assessment regarding patient complaint or injuries.
- **Check interventions such as adequacy of oxygen delivery/artificial ventilation, management of bleeding, and adequacy of other interventions.**

> **Clinical Significance**
> Patient compliance with taking medication in accordance with his/her physician is about 50% in the United States.

? CHAPTER QUESTIONS

1. In a blood pressure reading of 120/80, the 120 refers to the diastolic pressure and the 80 refers to the systolic pressure.

   a. True
   b. False

2. The *L* in SAMPLE stands for:

   a. length of illness
   b. last doctor's visit
   c. length of chief complaint
   d. last oral intake

3. The term used to describe a weak, rapid pulse is:

   a. mottled
   b. reedy
   c. thready
   d. bounding

4. The skin color that indicates inadequate breathing or inadequate perfusion is:

   a. flushed
   b. blue-gray
   c. jaundice
   d. yellow

5. Mechanism of injury refers to:

   a. the specific injury that the patient has received
   b. how the patient was injured
   c. the degree of your anticipation that the patient has received an injury
   d. injuries specifically caused by machinery or industrial equipment

6. When responding to a motor vehicle crash, significant mechanism of injury would include:

   a. vehicle rollover
   b. deformity to the vehicle greater than 12 in into the passenger compartment
   c. leaking fuel tank
   d. death of an occupant in the same vehicle
   e. all of the above

7. Patient assessment has several main purposes. These include:

   a. to obtain the patient's medical insurance information
   b. to diagnose the reason for the patient's symptoms
   c. to monitor the patient's condition
   d. both b and c are correct

8. The main purpose of the primary assessment is to:

   a. identify and manage immediately life-threatening injuries or conditions
   b. communicate patient information to the medical facility staff
   c. determine whether the patient is injured or has a medical illness
   d. examine the patient and gather a patient history

9. The four components of patient assessment include:

   a. the rapid trauma assessment
   b. baseline vitals
   c. the primary assessment
   d. transport
   e. all of the above

10. It is important to form a general impression of every patient you care for, as it provides valuable information about the patient's condition. Forming a general impression includes:

    a. obtaining the patient's chief complaint
    b. assessment of the patient's mental status
    c. estimation of the patient's weight
    d. the application of high-concentration oxygen

11. During the primary assessment you should be looking for conditions that require immediate management as they are found. These may include:

    a. possible internal injuries to the abdomen

    b. possible fractures to the extremities

    c. open wounds to the chest that may disrupt thoracic pressure

    d. capillary bleeding

12. The mnemonic used to assess a patient's mental status is:

    a. DCAP-BTLS

    b. AEIOU-TIPS

    c. AVPU

    d. OPQRST

13. You may need to make adjustments when gauging the mental status of a child or an infant. These include:

    a. knowing that crying may replace speech as a response

    b. watching and listening to the child's reaction to a shout

    c. noting whether the child follows movement with his eyes

    d. all of the above

14. As you approach your patient, he calls out "please help me—my leg hurts really bad." You would classify his level of responsiveness as:

    a. unresponsive

    b. alert

    c. responds to verbal stimulus

    d. responds to painful stimulus

15. During your assessment, the patient no longer responds to you when you speak to him. However, when you pinch the shoulder skin he tries to move away. Which of the following is true regarding his level of responsiveness?

    a. The patient has become unresponsive.

    b. He has responded with purposeful movement to painful stimulus.

    c. His response to the painful stimulus means he is still alert.

    d. He has responded with nonpurposeful movement to painful stimulus.

16. An unresponsive medical patient requires airway management. Which of the following is true regarding airway control of the unresponsive patient?

    a. An airway adjunct should still be used to keep the airway of a conscious, alert patient open.

    b. The head-tilt-chin-lift maneuver can be used on both medical and trauma patients.

    c. Manual airway maneuvers prevent the tongue and epiglottis from blocking the airway of an unresponsive patient.

    d. Manual airway maneuvers are not necessary if you are using an airway adjunct.

17. A gurgling sound may indicate a liquid substance in the airway. You should immediately:

    a. insert an airway adjunct

    b. turn the patient on his side to let the contents drain out of the mouth

    c. open the mouth and suction out the contents

    d. tilt the head back farther to more completely open the airway

18. Which of the following is true regarding crowing and stridor?

    a. Both are rattling sounds produced on exhalation.
    b. Airway adjuncts should be used in a child with suspected infection of the epiglottis.
    c. Both are commonly associated with swelling or muscle spasms of the airway.
    d. They are usually relieved by proper positioning of the airway, and airway adjuncts.

19. As soon as the patient's airway is opened, assess the breathing status to:

    a. determine the need for early oxygen therapy
    b. determine if the breathing is adequate or inadequate
    c. provide positive-pressure ventilation with supplemental oxygen if needed
    d. all of the above

20. As an EMT, your initial evaluation of the scene is called the:

    a. primary assessment
    b. secondary assessment
    c. hazard assessment
    d. scene size-up

21. You have three basic goals during scene size-up. These include all of the following *except*:

    a. determining if additional assistance is needed
    b. determining the patient's chief complaint
    c. identifying hazards and ensure safety
    d. determining what led to your being called to the scene

22. Scene safety should be assessed:

    a. during your assessment of the patient
    b. when you first make contact with the patient
    c. throughout the call
    d. when you first arrive at the scene

23. The process of ensuring scene safety should begin with:

    a. arrival on-scene
    b. dispatch information
    c. the arrival of law enforcement
    d. first contact with patient

24. EMTs should consider scene safety when responding to:

    a. domestic violence calls
    b. motor vehicle crashes
    c. all EMS responses
    d. chest pain calls

Suggested Reading

US Department of Transportation, National Highway Traffic Safety Administration. *EMT-Basic National Standard Curriculum.* Washington, DC: US Department of Transportation, National Highway Traffic Safety Administration; 1994.

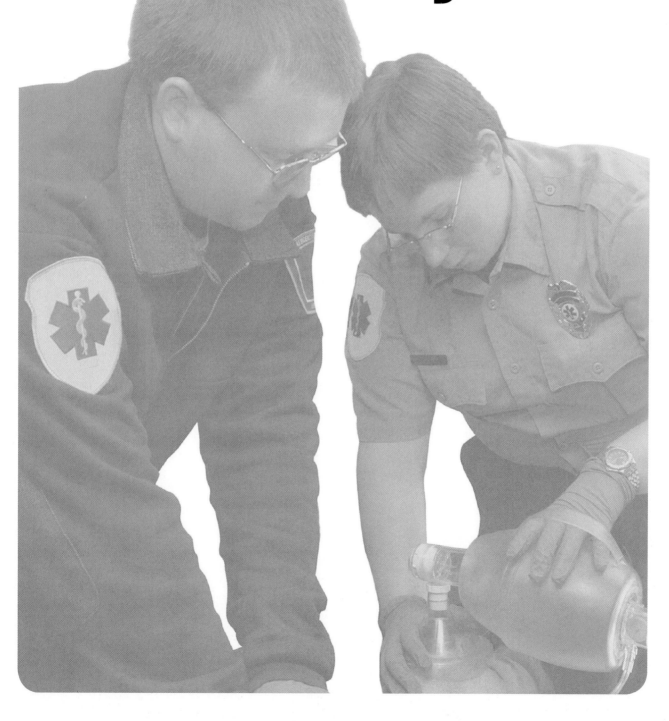

Section 4
Airway

Chapter 9
Airway Management, Ventilation, and Oxygen Therapy

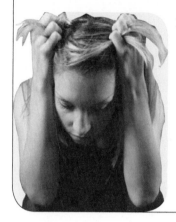

It is 11:30 PM in a suburban town. A 40-year-old woman has just gone to bed when she begins to complain of difficulty in breathing. The patient's husband summons emergency medical services (EMS). A few moments later, you are dispatched to this location for a person having respiratory difficulty from asthma. When you arrive you find a woman 40 years old sitting in her kitchen, obviously breathing heavy (in severe distress), sitting tripod with accessory muscle use, trying to speak but is unable because she is only able to speak in one-word sentences. She says, "I......can't.......breathe, my.........asthma." What would be your next action?

RESPIRATORY ANATOMY REVIEW

Upper Airway

- Nose and mouth (Fig. 9-1)
- Pharynx—U-shaped muscular structure located between the oral and nasal cavity, posterior to the larynx
  - Oropharynx—Encompassed by the soft palate above and the epiglottis below
  - Nasopharynx—Situated behind the nasal cavity, above the soft palate
- Epiglottis—A leaf-shaped structure that prevents food and liquid from entering the trachea during swallowing
- Trachea (windpipe)
- Cricoid cartilage—Firm cartilage ring forming the lower portion of the larynx
- Larynx (voice box)

Lower Airway

- Bronchi—Two major branches of the trachea to the lungs. Bronchus subdivides into smaller air passages ending at the alveoli.
- Lungs.
- Diaphragm.

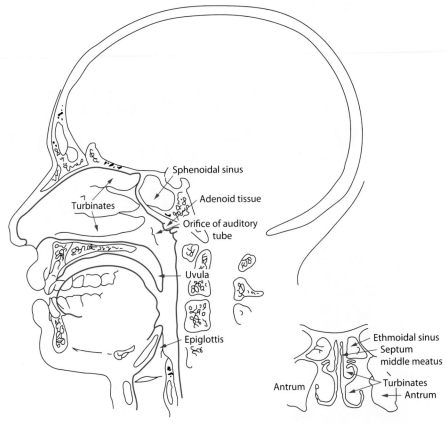

Figure 9-1   Respiratory anatomy.

- Inhalation (active).
  - Diaphragm and intercostal muscles contract, increasing the size of the thoracic cavity.
  - Diaphragm moves slightly downward.
  - Ribs move upward/outward.
  - Air flows into the lungs.
- Exhalation (passive).
  - Diaphragm and intercostal muscles relax, decreasing the size of the thoracic cavity.
  - Diaphragm moves upward.
  - Ribs move downward/inward.
  - Air flows out of the lungs.

RESPIRATORY PHYSIOLOGY

See Figure 9-2.

- Alveolar/capillary exchange (site of gas exchange).
- Oxygen-rich air enters the alveoli during each inspiration.
- Oxygen-poor blood in the capillaries passes into the alveoli.
- Oxygen enters the capillaries as carbon dioxide enters the alveoli.
- Capillary/cellular exchange.
  - Cells give up carbon dioxide to the capillaries.
  - Capillaries give up oxygen to the cells.

Clinical Significance

Although these ranges are considered normal for the adult, child, and infant, it is important to remember that abnormal findings, such as perioral cyanosis, tripoding, tachypnea, and altered mental status, in conjunction with these ranges, are clinical findings of respiratory distress/failure.

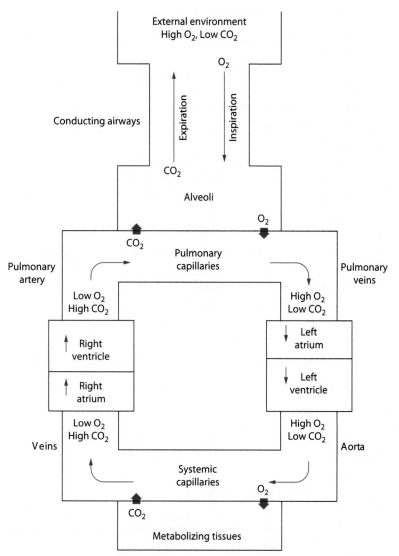

Figure 9-2 Respiratory physiology. (*Reproduced with permission from Levitzky MG. Pulmonary Physiology. 7th ed. New York: McGraw-Hill; 2007*)

ADEQUATE BREATHING

Normal Rate

- Adult—12 to 20/min
- Child—15 to 30/min
- Infant—25 to 50/min

Rhythm

- Is the rhythm regular or irregular?

Quality

- Breath sounds—Present and equal
- Chest expansion—Adequate and equal
- Minimum effort of breathing—Use of accessory muscles (predominantly in infants and children)

Depth (Tidal Volume)

- Adequate tidal volume for the adult patient is approximately 500 cc.

EVALUATION OF INADEQUATE BREATHING

- Rate—Outside of normal ranges.
- Rhythm—Irregular?
- Quality.
  - Breath sounds—Diminished or absent
  - Chest expansion—Unequal or inadequate
  - Increased effort of breathing—Use of accessory muscles (predominantly in infants and children)
- Depth (tidal volume)—Inadequate/shallow.
- The skin may be pale or cyanotic (blue), and cool and clammy.
- There may be retractions above the clavicles, between the ribs, and below the rib cage, especially in children.
- Nasal flaring may be present, especially in children.
- In infants, there may be "see-saw" breathing where the abdomen and chest move in opposite directions.
- Agonal respirations (occasional gasping breaths) may be seen just before death.

PEDIATRIC ANATOMY CONSIDERATIONS

- Mouth and nose—In general, all structures are smaller and more easily obstructed than in adults.
- Pharynx—Infants' and children's tongues take up proportionally more space in the mouth than adults.
- Trachea (windpipe).
  - Infants and children have narrower tracheas that are obstructed more easily by swelling.
  - The trachea is softer and more flexible in infants and children.
  - Cricoid cartilage—Like other cartilage in the infant and child, the cricoid cartilage is less developed and less rigid.
  - Diaphragm—Chest wall is softer; infants and children tend to depend more heavily on the diaphragm for breathing.

ADEQUATE AND INADEQUATE ARTIFICIAL VENTILATION

- An emergency medical technician (EMT) is artificially ventilating a patient adequately when:
  - The chest rises and falls with each artificial ventilation.
  - The rate is sufficient, approximately 10 to 12 per minute for adults and 12 to 20 times per minute for children and infants.
  - Heart rate returns to normal with successful artificial ventilation.
- Artificial ventilation is inadequate when:
  - The chest does not rise and fall with artificial ventilation.
  - The rate is too slow or too fast.

- In pediatric patients heart rate does not return to normal with artificial ventilation.
- Skin color does not improve.

OPENING THE AIRWAY

- Head-tilt-chin-lift when no neck injury suspected (Fig. 9-3)
- Jaw-thrust when EMT suspects spinal injury (Fig. 9-4)
- Assess need for suctioning

TECHNIQUES OF SUCTIONING

- Utilize proper body substance isolation.
- Purpose of suctioning include:
  - Remove blood, other liquids, and food particles from the airway.

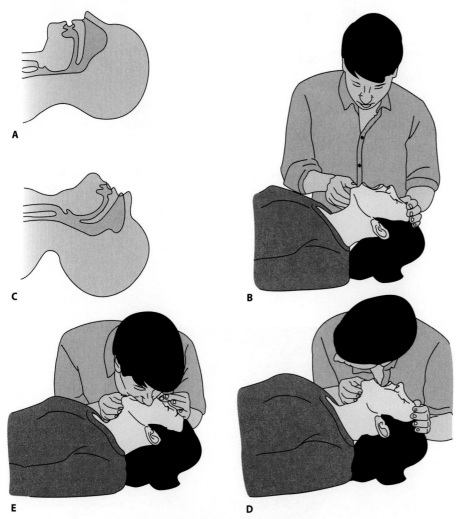

Figure 9-3 Head-tilt-chin-lift. *(Reproduced with permission from Stone CK, Humphries RL. Current Diagnosis and Treatment: Emergency Medicine. 6th ed. New York: McGraw-Hill; 2007)*

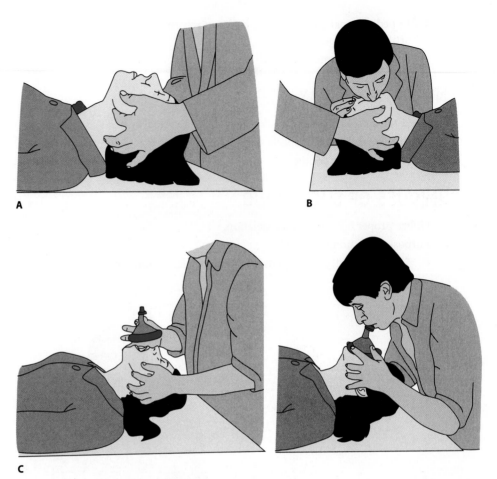

A   **B**

C

Figure 9-4A   Modified jaw thrust. *(Reproduced with permission from Stone CK, Humphries RL. Current Diagnosis and Treatment: Emergency Medicine. 6th ed. New York: McGraw-Hill; 2007)*

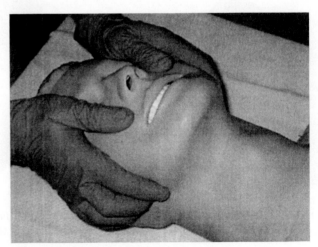

Figure 9-4B   Modified jaw thrust. *(Used with permission of Peter DiPrima.)*

- Some suction units are inadequate for removing solid objects like teeth, foreign bodies, and food.
- A patient needs to be suctioned immediately when a gurgling sound is heard with artificial ventilation.

TYPES OF SUCTION UNITS

- Mounted (Fig. 9-5A)
- Portable suction units (Fig. 9-5B)
- Hand operated (Fig. 9-5C)

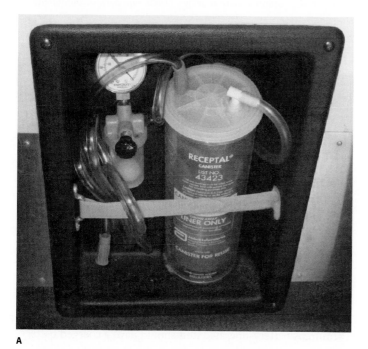

A

Figure 9-5A   Onboard suction unit. *(Used with permission of Peter DiPrima.)*

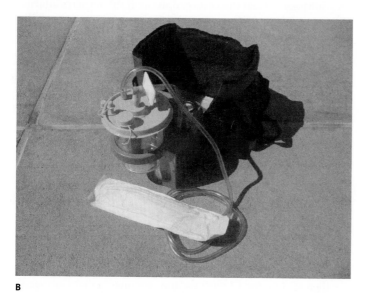

B

Figure 9-5B   Portable suction unit. *(Used with permission of Peter DiPrima.)*

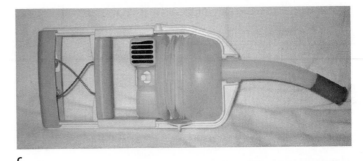

c

Figure 9-5C   Manual suction device. *(Used with permission of Peter DiPrima.)*

SUCTION CATHETERS

- Hard or rigid ("tonsil sucker," "tonsil tip") Yankauer
  - Used to suction the mouth and oropharynx of an unresponsive patient.
  - Should be inserted only as far as you can see.
  - Use rigid catheter for infants and children, but take caution not to touch back of airway.
- Soft (French)
  - Useful for suctioning the nasopharynx and in other situations where a rigid catheter cannot be used.
  - Should be measured so that it is inserted only as far as the base of the tongue.

Techniques of Use

- Suction device should be inspected on a regular basis before it is needed. A properly functioning unit with a gauge should generate 300 mm Hg vacuum. A battery-operated unit should have a charged battery.
- Turn on the suction unit.
- If there is no measuring gauge, allow suction tubing to begin suctioning on your finger. Turn the suction unit off; if tubing stays attached, there is adequate suction.
- Attach a catheter.
- Use rigid catheter when suctioning mouth of an infant or child.
- Often will need to suction nasal passages; should use a bulb suction or French catheter with low-to-medium suction.
- Insert the catheter into the oral cavity without suction. Insert only to the base of the tongue (as far as you can see).
- Apply suction. Move the catheter tip side to side.
- Suction for no more than 15 seconds at a time.
  - In infants and children, shorter suction time should be used.
  - If the patient has secretions or emesis that cannot be removed quickly and easily by suctioning, the patient should be log rolled and the oropharynx should be cleared.
  - If patient produces frothy secretions as rapidly as suctioning can remove, suction for 15 seconds, artificially ventilate for 2 minutes, then suction for 15 seconds, and continue in that manner. Consult medical direction for this situation.
  - If necessary, rinse the catheter and tubing with water to prevent obstruction of the tubing from dried material.

TECHNIQUES OF ARTIFICIAL VENTILATION

- Methods for ventilating a patient by the EMT are as follows:
  - Two-person bag-valve-mask (Fig. 9-6A)
  - Flow-restricted, oxygen-powered ventilation device
  - One-person bag-valve-mask (Fig. 9-6B)
- Use of body substance isolation.
- Mouth-to-mouth—Review technique learned in BCLS course.
- Mouth-to-mask (Fig. 9-6C).
- Bag-valve-mask—The mask should be connected to high-flow oxygen = 15 L/min (Fig. 9-7).
- The bag-valve-mask consists of a self-inflating bag, one-way valve, face mask, and oxygen reservoir. It needs to be connected to oxygen to perform effectively.
- Bag-valve-mask pros/cons include:
  - Maximum volume is approximately 1600 mL.
  - Provides less volume than mouth-to-mask.
  - Bag-valve-mask ventilation is challenging for a single EMT because maintaining an airtight seal requires considerable practice for competency.
  - Two EMTs using the device will be more effective.
  - Position self at the top of patient's head for optimal performance.
  - Adjunctive airways (oral or nasal) may be necessary in conjunction with bag-valve-mask.
  - May produce gastric inflation with positive-pressure ventilation.
- The bag-valve-mask should have:
  - A self-refilling bag.
  - A nonjam valve that allows a maximum oxygen inlet flow of 15 L/min.
  - No pop-off valve or the pop-off valve must be disabled. Failure to do so may result in inadequate artificial ventilations.
  - Standardized 15/22 mm fittings.

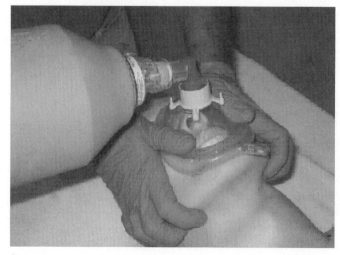

A

Figure 9-6A   Bag-valve-mask (BVM) with modified jaw-thrust maneuver (two rescuers). *(Used with permission of Peter DiPrima.)*

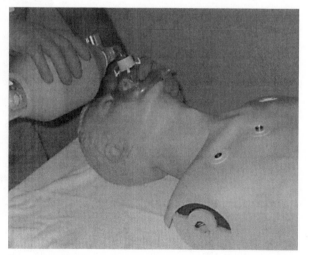

B

Figure 9-6B   Bag-valve-mask (BVM) with the head-tilt-chin-lift (one rescuer). *(Used with permission of Peter DiPrima.)*

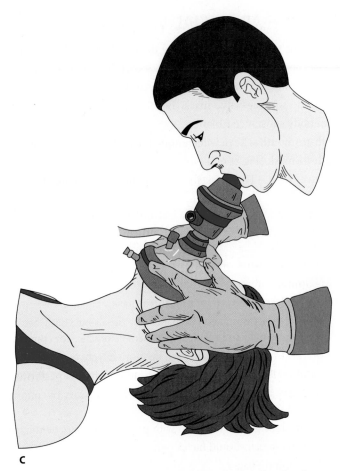

C

Figure 9-6C Adult bag-valve-mask (BVM). *(Reproduced with permission from Tintinalli JE, Kelen GD, Stapczynski JS. Tintinalli's Emergency Medicine: A Comprehensive Study Guide, 6th ed. New York: McGraw-Hill; 2003)*

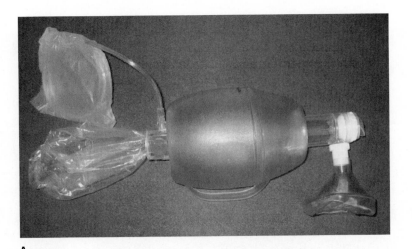

A

Figure 9-7A Adult bag-valve-mask. *(Used with permission of Peter DiPrima.)*

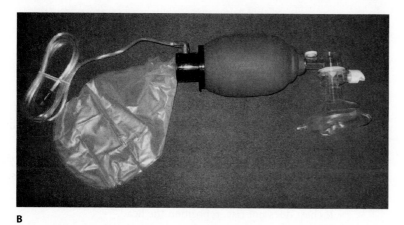

B

Figure 9-7B   Pediatric bag-valve-mask. *(Used with permission of Peter DiPrima.)*

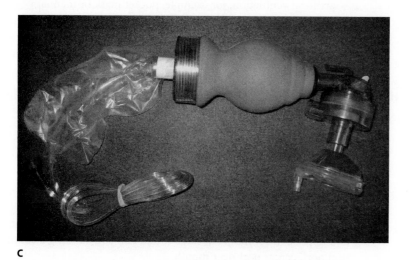

C

Figure 9-7C   Infant bag-valve-mask. *(Used with permission of Peter DiPrima.)*

- An oxygen inlet and reservoir to allow for high concentration of oxygen.
- A true valve for non-rebreather.
- Ability to perform in all environmental conditions and temperature extremes.
- Availability in infant, child, and adult sizes.

Using the Bag-Valve-Mask and the Head-Tilt-Chin-Lift

- Use when trauma is not suspected; after opening airway, select correct mask size (adult, infant, or child).
    - Position thumbs over top half of mask, and index and middle fingers over bottom half.
    - Place apex of mask over bridge of nose, then lower mask over mouth and upper chin.

Clinical Significance

During cardiopulmonary resuscitation (CPR), tidal volumes of approximately 500 to 600 cc are sufficient. Equivalent to 6 to 7 mL/kg.

- If mask has large round cuff surrounding a ventilation port, center port over mouth.
- Use ring and little fingers to bring jaw up to mask.
- Connect bag to mask if not already done.
- Have assistant squeeze bag with two hands until chest rises.
- If alone, form a "C" around the ventilation port with thumb and index finger; use middle, ring, and little fingers under jaw to maintain chin lift and complete the seal.
- Key is to observe adequate chest rise. Repeat a minimum of every 5 to 6 seconds for adults and every 3 seconds for children and infants.
- If chest does not rise and fall, reevaluate.
  — If chest does not rise, reposition the head.
  — If air is escaping from under the mask, reposition fingers and mask.
  — Check for obstruction.
  — If chest still does not rise and fall, use alternative method of artificial ventilation, for example, pocket mask or manually triggered device.
- If necessary, consider use of adjuncts, such as an oropharyngeal or nasopharyngeal airway.

Using the Bag-Valve-Mask and Modified Jaw Thrust

- Use with suspected trauma.
  - After opening airway, select the correct mask size (adult, infant, or child).
  - Immobilize head and neck, that is, have an assistant hold head manually or use your knees to prevent movement.
  - Position thumbs over top half of mask, and index and middle fingers over bottom half.
  - Place apex of mask over bridge of nose, then lower mask over mouth and upper chin. If mask has large round cuff surrounding a ventilation port, center port over mouth.
  - Use ring and little fingers to bring jaw up to mask *without* tilting head or neck.
  - Connect bag to mask if not already done.
  - Have assistant squeeze bag with two hands until chest rises.
  - Repeat every 5 to 6 seconds for adults and every 3 to 5 seconds for children and infants, continuing to hold jaw up without moving head or neck.
  - If chest does not rise, reevaluate.
    — If abdomen rises, reposition jaw.
    — If air is escaping from under the mask, reposition fingers and mask.
    — Check for obstruction.
    — If chest still does not rise, use alternative method of artificial ventilation, such as a pocket face mask.

Flow-Restricted, Oxygen-Powered Ventilation Devices

- Flow-restricted, oxygen-powered ventilation devices (for use in adults only) should provide:
  - A peak flow rate of 100% oxygen at up to 40 L/min.

- An inspiratory pressure relief valve that opens at approximately 60-cm water and vents any remaining volume to the atmosphere or ceases gas flow.
- An audible alarm that sounds whenever the relief valve pressure is exceeded.
- Satisfactory operation under ordinary environmental conditions and extremes of temperature.
- A trigger positioned so that both hands of the EMT can remain on the mask to hold it in position.

- *Use when no neck injury is suspected.*
  - After opening airway, insert correct size oral/nasal airway and attach adult bag-valve-mask.
  - Position thumbs over top half of mask, and index and middle fingers over bottom half.
  - Place apex of mask over bridge of nose, then lower the mask over mouth and upper chin.
  - Use ring and little fingers to bring jaw up to mask.
  - Connect flow-restricted, oxygen-powered ventilation device to mask.
  - Trigger the flow-restricted, oxygen-powered ventilation device until chest rises.
  - Repeat every 5 to 6 seconds in the adult patient only.
  - If necessary, consider use of adjuncts.
  - If chest does not rise, reevaluate.
  - If abdomen rises, reposition head.
  - If air is escaping from under the mask, reposition fingers and mask.
  - If chest still does not rise, use alternative method of artificial ventilation such as pocket mask.
  - Check for obstruction.

- *Use when there is suspected neck injury.*
  - After opening airway, attach adult mask.
  - Immobilize head and neck; for example, have an assistant to hold head manually or use your knees to prevent movement.
  - Position thumbs over top half of mask, and index and middle fingers over bottom half.
  - Place apex of mask over bridge of nose, then lower mask over mouth and upper chin.
  - Use ring and little fingers to bring jaw up to mask without tilting head or neck.
  - Connect flow-restricted, oxygen-powered ventilation device to mask, if not already done.
  - Trigger the flow-restricted, oxygen-powered ventilation device until chest rises.
  - Repeat every 5 to 6 seconds.
  - If necessary, consider use of adjuncts.
  - If chest does not rise and fall, reevaluate.
  - If chest does not rise and fall, reposition jaw.
  - If air is escaping from under the mask, reposition fingers and mask.
  - If chest still does not rise, use alternative method of artificial ventilation.
  - Check for obstruction.

Bag to Stoma or Tracheotomy Tube

- Tracheotomy—An artificial permanent opening in the trachea.
- If unable to artificially ventilate, try suction, then artificial ventilation through mouth and nose; sealing stoma may improve ability to artificially ventilate from above or may clear obstruction.

Bag-Valve-Mask to Stoma

- Use infant and child mask to make seal. The technique is otherwise very similar to artificially ventilating through mouth. Head and neck do not need to be positioned.

AIRWAY ADJUNCTS

Oropharyngeal (Oral) Airways

- Oropharyngeal airways may be used to assist in maintaining an open airway on unresponsive patients without a gag reflex (Fig. 9-8).

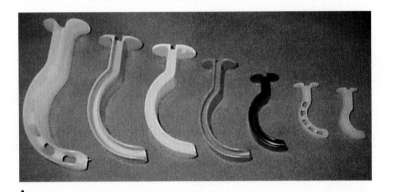

A

Figure 9-8A   Oropharyngeal airways. *(Used with permission of Peter DiPrima.)*

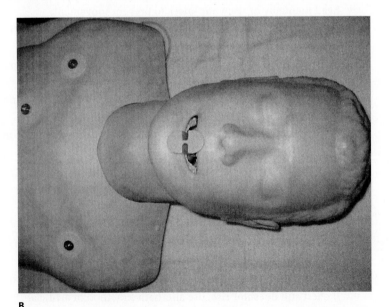

B

Figure 9-8B   Oropharyngeal airway placed. *(Used with permission of Peter DiPrima.)*

- ○ Select the proper size—Measure from the corner of the patient's lips to the bottom of the earlobe or angle of jaw.
- ○ Open the patient's mouth.
- ○ In adults, to avoid obstructing the airway with the tongue, insert the airway upside down, with the tip facing toward the roof of the patient's mouth.
- ○ Advance the airway gently until resistance is encountered. Turn the airway 180 degrees so that it comes to rest with the flange on the patient's teeth.
- ○ Another method of inserting an oral airway is to insert it right side up, using a tongue depressor to press the tongue down and forward to avoid obstructing the airway. This is the preferred method for airway insertion in an infant or child.

Nasopharyngeal (Nasal) Airways

- Nasopharyngeal airways (Fig. 9-9) are less likely to stimulate vomiting and may be used on patients who are responsive but need assistance keeping the tongue from obstructing the airway. Even though the tube is lubricated, it may be painful.
- Select the proper size—Measure from the tip of the nose to the tip of the patient's ear. Also consider diameter of airway in the nostril.
- Lubricate the airway with a water-soluble lubricant.
- Insert it posteriorly. Bevel should be toward the base of the nostril or toward the septum.
- If the airway cannot be inserted into one nostril, try the other nostril.
- Never force the airway adjunct into the nostril.

> ▶Note:
> Patients with an intact gag reflex will gag and vomit.

Use of Oxygen Cylinders

- Oxygen cylinders come in different sizes.
  - ○ D cylinder has 350 L (portable cylinder)
  - ○ E cylinder has 625 L (portable cylinder)
  - ○ M cylinder has 3000 L (onboard tank)
  - ○ G cylinder has 5300 L (onboard tank)
  - ○ H cylinder has 6900 L (onboard tank)

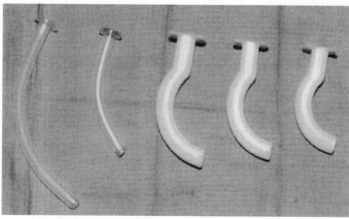

Nasal airways   Oral airways

Figure 9-9 Oral and nasal airways. *(Reproduced with permission from Brunicardi FC, Andersen DK, Billiar TR, et al (eds). Schwartz's Principles of Surgery, 8th ed. New York: McGraw-Hill; 2005)*

- Careful handling of the tanks is required because their contents are under pressure.
- Oxygen is an oxidizer and supports combustion. It is one of the four sides of the fire tetrahedron (oxygen, chemical reaction, fuel, and heat).
- Tanks should be positioned to prevent falling and blows to the valve-gauge assembly, and should always be secured during transport.
- Full tank has approximately 2000 psi and it varies with ambient temperature.
- Dry oxygen is typically not harmful short-term; keep in mind certain respiratory emergencies require treatment with humidified oxygen such as smoke inhalation, toxic inhalation, croup (pediatric patients), and asthma patients.

Operating Procedures

- Remove protective seal.
- Burp the tank by quickly opening, and then shutting, the valve.
- Attach regulator-flow meter to tank.
- Attach oxygen device to flow meter.
- Open flow meter to desired setting.
- Apply oxygen device to patient.
- When complete, remove device from patient, then turn off valve and remove all pressure from the regulator.

EQUIPMENT FOR OXYGEN DELIVERY

Non-rebreather Mask

- Preferred method of giving oxygen to pre-hospital patients.
- Up to 90% oxygen can be delivered.
- Non-rebreather bag must be full before mask is placed on patient.
- Flow rate should be adjusted so that when the patient inhales, bag does not collapse.

Indications for Oxygen Administration Using a Non-rebreather

- Patients who are cyanotic, cool, clammy, or short of breath need oxygen. Concerns about the dangers of giving too much oxygen to patients with a history of chronic obstructive pulmonary disease and infants and children have not been shown to be valid in the pre-hospital setting. Patients with chronic obstructive pulmonary disease and infants and children who require oxygen should receive high-concentration oxygen.
- Masks come in different sizes for adults, children, and infants. Be sure to select the correct mask size.

Contraindications

- None

Special Considerations

- Patients with laryngectomies (stomas).
- A breathing tube may be present. If it is obstructed, suction it.

▶Note:

Duration of oxygen flow formula
(Gauge pressure in pounds per square inch [psi] − safe residual pressure) × constant/flow rate in L/min
Safe residual pressure = 200 psi
Cylinder constant =
D = 0.16
E = 0.28
M = 1.56
G = 2.41
H = 3.14
K = 3.14

▶Note:

Nasal cannula should be used only when patients will not tolerate a non-rebreather mask, despite coaching from the EMT.

- Some patients have partial laryngectomies. If, upon artificially ventilating stoma, air escapes from the mouth or nose, close the mouth and pinch the nostrils.
- Pediatric patients.
  - Place the head in correct neutral position for the infant and extend a little past neutral for a child.
  - Avoid excessive hyperextension of the head and avoid excessive bag pressure—use only enough to make chest rise.
  - Ventilate with bag-valve-mask until adequate chest rise occurs. Do not use pop-off valve; must be disabled (placed in closed position) in order to adequately ventilate the child or infant.
  - Gastric distention is more common in children.
  - An oral or nasal airway may be considered when other procedures fail to provide a clear airway.

Facial Injuries

- Because the blood supply to the face is so rich, blunt injuries to the face frequently result in severe swelling.
- For the same reason, bleeding into the airway from facial injuries can be a challenge to manage.
- Obstructions.
  - Ask "are you choking?"
  - Give abdominal thrusts/Heimlich maneuver or chest thrusts for pregnant or obese victims. Repeat abdominal thrusts until patient becomes unresponsive.
  - When the patient becomes unresponsive, begin CPR.
  - Look into mouth when opening the airway during CPR. Use finger sweep only to remove visible foreign body.
- Dental appliances.
  - Dentures—Ordinarily dentures should be left in place. Dentures maintain a natural curvature of the face and will assist in proper ventilation. When dentures are removed, ventilation can become difficult due to the anatomical changes in the face.
  - Partial dentures (plates) may become dislodged during an emergency. Leave in place, but be prepared to remove it if it becomes dislodged.

? CHAPTER QUESTIONS

1. The primary function of the respiratory system is:

   a. the transportation of oxygen to the body cells
   b. the transportation of waste products from the cells to the lungs
   c. filtering the air that enters the lungs
   d. taking oxygen from the air and supplying it to the blood

2. A common cause of airway obstruction in the patient with an altered mental status is:

   a. the tongue
   b. food
   c. dentures
   d. secretions

3. Air entering the body through the mouth and nostrils travels into the:

   a. nasopharynx
   b. oropharynx
   c. laryngopharynx
   d. pharynx

4. The trachea is protected by a small flap of tissue called the:

   a. larynx
   b. epiglottis
   c. esophagus
   d. vallecula

5. The patient's vocal chords are contained in the:

   a. epiglottis
   b. larynx
   c. pharynx
   d. Adam's apple

6. The only completely circular cartilaginous ring of the upper airway is the:

   a. laryngeal cartilage
   b. hyoid membrane
   c. thyroid cartilage
   d. cricoid cartilage

7. The trachea descends into the chest cavity and branches into two main tubes, called:

   a. alveoli
   b. bronchioles
   c. bronchi
   d. alveolar ducts

8. The muscle that separates the chest cavity from the abdominal cavity is the:

   a. intercostal muscle
   b. pleura
   c. pectoralis muscle
   d. diaphragm

9. When a patient inhales:

   a. the diaphragm and the intercostal muscles relax
   b. the diaphragm relaxes and the intercostal muscles contract
   c. the diaphragm and the intercostal muscles contract
   d. the diaphragm contracts and the intercostal muscles relax

10. Inadequate oxygen being delivered to the cells is called:

    a. cyanosis
    b. deoxygenation
    c. hypoperfusion
    d. hypoxia

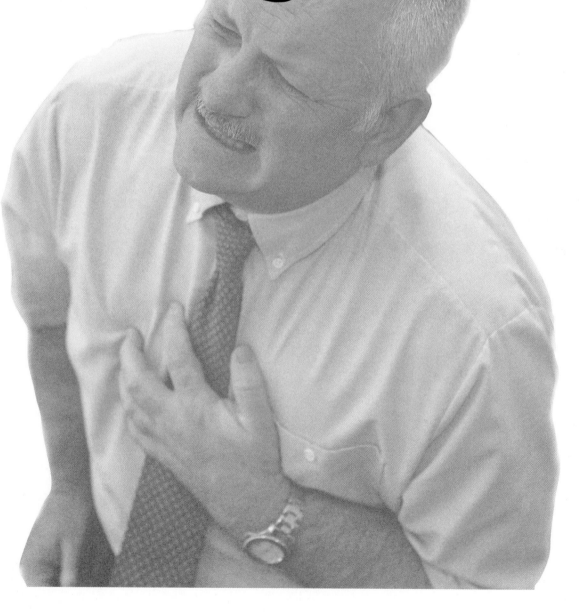

Section 5
Medical Emergencies

Chapter 10
Respiratory Emergencies

Upon arriving on-scene, you are met by an elderly woman who is screaming, "What took you so long to get here? My husband's inside dying! Hurry! Get in there and help him!" You enter the apartment with caution and determine your scene to be safe. As you enter, you see an elderly man sitting by the window, in a tripod sitting position, in obvious respiratory distress. You hear audible wheezing and the patient is cyanotic. He says, "I...cannot...breathe!" You and your partner begin your assessment and determine the patient has an extensive medical history, which includes chronic obstructive pulmonary disease. What initial treatment do you want to render?

REVIEW OF THE RESPIRATORY SYSTEM ANATOMY AND PHYSIOLOGY

Figure 10-1 is a schematic diagram showing the anatomy of the respiratory system.

- "Eupnea" describes normal, unlabored breathing.
- "Dyspnea"—difficulty breathing.
- "Tachypnea"—rapid breathing.
- "Bradypnea"—slow breathing.
- "Apnea"—absent breathing.
- **Hypoxic drive** is a form of respiratory drive in which the body uses oxygen chemoreceptors instead of carbon dioxide receptors to regulate the respiratory cycle.

Diaphragm Physiology

- Inhalation (active process)
  - Diaphragm and intercostal muscles contract, increasing the size of the thoracic cavity.
  - Diaphragm moves slightly downward, flares lower portion of rib cage.
  - Ribs move upward/outward.
  - Air flows into the lungs.
- Exhalation (passive process)
  - Diaphragm and intercostal muscles relax, decreasing the size of the thoracic cavity.
  - Diaphragm moves upward.
  - Ribs move downward/inward.
  - Air flows out of the lungs.

Clinical Significance

According to the CDC, National Vital Statistics Reports, Vol. 61, No. 6, October 10, 2012: Over 200,000 people die from respiratory emergencies each year in the United States.

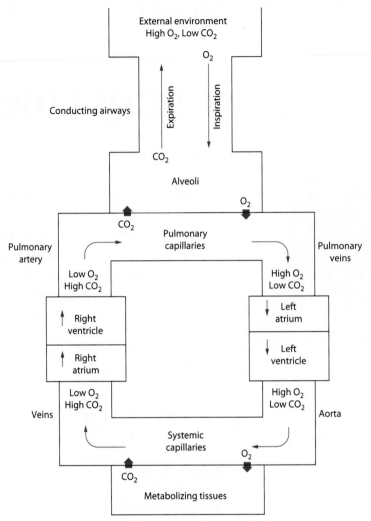

Figure 10-1 Anatomy of the respiratory system. *(Reproduced with permission from Levitsky MG. Pulmonary Physiology. 7th ed. New York: McGraw-Hill; 2007)*

Respiratory Physiology

Alveolar/Capillary Exchange

- Oxygen-rich air enters the alveoli during each inspiration.
- Oxygen-poor blood in the capillaries passes into the alveoli.
- Oxygen enters the capillaries as carbon dioxide enters the alveoli.

Capillary/Cellular Exchange

- Cells give up carbon dioxide to the capillaries.
- Capillaries give up oxygen to the cells.

ASSESSMENT OF THE RESPIRATORY SYSTEM

Primary Assessment

- General impression
  - What is the position the patient was found in?

- ○ What is the skin color?
- ○ Mental status (alert, verbal, painful, unresponsive [AVPU])
- ○ Ability to speak—Is the patient able to speak in full sentences?
- ○ Respiratory effort—Is breathing labored?

Airway

- Proper ventilation cannot take place without an adequate airway.

Breathing

- Signs of life-threatening problems
- Alterations in mental status
- Severe central cyanosis, pallor, or diaphoresis
- Absent or abnormal breath sounds
- Speaking limited to one or two words
- Tachycardia
- Use of accessory muscles or presence of retractions

History and Secondary Assessment

- SAMPLE (*s*igns/symptoms, *a*llergies, *m*edications, *p*ast medical problems, *l*ast oral intake, *e*vents) history
  - ○ Gather a past and present history.
  - ○ OPQRST (onset, provokes, quality, radiates, severity, time) history.
  - ○ Paroxysmal nocturnal dyspnea (sudden onset of dyspnea occurring suddenly at night, usually an hour or two after the individual has fallen asleep) and orthopnea (form of dyspnea in which the person can breathe comfortably only when standing or sitting erect).
  - ○ Coughing and hemoptysis (coughing up blood from the larynx, trachea, bronchi, or lungs).
  - ○ Associated chest pain.
  - ○ Smoking history or exposure to secondary smoke.
  - ○ Similar past episodes.

Physical Examination

- Inspection
  - ○ Look for asymmetry, increased diameter, or paradoxical motion of the chest.
- Palpation of the thoracic cavity
  - ○ Feel for subcutaneous emphysema or tracheal deviation in the neck.
  - ○ Percussion.
  - ○ Auscultation.

Normal Breath Sounds

- Bronchial, bronchovesicular, and vesicular

Abnormal Breath Sounds

- Snoring.
- Stridor—Sign of an upper airway obstruction and is described as a high-pitched or harsh sound which is heard on inspiration.

- Wheezing—Whistling sound heard during inspiration and/or expiration.
- Rhonchi—Low-pitched squeaking noise heard during auscultation.
- Rales/crackles—described as fine or coarse and is heard on auscultation. It is produced by air passing over retained secretions.

Extremities

- Look for peripheral cyanosis.
- Look for swelling and redness, indicative of a venous clot.
- Look for finger clubbing, which indicates chronic hypoxia.

Vital Signs

- Heart rate
  - Tachycardia
- Blood pressure
  - Pulsus paradoxus (a pulse that weakens abnormally during inspiration)
- Respiratory rate
  - Observe for trends.

Pulse Oximetry

Pulse oximetry is a noninvasive monitoring system that provides continuous information about arterial oxygen saturation without subjecting the patient to a painful arterial stick. Using light to measure arterial oxygen saturation (SaO_2), the pulse oximeter tracks the patient's SaO_2 level noninvasively and continuously monitors pulse rate and amplitude too. Pulse oximetry works by placing a pulsating arteriolar vascular bed between a dual light (red and infrared) source and a photo detector. The photo detector records the relative amount of each color absorbed by arterial blood and transmits the data to a monitor, which displays the information with each heartbeat. If the SaO_2 level or pulse rate exceeds or drops below user's preset limits, visual and audible alarms go off. Normal value for a pulse oximeter is 97% to 100%.

MANAGEMENT OF RESPIRATORY DISORDERS

Basic Principles

- Maintain the airway.
- Protect the cervical spine if trauma is suspected.
- Any patient with respiratory distress should receive high-concentration oxygen.
- Any patient suspected of being hypoxic should receive high-concentration oxygen.
- Oxygen should never be withheld from a patient suspected of suffering from hypoxia.

Common Causes of Airway Compromise

- Tongue, foreign matter, trauma, burns
- Allergic reaction, infection

Assessment

- Differentiate cause and correct when possible.

EMERGENCY MANAGEMENT OF A PATIENT WITH POSSIBLE AIRWAY COMPROMISE

Conscious Patient

- If the patient is able to speak, encourage coughing.
- If the patient is unable to speak, perform abdominal thrusts.

Unconscious Patient

- Open the airway and attempt to give two ventilations. If they fail, reposition the head and reattempt.
- If they fail, administer cardiopulmonary resuscitation (CPR).
- Attempt finger sweeps only if foreign body is visualized.
- If foreign body is removed, resume ventilation.
- If unsuccessful, continue CPR and finger sweeps if bolus is visualized.

ADULT RESPIRATORY DISTRESS SYNDROME

Common causes of adult respiratory distress syndrome (ARDS) include:

- Sepsis
- Aspiration
- Pneumonia
- Pulmonary injury
- Burns/inhalation injury
- Oxygen toxicity
- Drugs
- High altitude
- Hypothermia
- Near-drowning syndrome
- Head injury
- Pulmonary emboli
- Tumor destruction
- Pancreatitis
- Invasive procedures (bypass, hemodialysis)
- Hypoxia, hypotension, or cardiac arrest

Pathophysiology

- High mortality.
- Multiple organ failure.
- Affects interstitial fluid.
- Causes increase in fluid in the interstitial space, disrupts diffusion and perfusion.

Assessment

- Symptoms related to underlying cause.
- Abnormal breath sounds heard such as crackles or rales.

Management

- Manage the underlying condition.
- Provide supplemental high-concentration oxygen.
- Support respiratory effort.
- Provide positive-pressure ventilation if respiratory failure is imminent.
- Monitor vital signs.

TYPES OF OBSTRUCTIVE LUNG DISEASE

- Emphysema
- Chronic bronchitis
- Asthma

Causes

- Genetic disposition
- Smoking and other risk factors

EMPHYSEMA

Pathophysiology

- Exposure to noxious substances. Exposure results in the destruction of the walls of the alveoli. Weakens the walls of the small bronchioles and results in increased residual volume.
- Cor pulmonale—Hypertrophy or failure of the right ventricle.
- Polycythemia—Increase in red blood cells.
- Increased risk of infection and dysrhythmia.

Assessment

- History
  - Recent weight loss, dyspnea with exertion
  - Cigarette and tobacco usage
- Lack of cough
- Physical examination
  - Barrel chest
  - Prolonged expiration and rapid rest phase
  - Thin
  - Pink skin due to extra red cell production
  - Hypertrophy of accessory muscles
  - "Pink puffers"

CHRONIC BRONCHITIS

Pathophysiology

- Results from an increase in mucus-secreting cells in the respiratory tree.
- Alveoli relatively unaffected.
- Decreased alveolar ventilation.

Assessment

History
- Frequent respiratory infections
- Productive cough

Physical Examination
- Often overweight
- Rhonchi present on auscultation
- Jugular vein distention (JVD)
- Ankle edema (pedal edema)
- Hepatic congestion (ascites)
- "Blue bloater"

ASTHMA
- Chronic inflammatory disorder.
- Results in widespread but variable air-flow obstruction.
- The airway becomes hyperresponsive.
- Induced by a trigger, which can vary by individual.
- Trigger causes release of histamine, causing bronchoconstriction and bronchial edema.
- Approximately 6 to 8 hours later, immune system cells invade the bronchial mucosa and cause additional edema.

Assessment
- Identify immediate threats and treat as needed.
- SAMPLE and OPQRST history.
- History of asthma-related hospitalization?
- History of respiratory failure/ventilator use?
- Physical examination.
- Presenting signs may include dyspnea, wheezing, and cough.
- Wheezing is not present in all asthmatics.
- Speech may be limited to one to two consecutive words.
- Look for hyperinflation of the chest and accessory muscle use.
- Carefully auscultate breath sounds and measure peak expiratory flow rate.

Management/Treatment Goals
- Correct hypoxia.
- Reverse bronchospasm.
- Maintain the airway.
- Support breathing.
- High-flow oxygen or assisted ventilations as indicated.
- Administer medications such as nebulized albuterol sulfate (per local protocol).

How to administer nebulized medication

1. If using a multidose bottle of medicine when you use a nebulizer, use a dropper to administer the correct dosage of medication into the cup with saline solution. If the medicine is in single-use vials, twist the top off the plastic vial and squeeze the contents into the nebulizer cup.

2. Connect the mouthpiece, or mask, to the T-shaped elbow. Fasten the unit to the cup. For children older than 2 years, using a mouthpiece is recommended because it will deliver more medication than a mask.

3. Connect the nebulizer tubing to the port on the oxygen regulator.

4. Turn the oxygen on to a liter flow of 2 to 4 L/min and check the nebulizer for misting. When using a finger valve, cover the air hole to force air into the nebulizer. If you are not using a finger valve, the nebulizer will mist continually.

5. To administer a nebulizer correctly, hold it in an upright position. This will prevent spillage.

6. When you administer a nebulizer, have the patient sit in a comfortable, upright position. Place the mouthpiece in the patient's mouth between their teeth and have them close their lips around it. When using a mask, be sure it fits well so the mist doesn't get into the patient's eyes.

7. Have the patient gently exhale. As the mist starts, have them inhale slowly through their mouth. Have the patient take over 3 to 5 seconds for each breath while keeping your finger over the valve hole.

8. Have them hold their breath for up to 10 seconds before exhaling. This allows the medication time to deposit in the airway.

9. At the end of a deep breath, uncover the finger valve hole to stop the mist.

10. When you use a nebulizer, occasionally tap the side of the nebulizer to help the medication drop to where it can be misted.

11. Continue until the medicine is gone from the cup. The nebulizer will most likely begin sputtering when it is empty.

Pneumothorax

The presence of air between the outside of the lung and the inside of the chest wall, in an area called the "pleural cavity." Normally the result of trauma! The amount of air present will determine the severity of the pneumothorax and the amount of lung tissue that has "collapsed," which will, in turn, determine the degree of dyspnea experienced by the patient. The source of the air, in the pleural cavity can be external or internal (a hole in the chest wall or a hole in the lungs). If from a hole in the lungs, the hole may be secondary to some disease process (without trauma) and in such cases the pneumothorax is referred to as a "spontaneous pneumothorax." The hole (whether internal or external) may have a flap of tissue attached to its perimeter, creating a valve that will permit the movement of air in only one direction. This may lead to a condition called "tension pneumothorax," an immediate life-threatening condition. Tension pneumothorax, at its most threatening stage, is indicated by tracheal shift, as the tension pushes the lungs to one side or the other and the lungs drag the trachea over to the same side. A "life threat" is created when the mediastinum is also dragged to one side, which shifts the heart and may cause a "crimp" in the aorta and/or the vena cava, disrupting blood flow to or from the heart. If you observe tracheal shift, left or right of center, notify an advanced life support provider. Patients with pneumothorax will complain of mild-to-severe dyspnea (depending on the amount of collapsed lung tissue) with either a gradual or sudden onset (depending on the "size of the hole"). Breath sounds will either be diminished or absent over the site of the pneumothorax. For any patient with suspect pneumothorax, be alert to any change in tracheal position.

Pleural Effusion

Defined as a collection of fluid in the pleural cavity that may be the result of irritation, infection, or some other disease process. The presence of the fluid limits the movement of the lungs, and, if the amount of fluid is significant enough, may cause a "collapsed lung" or partial "collapse," in the area of the fluid. Patients will report dyspnea; lung sounds may be "distant" in the area of the effusion.

Pulmonary Embolism

An embolus is an obstruction in the circulatory system that interrupts blood flow. A pulmonary embolus is an "obstruction" (interruption) of blood flow to the lungs. Pulmonary embolism is a process where a blood clot (thrombus) breaks loose from its origin (usually the site of a "deep vein thrombosis" [DVT] in the leg) and becomes an embolus. This "traveling thrombus" (embolus) makes its way through the vena cava to the right side of the heart, and is immediately pumped out of the heart to the lungs through the pulmonary artery. This artery becomes smaller and smaller until the embolus is eventually lodged "in place" and interrupts the blood flow to the lungs. The patient reports a very sudden onset of dyspnea and acute pleuritic pain. You may observe cyanosis and/or tachypnea.

Hyperventilation Syndrome

Hyperventilation is a condition resulting in blood chemistry where arterial carbon dioxide levels fall below normal. It can be the result of fast shallow breathing (tachypnea,) as might be the case in aspirin (ASA) overdose, or slow deep breathing (bradypnea) as might be presented in some type of head injury. It is usually caused by some disease process, and as such, is to be considered as an indicator of some major, life-threatening illness. Hyperventilation syndrome occurs in the absence of any other associated disease process and is usually the result of some psychological influence. The patient usually presents tachypneic and reports dyspnea, in spite of the tachypnea. The determination of the underlying cause is *not* one that should be made in the field. This patient should be treated with high-concentration oxygen, as with any other patient in respiratory distress, and the diagnosis left to the professional health-care providers at the advanced level. If, however, you are convinced through a thorough history taking, that this event is psychologically triggered, and would like to try to "talk the patient" through the event, please feel free to do so, while the patient is being treated with high-flow oxygen. By encouraging the patient to breathe normally you may be able to break the psychological trigger, and hyper-oxygenated air, inhaled (and exhaled) normally during a hyperventilation syndrome event, will not otherwise exacerbate the syndrome condition. Breathing into paper bags, or using oxygen masks without the oxygen flowing, is inappropriate at this level of care.

There are a several other medical conditions that may present as dyspnea, and they warrant mention here. They include:

1. The **common cold**, a condition that may lead to mild-to-moderate dyspnea.

2. **Pneumonia**, a bacterial or viral infection, usually with an associated fever, where fluid accumulates in the interstitial space between the alveolus and its capillary, resulting in an ineffective exchange of oxygen and carbon dioxide. This patient will most likely present with moderate dyspnea and tachypnea.

3. **Croup**, an inflammation of the lining of the larynx, typically seen in children less than 3 years of age. It is characterized by a "seal bark" type cough and responds well to the administration of humidified air (oxygen).

4. **Epiglottitis**, a bacterial infection of the epiglottis that can produce moderate-to-severe swelling. When encountered in children (up to 12 years of age) can significantly threaten a patent airway, because of the degree of swelling compared to the size of the adolescent airway anatomy. Patients in this age range need to be approached cautiously because any action (by the provider) perceived as "threatening" by the patient, may exacerbate the condition beyond the ability of the basic life support provider to maintain a patent airway. A thorough history prior to approaching any child, when practical, will help avoid the problem.

? CHAPTER QUESTIONS

Your patient is a 69-year-old man who presents sitting at the kitchen table in moderate respiratory distress. His elbows are on the table allowing him to be seated in a tripod position, and he appears to be really working at breathing. Although this problem came on gradually today, his family states that he has had lung disease for a long time. He is a lifetime smoker and is on home oxygen at 2 L/min via nasal cannula. He takes the following medications:

- Atrovent MDI
- Proventil MDI

He appears very thin and barrel chested with a pink complexion. You immediately notice pronounced accessory muscles in his neck and chest along with retractions. He labors to breathe, pursing his lips during exhalation. His vital signs are pulse 90 regular, BP 140/80, respiratory rate of 40 labored, skin warm and pink, diffuse wheezes, and his SpO_2 is 90%.

1. Your pre-hospital diagnosis is:

   a. asthma

   b. congestive heart failure

   c. chronic bronchitis

   d. emphysema

2. This disease is characterized by:

   a. alveolar wall destruction

   b. hyper mucous secretion

   c. decreased left ventricular function

   d. decreased tidal volume

3. His pink complexion is caused by:

   a. decreased carbon dioxide
   b. increased oxygen levels
   c. increased production of red blood cells
   d. decreased tidal volume

4. Immediate management of this patient includes:

   a. continued oxygen at 2 L/min via nasal cannula
   b. bronchodilation
   c. IV fluid replacement with NS
   d. all of the above

Chapter 11
Cardiovascular and Hematological Emergencies

While evaluating a 55-year-old man complaining of crushing substernal chest pressure, the patient states he feels like he is going to "black out." The patient is pale, cool, and diaphoretic. He describes a feeling of impending doom. You summon an advanced life support unit through emergency medical services (EMS) dispatch and they have a 10-minute arrival time. The patient is placed in the supine position and you begin your primary assessment. What is your treatment regimen for this cardiac patient?

REVIEW OF CIRCULATORY SYSTEM—ANATOMY AND PHYSIOLOGY

Circulatory (Cardiovascular)

- Heart structure/function (Fig. 11-1)
  - Atrium
    - Right—Receives blood from the veins of the body and the heart and pumps oxygen-poor blood to the right ventricle.
    - Left—Receives blood from the pulmonary veins (lungs) and pumps oxygen-rich blood to the left ventricle.
  - Ventricle
    - Right—Pumps blood to the lungs.
    - Left—Pumps blood to the body.
  - Valves prevent backflow of blood.

Cardiac Conduction System

- Electrical impulses travel through the electrical conduction system (Fig. 11-2).
- Our heart is more than just a muscle.
- The heart has specialized contractile and conductive tissue:
  - *Automaticity*—Ability to generate an electrical impulse without stimulation from another source

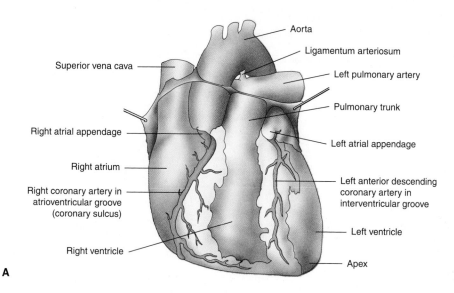

A

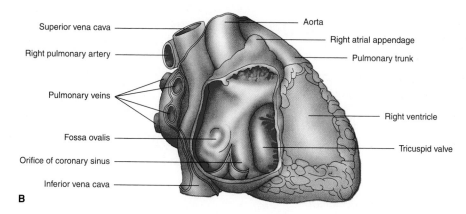

B

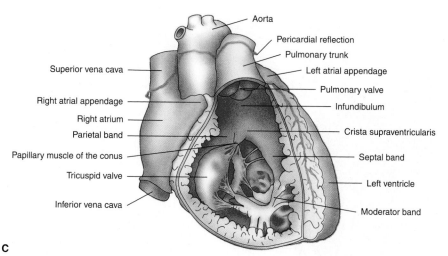

C

Figure 11-1 A-E Anatomy of the heart. *(Reproduced with permission from Cheitlin MD, Sokolow M, McIllroy MB. Clinical Cardiology. 6th ed. New York, NY: McGraw-Hill; 1993)*

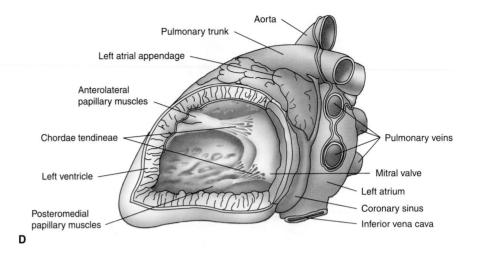

D

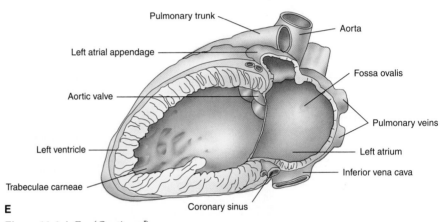

E

Figure 11-1 A-E   (*Continued*)

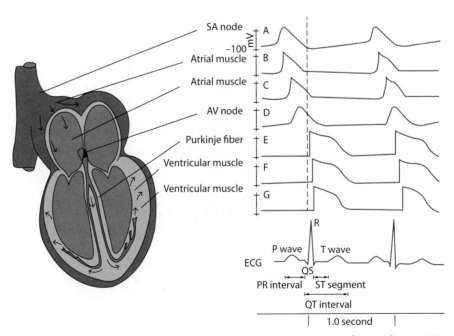

Figure 11-2   Cardiac conduction system. (*Reproduced with permission from Mohrman DE, Heller LJ. Cardiovascular Physiology. 6th ed. New York: McGraw-Hill: 2006*)

- *Excitability*—Ability to respond to an electrical stimulus (this is a property of all myocardial cells)
- *Conductivity*—Ability to propagate an impulse from cell to cell

Sinoatrial Node (Dominant Pacemaker of the Heart)

- Sinoatrial node (SA) is located in the right atrium near the entrance of the superior vena cava.
- Intrinsic rate is *60 to 100* beats/min.

Atrioventricular Node

- Responsible for creating a slight delay in conduction before sending the impulse to the ventricles.
- Impulse travel time is 0.08 to 0.16 seconds.
- No pacemaking properties in the node itself.
- Atrioventricular (AV) junction tissue has an intrinsic rate of *40 to 60* beats/min.

Bundle of His

- Bundle of fibers coming off the AV node, located at the top of the interventricular septum.
- Considered a part of the AV junction.
- Makes the electrical connection between the atria and ventricles.

Bundle Branches

- Created by the bifurcation of the bundle of His into left and right bundle branches.
- Carry electrical impulse at high velocity to the interventricular septum and each ventricle simultaneously.
- Rate of *20 to 40*/min.

Purkinje Fibers

- Terminal ends of the bundle branches.
- Network of fibers helping to spread the impulse throughout the ventricular walls.
- Rapid impulse of 0.08 to 0.09 seconds.
- Rate of *20 to 40*/min.

Blood Vessels

Arteries

- Function—Carry blood away from the heart to the rest of the body.
- Major arteries of the cardiovascular system include:
  - Coronary arteries—Vessels that supply the heart with blood
  - Aorta
    - Major artery originating from the heart and lying in front of the spine in the thoracic and abdominal cavities.
    - Divides at the level of the navel into the iliac arteries.
  - Pulmonary
    - Artery originating at the right ventricle.
    - Carries oxygen-poor blood to the lungs.

- Carotid
  — Major artery of the neck.
  — Supplies the head with blood.
  — Pulsations can be palpated on either side of the neck.
- Femoral
  — The major artery of the thigh.
  — Supplies the groin and the lower extremities with blood.
  — Pulsations can be palpated in the groin area.
- Radial
  — Major artery of the lower hand.
  — Pulsations can be palpated at the wrist thumb side.
- Brachial
  — An artery of the upper arm.
  — Pulsations can be palpated on the inside of the arm between the elbow and the shoulder.
  — Used when determining a blood pressure (BP) using a BP cuff (sphygmomanometer) and a stethoscope.
- Posterior tibial—Pulsations can be palpated on the posterior surface of the medial malleolus.
  — Dorsalis pedis.
  — An artery in the foot.
  — Pulsations can be palpated on the anterior surface of the foot.
- Arterioles—The smallest branches of an artery leading to the capillaries.

Capillaries

- Tiny blood vessels that connect arterioles to venules.
- Found in all parts of the body.
- Allows for the exchange of nutrients and waste at the cellular level.

Veins

- Function—Vessels that carry blood back to the heart
- Major veins
  - Pulmonary vein—Carries oxygen-rich blood from the lungs to the left atrium.
  - Venae cavae.
    — Superior.
    — Inferior.
    — Carries oxygen-poor blood back to the right atrium.
- Venules—The smallest branches of the veins leading to the capillaries

Blood Composition

- Red blood cells
  - Give the blood its color.
  - Carry oxygen to organs.
  - Carry carbon dioxide away from organs.
- White blood cells—Part of the body's defense against infections
- Plasma—Fluid that carries the blood cells and nutrients
- Platelets—Essential for the formation of blood clots

Physiology

Pulse

- Left ventricle contracts sending a wave of blood through the arteries.
- Can be palpated anywhere an artery simultaneously passes near the skin surface and over a bone.
- Peripheral pulses can be located at:
  - Radial
  - Brachial
  - Posterior tibial
  - Dorsalis pedis
- Central pulses can be located at:
  - Carotid
  - Femoral

Blood Pressure

- Systolic—The pressure exerted against the walls of the artery when the left ventricle contracts
- Diastolic—The pressure exerted against the walls of the artery when the left ventricle is at rest

Inadequate Circulation

- Shock (hypoperfusion)—A state of profound depression of the vital processes of the body
- Characterized by signs and symptoms such as pale, cyanotic, cool clammy skin, rapid but weak pulse, rapid and shallow breathing, restlessness, anxiety or mental dullness, nausea and vomiting, reduction in total blood volume, low or decreasing blood pressure, and subnormal temperature

SIGNS/SYMPTOMS OF CARDIAC COMPROMISE

- Squeezing, dull pressure, chest pain commonly radiating down the arms or to the jaw
- Sudden onset of sweating (this in and of itself is a significant finding)
- Difficulty breathing (dyspnea)
- Anxiety, irritability
- Feeling of impending doom
- Abnormal pulse rate (may be irregular)
- Abnormal blood pressure
- Epigastric pain
- Nausea/vomiting

EMERGENCY MANAGEMENT—PRIMARY PATIENT ASSESSMENT OF A CARDIAC PATIENT

Circulation—If Pulse Is Absent

- Effective chest compressions produce blood flow during cardiopulmonary resuscitation (CPR). Follow local protocol and the American Heart Association's (AHA) guidelines pertaining to resuscitation of a cardiac arrest patient.

Responsive Patient With a Known Cardiac History

- Perform primary assessment.
- Perform history and secondary assessment.
- Place patient in position of comfort.
- Cardiac
  - Complains of chest pain/discomfort.
  - Administer high-concentration oxygen, per local protocol.
  - Assess baseline vital signs.
  - Important questions to ask are:
    - Onset (Did the chest pain or discomfort occur during rest or exertion?)
    - Provocation (Does anything make the pain better or worse?)
    - Quality (Have the patient describe the discomfort—Dull, sharp, tearing, and so on. Remember not to ask leading questions.)
    - Radiation (Does the pain travel anywhere?)
    - Severity (Scale from 1 to 10.)
    - Time (How long has the patient been complaining of chest discomfort?)

Has the patient been prescribed nitroglycerin (NTG), and is the NTG with the patient? If so, is the blood pressure greater than 120 systolic?

- Administer one dose, repeat in 3 to 5 minutes if no relief and if authorized by medical direction (maximum of three doses).
- Reassess vital signs and chest pain after each dose.
- If the blood pressure is less than 120 systolic, continue with elements of focused assessment and transport promptly!

Automated External Defibrillation

You are called to the scene of a commercial dwelling where a 68-year-old patient has gone unconscious. When you arrive at the scene, a man comes frantically running out to the ambulance and says, "Please hurry. Bob was at a board meeting when he suddenly collapsed. The guys are inside doing cardiopulmonary resuscitation (CPR), and our manager is getting the automated external defibrillator (AED)!" You enter the boardroom and find two people performing CPR. One of the workers says they just defibrillated the patient and returned performing CPR. What would be your next step in this resuscitation?

IMPORTANCE OF AUTOMATED EXTERNAL DEFIBRILLATION TO THE EMT

- Fundamentals of early defibrillation—Successful resuscitation of out-of-hospital arrest depends on a series of critical interventions known as the chain of survival as outlined by the American Heart Association (AHA):
  - Early access
  - Early CPR

- Early defibrillation
- Early advanced cardiac life support (ACLS)
- Integrated postcardiac arrest care

DEFIBRILLATION

- Immediate defibrillation is appropriate for all rescuers responding to sudden *witnessed* collapse with an AED (Fig. 11-3) on site (for victims ≥1 year of age). Compressions before defibrillation should occur for 2 minutes or five cycles if cardiac arrest is not witnessed.
- One shock followed by immediate CPR, beginning with chest compressions. The rhythm is analyzed after five cycles of CPR or 2 minutes.
- For attempted defibrillation of children 1 to 8 years of age with an AED, the rescuer should use a pediatric dose-attenuator system if one is available. If the rescuer provides CPR to a child in cardiac arrest and does not have an AED with a pediatric dose-attenuator system, the rescuer should use a standard AED. For infants (<1 year of age), a manual defibrillator is preferred. If a manual defibrillator is not available, an AED with pediatric dose attenuation is desirable. If neither is available, an AED without a dose attenuator may be used.

Overview of Automated External Defibrillators

- Types of automated external defibrillators
  - Fully automated defibrillator operates without action by emergency medical technician (EMT), except to turn on power (used in public access defibrillation).
  - Semiautomated defibrillator uses a computer voice synthesizer to advise EMT as to what steps to take based on its analysis of the patient's cardiac rhythm.

ANALYSIS OF CARDIAC RHYTHMS

- Defibrillator computer microprocessor evaluates the patient's rhythm and confirms the presence of a rhythm for which a shock is indicated.
- Accuracy of devices in rhythm analysis has been high, both in detecting rhythms needing shocks and rhythms not needing shocks.
- Analysis is dependent on properly charged defibrillator batteries.

Clinical Significance

Studies have shown an increased rate of resuscitation when patients received $1\frac{1}{2}$ to 3 minutes of CPR prior to defibrillation.

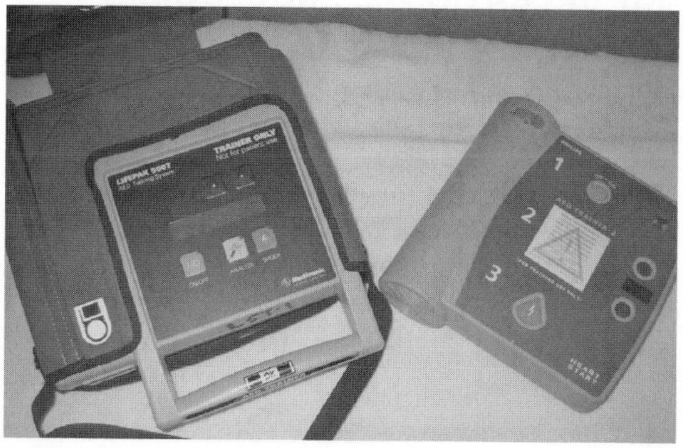

Figure 11-3 Examples of AEDs.

Causes of Inappropriate Delivery of Shocks

- Human error
- Mechanical error (machine failure)

LETHAL SHOCKABLE RYTHMS

Ventricular Tachycardia

- Attach defibrillator to unresponsive, pulseless, nonbreathing patients to avoid delivering inappropriate shocks (Fig. 11-4).

Interruption of CPR

- No person should be touching the patient when rhythm is being analyzed and when shocks are delivered.
- Chest compressions and artificial ventilations are stopped when the rhythm is being analyzed and when shocks are delivered.

ADVANTAGES OF AUTOMATED EXTERNAL DEFIBRILLATION

- Easier to learn than CPR; however, must memorize treatment sequence.
- EMS delivery system should have:
  - Necessary links in chain of survival
  - Medical direction
  - EMS system with audit and/or quality improvement program in place
  - Mandatory continuing education with skill competency review for EMS providers
  - Continuing competency skill review every 3 months for EMTs
  - Remote defibrillation through adhesive pads
    - Defibrillation is "hands-off."
    - Safer method.
    - Better electrode placement.
    - Has larger pad surface area.
    - Provokes less anxiety in EMT.
  - Rhythm monitoring—Option on some defibrillator models

STANDARD OPERATIONAL PROCEDURES

- Assuming no on-scene advanced life support (ALS), the patient should be transported when one of the following occurs:
  - The patient regains a pulse.
  - The patient is packaged and ready for transport.

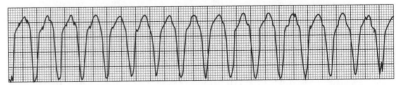

Figure 11-4   Ventricular tachycardia.

- One EMT operates defibrillator, one does CPR.
- EMT must be familiar with device used in operational EMS setting.
- All contact with patient must be avoided during analysis of rhythm.
- State "clear the patient" before delivering shocks.
- No defibrillator is capable of working without properly functioning batteries. Check batteries at beginning of shift. Carry extra batteries.

Age and Weight Guideline

- For infants, a manual defibrillator is preferred to an AED for defibrillation. If a manual defibrillator is unavailable, an AED equipped with a pediatric dose attenuator is preferred. If neither is available, you may use an AED without a pediatric dose attenuator.

Recurrent Ventricular Fibrillation

- Defibrillation with no available ACLS (Fig. 11-5).
- If pulse is not present:
  - Stop vehicle.
  - Start CPR if defibrillator is not immediately ready.
  - Analyze rhythm.
  - Deliver shock if indicated.
  - Continue resuscitation as per protocol.
- If transporting to hospital with a conscious patient having chest pain, who then becomes unconscious, pulseless, and apneic:
  - Stop vehicle.
  - Attach AED and turn defibrillator on, follow prompts.
  - Start CPR if defibrillator is not immediately ready.
  - Analyze rhythm.
  - Deliver one shock, if prompted by the AED.
  - Continue resuscitation as per AHA guidelines.
- If "no shock" message is delivered and no pulse is present:
  - Start or resume CPR.
  - Continue or begin transport.

WITNESSED ARREST

- Defibrillation is initial step; CPR should be performed if defibrillator is unavailable.
  - Pulse checks should not occur during rhythm analysis.
  - Coordination of ALS personnel or EMT-paramedics when EMTs are using automated external defibrillators.
    — EMS system design establishes protocols.

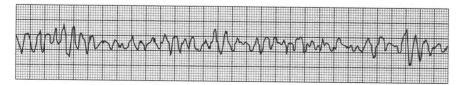

Figure 11-5   Ventricular fibrillation.

— AED usage does not require ALS on-scene.

— ALS should be notified of arrest events as soon as possible.

— Considerations for EMT transporting the patient or waiting for ALS to arrive on the scene to transport should be in local protocols established by medical direction.

o Safety considerations

— Water—Rain, pool, and the like

— Metal

o Postresuscitation care

— After automated external defibrillation protocol is completed, patient may:

– Have pulses

– Have no pulse with machine indicating "no shock indicated"

– Have no pulse with machine indicating shock

DEFIBRILLATOR MAINTENANCE

- Regular maintenance of defibrillators is necessary as outlined in the manufacturer's directions.
- EMS Shift Checklist for automated defibrillators must be accomplished on a daily basis by EMTs.
- Defibrillator failure is most frequently related to improper device maintenance; most common is battery failure. EMTs must assure proper battery maintenance and battery replacement schedules.

Training and Sources of Information

The AHA publishes a variety of guidelines and additional information on automated external defibrillation.

Maintenance of Skills

Most systems permit a maximum of 90 days between practice drills to reassess competency in usage of AEDs.

Medical Direction

- Successful completion of AED training in an EMT course does not permit usage of the device without approval by state laws/rules and local medical direction authority.
- Every event in which an AED is used must be reviewed by the medical director or a designated representative.
- Reviews of events using AEDs may be accomplished by:
  o Written report.
  o Review of voice-electrocardiogram (ECG) tape recorders attached to AEDs.
  o Solid-state memory sections and magnetic tape recordings stored in device.

Quality Improvement

Involves both individuals using AEDs and the EMS system in which the AEDs are used.

Sickle Cell Disease

Sickle cell disease in an inherited disorder that occurs in 7% of West Africans and African Americans. One in ten African Americans carries the abnormal gene. Many patients with sickle cell anemia die in their early 20s, but today 20% to 50% live into their 40s and 50s. A person who has the sickle cell trait has one sickle cell gene, and the disease remains clinically inactive. If two carriers have children, each child has a one in four chance of developing the disease. The disease also occurs in Puerto Rico, Turkey, India, the Mediterranean, and the Middle East.

In sickle cell anemia, a defective hemoglobin molecule, hemoglobin S, which results from an alteration in the molecular structure of hemoglobin, becomes insoluble when hypoxia occurs. As a result, these red blood cells become rigid and rough and sickle- or crescent-shaped. Sickled cells have a much shorter life span, less oxygen-carrying capacity, and are destroyed more quickly than normal red blood cells.

Each person with sickle cell disease has a different hypoxic threshold and different factors that cause a sickle cell crisis. Illness, cold exposure, high altitude, infection, respiratory or metabolic acidosis, overexertion, and stress are known to precipitate sickling crises in most people. It occurs most frequently at night. In response to the precipitating factors, the patient's altered hemoglobin molecules clump which causes the cells to change into sickled cells. These *sickled* cells build up in capillaries and smaller blood vessels, making the blood more viscous or thick. Normal circulation is impaired, causing pain, swelling, tissue infarction, and necrosis. Such blockage causes anoxic changes, which perpetuate the hypoxic state, creating a cycle that leads to further sickling and obstruction.

Sickle cell anemia causes long-term complications. An adult with this disease may develop chronic obstructive pulmonary disease, congestive heart failure, heart murmurs, or organ infarction, such as retinopathy or nephropathy. Splenic infarctions are common and often cause significant necrosis early in life and malfunctioning spleen. Infection or repeated occlusion of small blood vessels and consequent infarction or necrosis of major organs commonly causes premature death. Cerebral arterial occlusions lead to cerebrovascular accidents and are the most common cause of death in severe sickle cell disease. Sickle cell symptoms do not usually manifest until 6 months of age because fetal hemoglobin protects the infant for the first few months.

Signs and Symptoms of Sickle Cell Anemia and Crisis

- Pain
  - In children: hands, feet, and abdomen
  - In adults: long bones, large joints, and spine
- Weakness
- Chronic fatigue
- Pallor
- Unexplained dyspnea
- Dyspnea on exertion
- Tachycardia
- Jaundice
- Joint swelling
- Aching bones

- Chest pain
- Ischemic leg ulcers
- Depressed immunity
- Hepatomegaly in adults
- Splenomegaly in children
- Heart murmurs
- Children: small for their age with delayed puberty
- Adults: spider-like body (narrow shoulders and hips, long extremities, curved spine, and barrel chest)
- History of pulmonary infarctions
- Diagnosed cardiomegaly

Treatment

- Maintain airway, breathing, circulation
- Administer high-concentration oxygen
- Keep warm
- Provide emotional support

? CHAPTER QUESTIONS

1. When assessing a responsive adult patient with possible cardiac compromise, you should:

   a. insert an airway adjunct
   b. apply oxygen at 15 L/min via non-rebreather mask
   c. ventilate with high-concentration oxygen
   d. begin CPR

2. The mnemonic used to obtain a description of the patient's chest pain is:

   a. SAMPLE
   b. AVPU
   c. DCAP-BTLS
   d. OPQRST

3. When asking about the quality of chest pain, you are asking:

   a. if the pain is sharp, dull, burning, or squeezing
   b. what the patient was doing at the time the pain began
   c. for the patient to rate the pain on a scale of 1 to 10
   d. if the pain travels to any other part of the body

4. When using the mnemonic OPQRST, the *P* stands for:

   a. pressure
   b. pallor
   c. perspiration
   d. provocation

5. You assess your cardiac compromise patient for peripheral edema because:

    a. this condition suggests heart failure

    b. the patient might be going into shock from fluid shifting

    c. this may indicate cardiac tamponade

    d. this condition indicates hypoxia

6. When caring for a patient with cardiac compromise, you should place him in:

    a. a position of most comfort to him

    b. the Trendelenburg position

    c. the left lateral recumbent position

    d. a supine position

7. NTG eases chest pain by:

    a. constricting blood vessels and sending more blood back to the heart

    b. increasing the amount of oxygen absorbed by the blood in the lungs

    c. increasing the diameter of blood vessels and decreasing the workload of the heart

    d. relaxing the patient and reducing anxiety

8. Which of the following is true regarding the administration of nitroglycerin?

    a. Nitroglycerin is contraindicated if the patient's systolic BP is below 100 mm Hg.

    b. After the first dose, give two tablets for the second dose 3 to 5 minutes later.

    c. You may need to double the dose of nitroglycerin for patients taking Viagra.

    d. Even if the patient has taken several nitroglycerin tablets prior to your arrival, you may give up to three more doses.

9. When assisting a patient in taking nitroglycerin tablets for chest pain, you must make sure:

    a. the patient swallows the tablet with water

    b. you have contacted the patient's doctor

    c. the medication has not expired

    d. the medication is prescribed to another family member

10. You must reassess your patient within 2 minutes after administering nitroglycerin as one of the side effects is:

    a. a brief feeling of shortness of breath

    b. a sudden decrease in heart rate

    c. a decrease in blood pressure

    d. numbness and tingling in the extremities

11. When comparing angina pectoris and myocardial infarction (MI), remember:

    a. nitroglycerin may give incomplete or no relief of MI pain

    b. pain from an MI radiates, while pain from angina does not

    c. angina usually includes other symptoms such as pale, sweaty skin

    d. pain from both usually subsides within 10 minutes, or after activity stops

12. Which of the following is true regarding AEDs?

   a. Manual defibrillators can deliver the first shock more quickly than AEDs.
   b. The AED operator must know how to recognize various heart rhythms.
   c. AEDs allow "hands-free" defibrillation, which is safer for EMS personnel.
   d. AEDs require paramedics to operate them.

13. On which of the following patients would the AED *not* be applied?

   a. A traumatic cardiac arrest patient involved in a motor vehicle crash
   b. A 54-year-old female patient, pulseless, apneic, who collapsed in the kitchen
   c. A 64-year-old man, conscious and breathing, with a heart rate of 188/min
   d. A 6-year-old girl electrocuted with no pulse and no breathing

14. As soon as you find your adult patient is in cardiac arrest, and you establish the patient has been down for 5 minutes, you should immediately:

   a. apply the AED and begin the defibrillation process
   b. obtain the patient's history from family or bystanders if possible
   c. begin ventilating the patient with high-concentration oxygen and start chest compressions at a ratio of 30 compressions to 2 ventilations
   d. manage the airway by inserting an oropharyngeal airway

15. While transporting a patient with no pulse, remember:

   a. to arrange for an advanced life support rendezvous if possible
   b. if the patient regains a pulse, then goes back into cardiac arrest, you may administer the maximum number of shocks allowed again
   c. no matter what the maximum number of shocks you may give per protocol, medical control can order you to make additional attempts at defibrillation
   d. all of the above

Chapter 12
Neurological Emergencies: Stroke, Seizures, and Syncope

You respond to an assignment involving an elderly male with altered mental status. His wife called emergency medical services (EMS) because the patient has had an abrupt change in mental status. You try to evaluate the patient but he is having a difficult time speaking.

Evaluating this patient who is exhibiting signs and symptoms of a stroke, what three signs/symptoms are evaluated using the Cincinnati Pre-hospital Stroke Scale?

STROKE FACTS

- Third leading cause of death in the United States.
- 700,000 people in the United States suffer a stroke.
- The leading cause of disability in the United States.

Your brain has *three* main components (Fig. 12-1):

1. Cerebrum (which consists of the left and right cerebral hemispheres)
2. Cerebellum
3. The brain stem

The cerebral hemispheres of the brain make up the largest part of the brain. The cerebellum is the structure located behind the brain stem, and the brain stem is the lowest section of the brain and is connected to the spinal cord.

STROKE

- Sudden interruption of blood flow to the brain
- Also known as *cerebral vascular accident (CVA)* or "brain attack"
- Prior risk factors are:
  - Hypertension (HTN)
  - Cigarette smoking
  - Transient ischemic attack (TIA)
  - Diabetes mellitus
  - Hypercoagulopathy
  - Carotid bruit
  - High red blood cell count
  - Age, gender, race

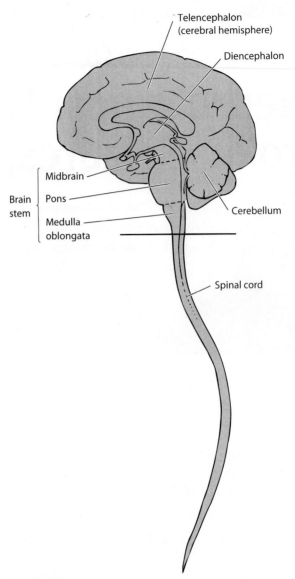

Figure 12-1   Anatomy of the brain. *(Reproduced with permission from Waxman SG. Clinical Neuroanatomy. 25th ed. New York: McGraw-Hill; 2003)*

- ○   Prior stroke
- ○   Heredity

WARNING SIGNS OF A STROKE

- Numbness, weakness, or paralysis of the face, arm, or leg
- Vision that suddenly blurs or decreases (in one or both eyes)
- Trouble speaking or understanding, or sudden confusion
- Dizziness, loss of balance, or an unexplained fall
- Difficulty swallowing
- Sudden, severe headache that is unexplained

STROKE CLASSIFICATION

- Stroke can be divided into two main classifications (Table 12-1).

TABLE 12-1: Comparison of Strokes

Ischemic Strokes	Hemorrhagic Strokes
Most common	Least common
Cause: Usually the result of an atherosclerosis or tumor	Cause: Usually the result of a cerebral aneurysm, AV malformation, HTN
Develop slowly	Develop abruptly
Long history of vessel disease	Commonly occur during stress or exercise
May be associated with valvular heart disease and atrial fibrillation	Associated with cocaine use and other sympathomimetic amines
History of angina, previous strokes	May be asymptomatic before rupture

Ischemic Stroke

- Caused by blood clots and accounts for 85% of all strokes.
- Only type of stroke where fibrinolytics are administered.
- Ischemic strokes are divided into two classes:
  - Cerebral thrombosis
  - Cerebral embolism

Hemorrhagic Stroke

- Caused by a ruptured vessel.
- There are two classes or subcategories:
  - Intracerebral hemorrhage
  - Subarachnoid hemorrhage
- Hemorrhagic stroke accounts for approximately one out of five strokes and is caused by a blood vessel breaking and leaking blood into or around the brain. This type of stroke is generally more serious than an ischemic stroke (one caused by a blocked blood vessel). The nerve cells normally nourished by the hemorrhaging blood vessel, deprived of oxygen and other nutrients, can perish very quickly. The death of these cells leads to varying states of disability.
- *Intracerebral hemorrhage (ICH)*—Refers to the bleeding that occurs into the substance of the brain itself. Intracerebral hemorrhage accounts for 10% of all strokes. Over 30% of patients with ICH will die. About 80% of hemorrhagic strokes are associated with a past medical history of chronic hypertension. Patients that survive an ICH often have a poor morbidity.
- *Subarachnoid hemorrhage (SAH)*—SAH is referred to as bleeding into the fluid that surrounds the brain. The cerebral spinal fluid (CSF) circulates around the subarachnoid space and serves to cushion the brain from injury. SAH accounts for 5% of strokes; 20% die.

Symptoms From Blockage in the Carotid Arteries

The carotid arteries stem off of the aorta (the primary artery leading from the heart) and lead up through the neck around the windpipe and on into the brain. When TIAs or stroke occur from blockage in the carotid artery, which they often do, symptoms may occur in either the retina of the eye or the cerebral hemisphere (the large top part of the brain). Symptoms include the following:

- When oxygen to the eye is reduced, people describe the visual effect as a shade being pulled down. People may develop poor night vision. About 35% of TIAs are associated with temporary loss of vision in one eye. Although such events are risk factors for future stroke, they pose a lower risk for a stroke and its complications than more widespread TIA symptoms.

- When the cerebral hemisphere is affected, a person can experience problems with speech and partial and temporary paralysis, drooping eyelid, tingling, and numbness, usually on one side of the body. The stroke victim may be unable to express thoughts verbally or to understand spoken words. If the stroke injuries are on the right side of the brain, the symptoms will develop on the left side of the body and vice versa.
- Uncommonly, patients may experience seizures.

Symptoms From Blockage in the Basilar Artery

The other major site of trouble, the basilar artery, is formed at the base of the skull from the vertebral arteries, which run up along the spine and join at the back of the head. When stroke or TIAs occur here, both hemispheres of the brain may be affected so the symptoms occur on both sides of the body. The following symptoms may develop:

- Temporarily dim, gray, blurry, or lost vision
- Tingling or numbness in the mouth, cheeks, or gums
- Headache, usually in the back of the head
- Dizziness
- Nausea and vomiting
- Difficulty swallowing
- Weakness in the arms and legs, sometimes causing a sudden fall

Such strokes usually occur in the brain stem, which can have profound effects on breathing, blood pressure, heart rate, and other vital functions, but does not affect thinking or language.

Signs and Symptoms of Hemorrhagic Stroke

Cerebral Hemorrhage

Symptoms of a cerebral, or parenchymal hemorrhage typically begin very suddenly and evolve over several hours and include:

- Headache
- Nausea and vomiting
- Altered mental states
- Seizures

Subarachnoid Hemorrhage

When the hemorrhage is subarachnoid in nature, warning signs may occur from the leaky blood vessel a few days to a month before the aneurysm fully develops and ruptures. Warning signs may include:

- Abrupt headaches
- Nausea and vomiting
- Sensitivity to light
- Various neurological abnormalities (seizures, eg, occur in about 8% of patients)

When the aneurysm ruptures, the stroke victim may experience the following:

- A terrible headache
- Neck stiffness
- Vomiting

- Altered states of consciousness
- Eyes may become fixed in one direction or lose vision
- Stupor, rigidity, and coma

MANAGEMENT GOALS FOR STROKE PATIENTS

- Rapid identification using the Cincinnati Pre-hospital Stroke Scale or Los Angeles Pre-hospital stroke scale (Table 12-2)
- Primary assessment.
  - Airway
  - Breathing
  - Circulation
- Transport to the closest stroke center.
- Alert hospital (stroke notification).
- Check glucose level, if it is appropriate for local protocol.

Seizures and Syncope

At a local café a 32-year-old man begins to have a seizure while waiting to be seated for dinner. A waiter calls 911 and summons help from other staff to clear the chairs and tables away from the patient who has now fallen on the floor. Two minutes go by and you and your partner arrive on-scene. The patient is found in the lobby supine, and presently having a generalized tonic-clonic seizure. What actions should you take initially in caring for this patient?

SEIZURE STATISTICS

According to the American Society of Epilepsy, more than 2 million people in the United States, and over 50 million people worldwide, suffer from epilepsy. In the United States, more than 300,000 people with epilepsy are under the age of 15, and more than 500,000 are over the age of 65. Epilepsy is the third most common neurological disorder in the United States after Alzheimer and stroke.

- Seizure is the sudden and temporary alteration in brain activity caused by a massive electrical discharge in a specific area of the brain.
  - Produces change in mental activity and behavior.

TABLE 12-2: Cincinnati Pre-hospital Stroke Scale (CPSS)

Sign/Symptom	How Tested	Normal	Abnormal
Facial droop	Have the patient show their teeth or smile	Both sides of the face move equally	One side of the face does not move as well as the other
Arm drift	The patient closes their eyes and extends both arms straight out for 10 seconds	Both arms move the same, or both do not move at all	One arm either does not move, or one arm drifts downward compared to the other
Speech	The patient repeats "The sky is blue in Cincinnati"	The patient says correct words with no slurring of words	The patient slurs words, says the wrong words, or is unable to speak

Data from *American Heart Association and Kothari RU, Pancioli A, Liu T, Brott T, Broderick J. Cincinnati Prehospital Stroke Scale: reproducibility and validity, Ann Emerg Med 1999 Apr;33(4):373–378.*

- ○ Convulsions.
- ○ Trancelike periods.
- Most common cause of seizures is epilepsy.
- Most common form of epileptic seizure is the grand mal or generalized tonic-clonic seizure.
- Recovery period is referred to as "postictal."

TYPES OF SEIZURES

The international classification of epileptic seizure identifies seizure types by the site of origin in the brain. The two main categories of seizures include partial seizures and generalized seizures. A partial seizure can evolve to a generalized seizure. There are several subtypes of each. Only the most common are described here.

Partial Seizures

- The site of origin is a localized or discreet area in one hemisphere of the brain.
- The two most common types of partial seizure are simple partial and complex partial.

Simple Partial

These produce symptoms associated with the area of abnormal neural activity in the brain—Motor signs, sensory symptoms, autonomic signs and symptoms (involuntary activity controlled by autonomic nervous system), and psychic symptoms (altered states of consciousness). There is no impairment of consciousness in simple partial seizures.

Complex Partial

Impairment of consciousness, characteristic of complex partial seizures (CPS), results in the inability to respond to or carry out simple commands or to execute willed movement, and a lack of awareness of one's surroundings and events. Automatisms may occur. An automatism is a more or less coordinated, involuntary motor activity. A simple complex seizure may begin as a simple partial seizure.

Generalized Seizures

At the onset, seizure activity occurs simultaneously in large areas of the brain, often in both hemispheres. Seizures can be convulsive or nonconvulsive. The two most common types are tonic-clonic and absence.

Tonic-Clonic (Grand Mal)

There is loss of consciousness during the seizure. The tonic phase, consisting of increased muscle tone (rigidity), is followed by the clonic phase, which involves jerking of the extremities. Autonomic symptoms may also be present.

Absence (Petit Mal)

This type occurs most often in children, usually beginning between the ages of 5 and 12 years and often stopping spontaneously in the teens. The loss of consciousness is so brief that the child usually does not even change position. Most absence seizures last 10 seconds or less. There is no postictal state, but the person usually lacks awareness of what occurs during the seizure.

Myoclonic

These seizures are so brief that they may go unnoticed. They involve sudden muscle contractions that occur much more rapidly than clonic activity and are often confused with tics. Myoclonic seizures occur at all ages and are associated with epileptic syndromes such as West syndrome and Lennox-Gastaut syndrome.

SYNDROME- AND SITUATION-RELATED EPILEPSY

Pediatric epilepsy is one of several symptoms that occur in West syndrome and Lennox-Gastaut syndrome.

West Syndrome

- Also called infantile spasm, is a rare disorder of infancy and early childhood.
- Epilepsy, hydrocephalus, congenital anomalies, and mental retardation characterize it.

Lennox-Gastaut Syndrome

- Usually develops between the ages of 1 and 8 years and is characterized by atonic, absence, and myoclonic seizures. Many of these children are developmentally delayed and have behavioral problems.
- In adults, several medical conditions may precipitate epilepsy, notably withdrawal from chronic alcohol and drug abuse, eclampsia, and stroke.

COMMON CAUSES OF SEIZURES

- Epilepsy
- Head injury
- Medical conditions other than epilepsy
- High fever (more prevalent in pediatric patients)
- Infection
- Poisoning
- Hypoglycemia
- Hyperglycemia
- Hypoxia
- Stroke
- Drug/alcohol withdrawal
- Dysrhythmia
- Hypertension
- Eclampsia
- Electrolyte imbalances
- Idiopathic (unknown)

STATUS EPILEPTICUS ("TRUE EMERGENCY")

- Classified as a seizure lasting greater than 10 minutes without a lucid interval
- Signs/symptoms include (five stages of a generalized tonic-clonic seizure)
    - *Aura*—Warning a seizure is going to happen
    - Tonic—*Muscle rigidity*

- *Hypertonic*—Severe or extreme muscle rigidity
- Clonic—*Convulsion*
- *Postictal*—Recovery period

COMMON PHYSICIAN-PRESCRIBED MEDICATIONS

- Tegretol or Carbatrol (carbamazepine)—First choice for partial, generalized tonic-clonic and mixed seizures.
  - Common adverse effects include fatigue, vision changes, nausea, dizziness, and rash.
- Zarontin (ethosuximide).
  - Adverse effects include nausea, vomiting, decreased appetite, and weight loss.
- Felbatol—Used to treat partial and some generalized seizures.
  - Side effects include decreased appetite, weight loss, inability to sleep, headache, and depression. The drug can rarely cause bone marrow or liver failure. Therefore, the use of the drug is limited, and the patients taking it must have blood cell counts and liver tests done regularly during therapy.
- Gabitril—Used with other epilepsy drugs to treat seizures.
  - Common side effects include dizziness, fatigue, weakness, irritability, anxiety, and confusion.
- Keppra—Used with other epilepsy drugs to treat partial seizures.
  - Side effects include tiredness, weakness, and behavioral changes.
- Lamictal—Used to treat partial and some generalized seizures.
  - Has few side effects, but rarely people report dizziness, insomnia, or rash.
- Lyrica—Used to treat partial seizures.
  - Side effects include dizziness, sleepiness (somnolence), dry mouth, peripheral edema, blurred vision, weight gain, and difficulty with concentration/attention.
- Neurontin—Used with other epilepsy drugs to treat partial and some generalized seizures.
  - Few lasting side effects. During the first weeks of treatment you may experience tiredness and dizziness.
- Phenytoin—Used to control partial seizures and generalized tonic-clonic seizures. Can also be given by vein (intravenously) in the hospital to rapidly control active seizures.
  - Side effects include dizziness, fatigue, slurred speech, acne, rash, and increased hair (hirsutism). Long-term use of the drug can cause bone thinning.
- Topamax—Used with other medications to treat partial or generalized tonic-clonic seizures.
  - Side effects include sleepiness, dizziness, speech problems, nervousness, memory problems, vision problems, and weight loss.
- Trileptal—Used to treat partial seizures.
  - Most common side effects are fatigue, dizziness, headache, blurred vision, or double vision.
- Depakene, Depakote (valproate, valproic acid)—Used to treat partial, absence, and generalized tonic-clonic seizures.
  - Common side effects include dizziness, nausea, vomiting, tremor, hair loss, weight gain, depression in adults, irritability in children,

reduced attention, and a decrease in thinking speed. Over the long term, the drug can cause bone thinning, swelling of the ankles, and irregular menstrual periods. More rare and dangerous effects include hearing loss, liver damage, decreased platelets (clotting cells), and pancreas problems.

- Zonegran—Used with other medications to treat partial seizures.
  - ○ Adverse effects include drowsiness, dizziness, unsteady gait, kidney stones, abdominal discomfort, headache, and rash.
- Valium and similar tranquilizers such as Klonopin or Tranxene—Also prescribed in an emergency setting. Effective in short-term treatment of all seizures. Used often in the emergency room to stop a seizure.

  - ○ Side effects include tiredness, unsteady walking, nausea, depression, and loss of appetite. In children, they can cause drooling and hyperactivity.

EMERGENCY MANAGEMENT

- Position the patient and protect from injury.
- Maintain airway.
- Suction as needed.
- Assist breathing as needed.
- Prevent injury.
- Administer high-concentration oxygen.
- Call for advanced life support (ALS)
- Begin transport

EMS is summoned to a local professional golf shop for an adult male who passed out. Upon arrival, EMS assesses the scene and determines the scene to be safe. They enter the store and find a 57-year-old morbidly obese patient sitting Fowler position against the wall. He is pale, cool, and extremely diaphoretic. Past/present medical history is gathered and the following is revealed:

Past Medical History
- Carotid endarterectomy
- Hypertension
- Previous syncopal episode

Present Medical History
- Denies chest pain.
- Denies shortness of breath.
- The patient is complaining of nausea and dizziness.

Vital Signs
- Blood pressure: 86/52
- Heart rate: 32 regular
- Respiratory rate: 16 normal, not labored

How should this EMS crew begin treating this patient?

SYNCOPE

- Sudden temporary loss of consciousness. Commonly confused by bystanders as a seizure because the patient usually experiences a convulsion-like activity for a short period.
- Temporary lack of blood flow to the brain.
- Usually occurs when the patient is upright.
- The patient usually regains consciousness when they become horizontal.
- *Look for an underlying cause; syncope could be a sign of serious underlying illness.*

CAUSES OF SYNCOPE

- Syncope is most commonly caused by conditions that do not directly involve the heart.

Noncardiac Causes

- Orthostatic hypotension.
- Dehydration.
- Blood pressure medications leading to low blood pressure.
- Diabetes.
- Parkinson.
- High altitude.
- Stroke.
- Migraine.
- Situational syncope, such as fainting from blood drawing, micturition syncope (urinating), defecating, coughing, and swallowing. This triggers a reflex of the involuntary nervous system (vasovagal stimulation) that slows the heart rate and dilates blood vessels in the legs causing one to feel nausea, sweating, or weakness prior to passing out.

Cardiac Causes

- Abnormal heart rhythms
- Abnormalities of the heart valves
- High blood pressure
- Tears in the aorta
- Cardiomyopathy

EMERGENCY MANAGEMENT

- Place the patient in the supine position or recovery position.
- Administer high-concentration oxygen via non-rebreather or bag-valve-mask.
- Consider immobilization.

? CHAPTER QUESTIONS

1. Seizure patients should be classified as a priority for transport, if:

   a. the patient has a history of epilepsy and has not taken antiseizure medication for more than 24 hours

   b. the seizure lasts longer than 5 minutes

   c. a second seizure occurs without a period of responsiveness between the seizure episodes

   d. the patient is still in the postictal state upon your arrival

2. Medications commonly used in the treatment of epilepsy include:

   a. Nitrostat

   b. Proventil

   c. epinephrine

   d. phenobarbital

3. If a seizure patient has been seizing for over 10 minutes, you should:

   a. apply high-concentration oxygen by non-rebreather mask and transport immediately

   b. insert a nasopharyngeal airway and begin positive-pressure ventilation

   c. protect the patient from injuring himself until the seizure stops

   d. begin CPR and transport immediately

4. A sudden, temporary loss of consciousness due to a temporary lack of blood flow to the brain is called:

   a. syncope

   b. a seizure

   c. stroke

   d. a TIA

5. Signs and symptoms of neurological deficit include:

   a. chest pain

   b. cool, clammy skin

   c. paralysis or weakness

   d. deep, regular respirations

6. General signs and symptoms of stroke include:

   a. severe headache

   b. sudden weakness or paralysis of face, arm, or leg

   c. difficulty speaking or slurred speech

   d. all of the above

7. Which of the following is correct regarding stroke, or cerebrovascular accident (CVA)?

    a. The cause is very different from that of a heart attack.

    b. Stroke may cause loss of bladder or bowel control, nausea, and vomiting.

    c. About 25% of all stroke victims die.

    d. The onset of the signs and symptoms is usually gradual, sometimes over days.

8. Which of the following statements is true regarding paralysis caused by stroke?

    a. It is common for both sides of the body to be paralyzed from stroke.

    b. It is difficult to distinguish stroke from spinal injury, as both can cause paralysis to both legs.

    c. Typically, paralysis from strokes affects only one side of the body.

    d. It is a good sign when weakness is only experienced in the extremities, as these patients will not deteriorate further.

Chapter 13
Immunological Emergencies

You have just administered 0.3 mg from an epinephrine preloaded auto-injector to a patient having a severe allergic reaction to shellfish. What are some of the side effects you should see after the administration of this medication?

Allergic reaction is a defense mechanism the body has that provides an exaggerated immune response to any substance. This is a true emergency. The allergic reaction can present with mild symptoms to severe (cardiac arrest).

- The foreign substance is known as an antigen.
- After the antigen is destroyed, the body produces antibodies and the patient becomes sensitized.
- Antibodies are proteins that circulate throughout the body in the blood.
- The primary function is to recognize any future exposure.
- Initial sensitization may have occurred hours, days, months, or years before the patient develops an antigen/antibody reaction.

Pathways for allergens to enter the body:

- Injection—Introduced by a bite, sting, needle, or infusion
- Ingestion—Introduced through the stomach
- Inhalation—Introduced through the respiratory tract
- Absorption—Introduced through the skin

ANAPHYLAXIS

Anaphylaxis is a severe systemic allergic reaction, generally acute in onset, but depends on individual sensitivity, dose, and rate of administration.

- Most anaphylactic episodes are mediated by immunoglobulin E (IgE) antibodies.
- Prior to the anaphylactic event, a sensitization stage must occur.
- The sensitization stage includes:
  - Antigen exposure.
  - Plasma cells produce IgE antibodies against the allergen.
  - IgE antibodies attach to mast cells and basophils.
  - More of the same allergen invades the body.
  - Allergen combines with IgE and attaches to the mast cells and basophils which trigger degranulation. This degranulation causes a release of histamine and other chemical mediators.

- Together these chemicals induce an inflammatory response producing:
  — Increased vascular permeability
  — Vasodilation
  — Smooth muscle contraction
  — Myocardial depression

All of these are responsible for the manifestation of hives (urticaria), edema, bronchospasm, and shock (hypoperfusion).

Possible Causes of an Allergic Reaction

- Venom from insect bites/stings—Bees, wasps, and the like (40-100 deaths occur each year from insect stings)
- Food—Nuts, crustaceans, peanuts, and so on
- Plants, pollen
- Medications (most common penicillin [PCN])
- Other substances such as latex
- Assessment includes:
  - Headache
  - Decreased mental status
  - Skin
    — Patients may state they have a warm tingling feeling in the face, mouth, chest, feet, and hands.
    — Itching (pruritus).
    — Hives (urticaria).
    — Red skin (flushing, erythema).
    — Swelling to face, neck, hands, feet, and/or tongue.
  - Respiratory system
    — Patients may state they feel a tightness in their throat (angio edema) or chest.
    — Cough.
    — Rapid breathing.
    — Labored breathing.
    — Noisy breathing.
    — Hoarseness (losing the voice)—"ominous symptom."
    — Stridor.
    — Wheezing (audible without stethoscope) secondary to severe bronchospasm.
    — Runny nose (rhinorrhea).
  - Cardiac
    — Increased heart rate
    — Decreased blood pressure
    — Sense of impending doom

Assessment findings that reveal shock (hypoperfusion) or respiratory distress indicate the presence of a severe allergic reaction.

Emergency Management

Patient has come in contact with the substance that caused past allergic reaction and complains of respiratory distress or exhibits signs and symptoms of shock (hypoperfusion).

Clinical Significance

Insects most commonly associated with triggering severe allergic reactions are members of the *Hymenoptera* class; these include bees, wasps, yellow jackets, hornets, and fire ants.

Clinical Significance

During a severe reaction any delay in care could result in death.

- Perform primary assessment.
- Perform focused history and physical examination.
- Common questions asked include:
  - History of allergies.
  - What was the patient exposed to?
  - How were they exposed?
  - What effects (signs/symptoms)?
  - Progression.
  - Interventions prior to EMS arrival.
- Assess baseline vital signs and SAMPLE history.
- Administer high-concentration oxygen if not already done in the primary assessment.
- Determine if the patient has prescribed preloaded epinephrine available. Facilitate administration of preloaded epinephrine.
- Contact medical direction.
- Record and reassess in 2 minutes.
- Record reassessment findings.
- If the patient does not have epinephrine auto-injector available, transport immediately, contact medical direction, and proceed with the administration of epinephrine (preloaded). Follow local protocol.
- Patient has contact with substance that causes allergic reaction without signs of respiratory distress or shock (hypoperfusion).
  - Continue with focused assessment.
  - Patient not wheezing or without signs of respiratory compromise or hypotension should not receive epinephrine.

Relationship to Airway Management

- These patients may initially present with airway/respiratory compromise, or airway/respiratory compromise may develop as the allergic reaction progresses.
- The airway should be managed according to the principles identified in the airway management lesson presented in Chap. 9.

Medications

Epinephrine Auto-Injector

- Medication name
  - Generic—Epinephrine
  - Trade—Adrenalin
- Indications—Must meet the following three criteria:
  - Emergency management of the patient exhibiting the assessment findings of an allergic reaction.
  - Medication is prescribed for this patient by a physician.
  - Medical direction authorizes use for this patient, or standing orders dependent on local protocol.
- Contraindications—There are no contraindications when used in a life-threatening situation.
- Medication form—Liquid administered via an automatically injectable needle and syringe system.

- Dosage
  - Adult—One adult auto-injector (0.3 mg)
  - Infant and child—One infant/child auto-injector (0.15 mg)
- Administration
  - Obtain order from medical direction either on-line or off-line.
  - Obtain the patient's prescribed auto-injector. Ensure:
    — Prescription is written for the patient experiencing allergic reactions.
    — Medication is not discolored (if able to see).
  - Remove safety cap from the auto-injector.
  - Place tip of auto-injector against the patient's thigh.
    — Lateral portion of the thigh, midway between the waist and the knee.
  - Push the injector firmly against the thigh until the injector activates.
  - Hold the injector in place until the medication is injected.
  - Record activity and time.
  - Dispose of injector in biohazard container.
- Actions
  - Dilates the bronchioles.
  - constricts peripheral blood vessels.
- Side effects (mimics a sympathetic nervous discharge)
  - Increases heart rate.
  - Pallor.
  - Dizziness.
  - Chest pain.
  - Headache.
  - Nausea.
  - Vomiting.
  - Excitability, anxiousness.
- Reassessment strategies
  - Transport.
  - Continue focused assessment, monitor the airway and breathing, and look for circulatory collapse.

? CHAPTER QUESTIONS

1. Anaphylactic shock is brought about by:

   a. fluid loss due to tissue swelling

   b. massive systemic vasodilatation

   c. decreased contractility of the heart

   d. pulmonary hemorrhage

2. An allergen may enter the body through:

   a. the respiratory tract

   b. skin

   c. the GI tract

   d. any of the above

3. During your primary assessment of a patient with an allergic reaction, you may find:

   a. a slow, bounding pulse

   b. strong distal pulses in the feet

   c. edema of the face, neck, lips, hands, and feet

   d. tiny bruises from ruptured capillaries

4. Once epinephrine has been administered to a patient, you should:

   a. routinely administer a second dose after 10 minutes, if available

   b. administer an over-the-counter antihistamine for long-term relief.

   c. see marked improvement and allow the patient to remain at home if he wants

   d. reassess the patient after 2 minutes

5. Epinephrine is the drug of choice for the emergency treatment of severe allergic reactions and:

   a. comes packaged in a vial with a separate syringe and needle

   b. quickly causes vasoconstriction and relaxes the smooth muscles in the lungs to improve breathing

   c. the same dose is administered to both children and adults

   d. works immediately and lasts for up to 2 hours

6. Steps included in administering epinephrine by auto-injector include:

   a. drawing up the medication into the syringe

   b. pushing the injector firmly into the patient's buttocks until the needle is deployed, and the medication is delivered

   c. holding the injector in place until all the medication has been injected

   d. placing the injector back into its container for reuse

Chapter 14
Toxicological Emergencies

A man calls 911 after arriving at his father's home and finding him unconscious in his car in an enclosed garage. The elderly man, suffering from terminal liver cancer, had written a suicide note, turned on his vehicle in the closed garage, and then remained in his car.

The patient's son removed the patient from the garage and placed the patient outside. The son began resuscitative efforts with the assistance of the emergency 911 operator. Upon arrival, the scene is determined to be safe by the local fire department and you notice firefighters performing rescue breathing via bag-valve-mask. What are some of the signs and symptoms you would see during a thorough patient assessment?

Thousands of people die each year from accidental or intentional poisonings.

EMERGENCY MANAGEMENT OF A POISONING/OVERDOSE

Important questions to consider asking the patient are:

- What was the substance?
- When did you ingest/become exposed?
- If ingestion, how much did you ingest?
- Over what time period?
- Were there any interventions?
- How much do you weigh?

Signs, Symptoms, and History of an Ingested Poisoning

- History of ingestion
- Nausea
- Vomiting
- Diarrhea
- Altered mental status
- Abdominal pain
- Chemical burns around the mouth
- Different breath odors

Emergency Management

- Remove pills, tablets, or fragments with gloves from patient's mouth, as needed, without injuring oneself.
- Consult medical direction for administration of activated charcoal.
- Bring all containers, bottles, labels, and the like of poisonous agents to receiving facility.

Signs and Symptoms of an Inhaled Poisoning

- History of inhalation of toxic substance
- Difficulty breathing
- Chest pain
- Cough
- Hoarseness
- Dizziness
- Headache
- Confusion
- Seizures
- Altered mental status

Emergency Management

- Have trained rescuers remove patient from poisonous toxic environment.
- Maintain airway.
- Give high-concentration oxygen, provide rescue breathing when necessary.
- Bring all containers, bottles, labels, and the like of poisonous agents to receiving facility.

Signs and Symptoms of a *Toxic Injection* Poisoning

- Weakness
- Dizziness
- Chills
- Fever
- Nausea
- Vomiting

Emergency Management

- Maintain airway and administer high-concentration oxygen.
- Be alert for vomiting, have suction available.
- Bring all containers, bottles, labels, and the like of poisonous agents to receiving facility.

Signs and Symptoms of an *Absorbed* Poisoning

- History of exposure
- Does the patient have liquid or powder on their skin?

- Burns
- Itching
- Irritation
- Redness

Emergency Management

- Skin—Remove contaminated clothing while protecting oneself from contamination.
- Powder—Brush powder off patient, and then continue as for other absorbed poisons.
- Liquid—Irrigate with clean water for at least 20 minutes (and continue en route to facility if possible).
- Eye—Irrigate with clean water away from affected eye for at least 20 minutes and continue en route to facility if possible.

Relationship to Airway Management

A patient's condition may deteriorate, so continue to assess patient for airway difficulties and manage as learned previously.

Medications Used for the Treatment of Poisoning

Medication Name: Activated Charcoal

- Generic—Activated charcoal (Fig. 14-1)
- Trade
  - SuperChar
  - Insta-Char
  - Actidose
  - Liqui-Char
- Indications—Poisoning by mouth
- Contraindications
  - Altered mental status
  - Ingestion of acids or alkalis
  - Unable to swallow
- Medication form
  - Premixed in water, frequently available in plastic bottle containing 12.5-g activated charcoal.
  - Powder should be avoided in field.

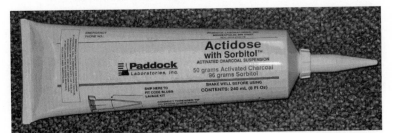

Figure 14-1   Activated charcoal. *(Used with permission of Peter DiPrima)*

- Dosage
  - Adults and children: 1-g activated charcoal/kg of body weight
  - Usual adult dose: 25 to 50 g
  - Usual infant/child dose: 12.5 to 25 g
- Administration
  - Obtain order from medical direction either on-line or off-line.
  - Container must be shaken thoroughly.
  - Since medication looks like mud, patient may need to be persuaded to drink it.
  - A covered container and a straw may improve patient compliance since the patient cannot see the medication this way.
  - If patient takes a long time to drink the medication, the charcoal will settle and will need to be shaken or stirred again.
  - Record activity and time.
- Actions
  - Binds to certain poisons and prevents them from being absorbed into the body.
  - Not all brands of activated charcoal are the same; some bind much more poison than others, so consult medical direction about the brand to use.
- Side effects
  - Black stools.
  - Some patients, particularly those who have ingested poisons that cause nausea, may vomit.
  - If the patient vomits, the dose should be repeated once.
  - Reassessment strategies—The emergency medical technician (EMT) should be prepared for the patient to vomit or further deteriorate.

CARBON MONOXIDE POISONING

- Carbon monoxide (CO) "the silent killer" is a product of incomplete combustion (Fig. 14-2).
  - Colorless gas
  - Odorless gas
  - Tasteless gas
- Carbon monoxide has a greater affinity to hemoglobin than oxygen. This binding of carbon monoxide to hemoglobin is known as carboxyhemoglobin (COHb).

Stages of CO Poisoning

1. About 20% to 30% COHb produces headache, weariness, drunken feeling.
2. About 30% to 40% COHb produces an increased pulse, increased respiration, ataxia (poor coordination), vomiting, and change in vision.
3. About 40% to 60% COHb produces weakness, amnesia, short attention span.
4. Greater than 60% COHb produces unconsciousness, convulsions, and often is fatal.

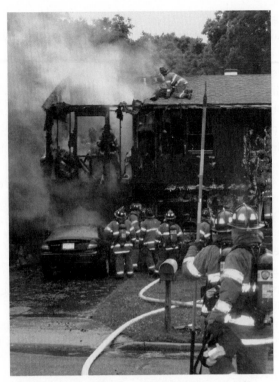

Figure 14-2   Firefighters operating without a self-contained breathing apparatus is a common cause of carbon monoxide poisoning in firefighters. *(Used with permission of Peter DiPrima)*

ACUTE CYANIDE POISONING

Signs/Symptoms

- Shut down of cellular respiration
- Rapid breathing
- Restlessness
- Dizziness
- Weakness
- Headache
- Nausea/vomiting
- Rapid heart rate
- Convulsions
- Decreased blood pressure
- Loss of consciousness
- Lung injury
- Respiratory failure leading to death

Treatment and Management

- Personal protective equipment
- Decontamination by trained personnel
- Airway
- Breathing
- Circulation

Drug and Alcohol Emergencies

You are called to scene of a local bar for a patron who is acting irrational, belligerent, and starting a fight with other patrons in the bar. Upon arrival, what scene safety issues should be observed prior to making any patient contact?

Drug abuse is the self-administration of a drug in a manner that is not in accordance with medical or social patterns.

STREET DRUGS OF ABUSE

1. *Gamma hydroxybutyrate (GHB).*
   - Central nervous system (CNS) depressant and hypnotic drug
   - Taken by mouth
   - Signs/symptoms—Headache, confusion, ataxia, hallucinations, delirium, euphoria, dizziness, $\Downarrow$ HR, $\Downarrow$ RR, extra pyramidal effects, seizure-like activity, and coma
   - Onset—15 to 30 minutes
   - Duration—1 to 2 hours with full recovery in about 8 hours
   - Management—Treat symptoms, airway control, restrain as patient will come up combative
   - Names—Gamma hydroxybutyric acid, Verve, Rejoov, Remforce, furanone, Blue Nitro

2. *Methamphetamines and amphetamines*—Strong CNS stimulants that influence and accelerate certain body functions such as increased heart and respiratory rate.
   - Sympathetic excitation
   - Signs/symptoms—Agitation, hypertension (HTN), mydriasis, trismus, diaphoresis, $\Uparrow$ Temp, $\Uparrow$ HR, $\Uparrow$ RR, arrhythmias, seizures
   - Onset—20 to 60 minutes
   - Duration—9 to 19 hours
   - Management—Treat symptoms
   - Names—Ecstasy, X, Crystal, Ice, Meth, Glass, MDMA, Ritalin, Dexedrine, Adderall

3. *Cocaine*—Strong CNS stimulants that influence and accelerate certain body functions such as increased heart and respiratory rate.
   - Local anesthetic, CNS and cardiac stimulant
   - Taken by mouth (PO), main-line, intranasal, rectal, vaginal
   - Signs/symptoms—Similar to amphetamines, CNS $\Uparrow$ → CNS $\Downarrow$, $\Uparrow$ Temp = $\Uparrow$ fatality HTN and $\Uparrow$ HR → $\Downarrow$ BP/shock, $\Uparrow$ RR, mydriasis, seizures, acute myocardial infarction (AMI), cardiovascular disease (CVA)
   - Onset—5 to 60 minutes
   - Duration—1 to 2 hours
   - Management—Treat symptoms
   - Names—Coke, crack, rock

4. *Heroin*—An opiate narcotic that is illegal and highly addictive.
   - CNS depressant, analgesic
   - Taken PO, main-line, intranasal, intradermal
   - Signs/symptoms—Miosis, $\Downarrow$ RR, $\Downarrow$ LOC, $\Downarrow$ HR, euphoria, lethargy
   - Onset—Rapid
   - Duration—Several hours
   - Management—Naloxone or a new longer-acting narcotic antagonist, consider a drip to maintain airway control
   - Names—Smack, black tar, horse

5. *Hallucinogens*—Chemical substances classified in this group are known as psychotomimetic and refer to drugs that mimic a psychological or psychotic state. *Hallucinogen* refers to the hallucinations that these types of drugs produce. This drug group has the ability to induce visual and/or auditory hallucinations.
   - CNS stimulants
   - Taken PO, inhalation
   - Signs/symptoms—$\Uparrow$ $\Uparrow$ activity, miosis or mydriasis, omnipotence, nystagmus, $\Uparrow$ BP, $\Uparrow$ HR, hallucinations, paranoia, increased activity and strength, seizures
   - Onset—Rapid
   - Duration—Several hours to days
   - Management—Treat symptoms
   - Names—PCP (phencyclidine), peyote, LSD (lysergic acid diethylamide), mescaline, Jimson weed, nutmeg

6. *Inhalants*—*Huffing* refers to deliberately breathing certain volatile substances which can intoxicate an individual.
   - Short-term effects of inhalant abuse
     - Headaches
     - Rashes around the nose and mouth
     - Weight loss
     - Irregular heart beat
     - Lack of appetite
     - Runny nose
     - Upper respiratory problems
     - Night sweats
     - Shortness of breath
     - Signs of acute poisoning
   - Long-term effects of inhalant abuse
     - Brain damage
     - Liver damage

7. *Imidazolines.*
   - Alpha-2 stimulant similar to clonidine that inhibits the release of norepinephrine
   - Taken PO
   - Signs/symptoms—Lethargy, $\Downarrow$ BP, shock, $\Downarrow$ HR, $\Downarrow$ RR, coma, possible seizures
   - Onset—30 to 60 minutes

- Duration—12 to 36 hours
- Management—Activated charcoal, treat symptoms
- Names—Visine, Murine, Afrin, Clonidine

8. *Serotonin syndrome.*
    - Adverse reaction to several types of medications.
    - Signs/symptoms—*Must include at least three of the following*: mental status changes, agitation, myoclonus, hyperreflexia diaphoresis, shivering, tremor, diarrhea, incoordination, ⇑ temperature.
    - Additional signs/symptoms—⇑ HR/RR, mydriasis, HTN, trismus, opisthotonus, flushing, ⇓ BP, abdominal pain, salivation, seizures, insomnia.
    - Onset—Varies
    - Duration—Varies
    - Management—Treat symptoms
    - Names—Amphetamine, cocaine, ecstasy

9. *Other current drugs*
    - *Coricidin HBP (CCC)*—Antihistamine for anticholinergic effects—hallucinations, tachycardia, lethargy, seizures (seizure), dry mouth, mydriasis.
    - *Robitussin DM*—CNS depressant, similar to narcotics, attaches to narcotic receptor sites in brain; consider naloxone or a new longer-acting narcotic antagonist—Agent Lemon/Lemonade /Robofire = Robitussin DM with ammonia, lighter fluid, and lemon flavor.
    - *Vicks VapoRub*—Used to bring down the effects of an Ecstacy high or just for camphor effects—CNS stimulant; leads to seizure and CNS depression—usually occur within 90 minutes; treat symptoms.
    - *Ritalin*—Used by non-attention deficit hyperactivity disorder (ADHD persons)—crush and snort it—amphetamine signs/symptoms.
    - *Prescription narcotics*—Readily abused and often crushed and snorted for a different high.

DRUG WITHDRAWAL

- Symptoms peak 24 to 72 hours
- Seizures possible
- Inadequate breathing
- Hypoperfusion
- Anxiety/agitation
- Confusion
- Tremors
- Profuse sweating
- Tachycardia
- Hypertension
- Hallucinations
- Nausea/vomiting
- Abdominal cramping

ALCOHOL

- *Alcohol* is a depressant, which means it slows the function of the central nervous system.
- Alcohol actually blocks some of the messages trying to get to the brain. This alters a person's perceptions, emotions, movement, vision, and hearing.
- In very small amounts, alcohol can help a person feel more relaxed or less anxious. More alcohol causes greater changes in the brain, resulting in intoxication. People who have overused alcohol may stagger, lose their coordination, and slur their speech. They will probably be confused and disoriented. Depending on the person, intoxication can make someone very friendly and talkative or very aggressive and angry. Reaction times are slowed dramatically, which is why people are told not to drink and drive. People who are intoxicated may think they are moving properly when they are not. They may act totally out of character.
- When large amounts of alcohol are consumed in a short period of time, alcohol poisoning can result. Alcohol poisoning is exactly what it sounds like—The body has become poisoned by large amounts of alcohol. Violent vomiting is usually the first symptom of alcohol poisoning, as the body tries to rid itself of the alcohol. Extreme sleepiness, unconsciousness, difficulty breathing, dangerously low blood sugar, seizures, and even death may result.

DELIRIUM TREMENS

- Life threatening, 5% to 15% mortality
- Suspect in any patient with delirium of unknown cause

Symptoms most commonly occur within 72 hours after the last drink, but may occur up to 7 to 10 days after the last drink. Symptoms may get worse rapidly, and can include:

- Body tremors
- Mental status changes
  - Agitation, irritability
  - Confusion, disorientation
  - Decreased attention span
  - Decreased mental status
    - Deep sleep that persists for a day or longer
    - Stupor, sleepiness, lethargy
    - Usually occurs after acute symptoms
  - Delirium (severe, acute loss of mental functions)
  - Excitement
  - Fear
  - Hallucinations (such as seeing or feeling things that are not present are most common)
  - Highly sensitive to light, sound, touch
  - Increased activity
  - Mood changes rapidly
  - Restlessness, excitement

- Seizures
  - Most common in first 24 to 48 hours after last drink
  - Most common in people with previous complications from alcohol withdrawal
  - Usually generalized tonic-clonic seizures
- Symptoms of alcohol withdrawal
  - Anxiety
  - Depression
  - Difficulty thinking clearly
  - Fatigue
  - Feeling jumpy or nervous
  - Feeling shaky
  - Headache, general, pulsating
  - Insomnia (difficulty falling and staying asleep)
  - Irritability or easily excited
  - Loss of appetite
  - Nausea
  - Pale skin
  - Palpitations (sensation of feeling the heart beat)
  - Rapid emotional changes
  - Sweating, especially the palms of the hands or the face
  - Vomiting

EMERGENCY MANAGEMENT

- Administer high-concentration oxygen via non-rebreather if breathing is adequate, or positive-pressure ventilation (PPV) if breathing is inadequate.
- Position patient, maintain high index of suspicion for C-spine injuries.
- Maintain body temperature.
- Access blood glucose.
- Request advanced life support (ALS).
- Access the need for restraints for combative patients per local protocol.
- Transport.

? CHAPTER QUESTIONS

1. Friends of your patient tell you that at a college fraternity party, he drank 15 shots of tequila without stopping. Friends called 911 when he wouldn't respond when they tried to wake him up. You expect your findings to include:

   a. hypoventilation, cyanosis, and coma

   b. diaphoresis, vomiting, and hyperthermia

   c. a 0.350 mg/dL blood alcohol level, seizure activity, and hypertension

   d. pulmonary edema, dysrhythmias, and dilated pupils

2. All of the following are patterns of alcohol abuse *except*:

   a. drinking early in the day
   b. drinking alone or in secret
   c. admitting a problem with alcohol when confronted
   d. denial of any inference of a drinking problem

3. Emergency management for an inhalation poisoning includes:

   a. starting PPV with supplemental O_2 immediately if breathing is inadequate
   b. applying O_2 via non-rebreather mask for apneic patients
   c. decontaminating completely with water from head to toe
   d. transporting the patient in the Trendelenburg position to facilitate blood flow to the brain

Chapter 15
Abdominal and Gastrointestinal Emergencies

Upon arriving at the scene, you find an elderly woman who states, "My granddaughter is sick. I don't know what's wrong with her." She then asks you to follow her upstairs to her bedroom. As you enter the room you find a 7-year-old girl lying in bed guarding her abdomen complaining of severe abdominal pain.

What type of questions should you ask the patient and her guardian?

ANATOMY OF THE ABDOMEN GASTROINTESTINAL SYSTEM EMERGENCIES

Figure 15-1 is a schematic diagram showing the anatomy of the abdomen.

- Esophageal varices—Swollen veins in the lower third of esophagus.
  - Caused by increased pressure in portal circulation.
  - Most common presentation—Painless gastrointestinal (GI) bleeding.
- Gastritis—Stomach lining inflammation.
  - Caused by increased gastric secretion associated with alcohol, drugs, stress.
  - Presents with epigastric pain, belching, indigestion.
  - Can lead to gastric ulcer.
  - Treatment involves administration of antacids and histamine$_2$-blocking drugs, such as cimetidine.
- Peptic ulcer disease—Ulcerations in the stomach, esophagus, or duodenum.
  - Caused by excess secretion of hydrochloric acid.
  - Also caused by breakdown of mucous lining by drugs or alcohol.
  - Presents with epigastric or upper left quadrant pain.
  - Pain often improves following meals or antacids.
  - If left untreated, can erode entire lining of the organ.
- Diverticulitis—Inflammation of the diverticuli.
  - Diverticula—Pouches on the large intestine.
  - Can become inflamed as with appendicitis.
  - Presents like a left-sided appendicitis with abdominal pain, fever, vomiting, anorexia, tenderness.
  - Treatment includes antibiotics, diet modification, and surgery.

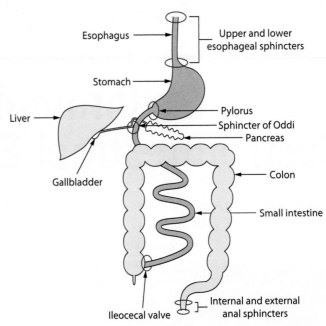

Figure 15-1   Abdominal anatomy simplified. (*Reproduced with permission from Barrett KE. Gastrointestinal Physiology. New York: McGraw-Hill; 2006*)

- Bleeding diverticulosis.
  - Bleeding from diverticuli on the large intestine.
  - Presents with painless rectal bleeding or with some left-side abdominal pain.
- Carcinoma of the colon—Malignant growth in the colon.
  - Diverse presentation including painless rectal bleeding, weight loss, or abdominal pain
- Appendicitis—Inflammation of the appendix from obstruction or from undetermined cause.
  - Patient often complains of acute onset of right lower quadrant pain beginning around the umbilicus with associated nausea, vomiting, fever, and anorexia.
  - Rupture can cause peritonitis characterized by guarding, rebound tenderness, and rigid abdomen.
  - Treatment includes prevention of shock and transport for surgical removal of appendix.
- Perforated abdominal viscus—Perforation of a hollow abdominal organ causing loss of stomach or intestine contents into the abdominal cavity.
  - Produces inflammation and infection of peritoneum and other organs
  - Most common causes are perforated ulcers or diverticulum.
  - Presents with sudden-onset abdominal pain and generalized tenderness; rebound often present; abdomen can be rigid.
- Bowel obstruction—Intestinal blockage.
  - Common causes include tumors, foreign bodies, prior surgery.
  - Presents with history of progressive anorexia, abdominal bloating, diffuse abdominal pain, nausea, vomiting, fever, chills.
- Upper GI hemorrhage.
  - Bleeding from esophagus, stomach, duodenum.

- Common causes include peptic ulcer disease, gastritis, esophagitis, tumors, esophageal varices.
- Signs/symptoms include hematemesis, dark stools, frequent diarrhea, orthostatic vital signs.
- Treatment—Supplemental O_2 and rapid transport.
- Lower GI hemorrhage.
  - Bleeding from distal small intestine, colon, rectum.
  - Common causes include tumors, diverticulosis, hemorrhoids, and rectal fissures.
  - Signs/symptoms include rectal bleeding (wine colored or bright red), increased stool frequency, crampy diffuse pain, and orthostatic vital signs.
- Pancreatitis.
  - Inflammation of the pancreas.
  - Caused by alcoholism or elevated blood fats.
  - Presents with sudden onset of midabdominal pain that radiates to the back and shoulders, nausea, and vomiting.
  - Treatment includes supportive care and transport.
- Cholecystitis.
  - Inflammation of the gallbladder.
  - Caused by gallstones lodging in duct that drains the bladder or in bile duct, causing liver or pancreatic congestion.
  - Presents with colicky pain in the upper right quadrant that worsens following meals and is unrelieved by antacids.
  - Treatment—Surgical removal of gallbladder.
- Hepatitis.
  - Inflammation or infection of the liver.
  - Results from viral infections and alcohol or substance abuse.
  - Presents with dull right upper quadrant tenderness unrelated to food digestion and often with malaise, decreased appetite, clay-colored stools, jaundice.
  - Treatment in nonviral cases involves removing offending agent, while in viral cases patient is observed and treated symptomatically.
- Aortic aneurysm.
  - Weakness in the wall of the descending aorta creates ballooning in wall which can increase in size and rupture.
  - Patient complains of diffuse abdominal pain and severe back pain or tearing sensation, if the artery is dissecting.
- Kidney stones.
  - Result from crystal aggregation in the collecting system of the kidney; crystallized urinary salts held together by organic matter.
  - Most common in men of 20 to 50 years old.
  - Most often seen in spring and fall.
  - Presenting symptoms can include excruciating flank pain, difficulty in urinating, hematuria, nausea, and vomiting.
  - Predisposing factors.
    - Urinary tract infections
    - Immobilization
    - Metabolic disorders (hypercalcemia)
    - Gout (increased uric acid)
    - Tumors

- Complications
  - — Inflammation, infection
  - — Partial or total urinary obstruction
- Urinary tract infections (UTIs).
  - Bladder infection (cystitis) is most common.
  - Most common in sexually active females.
  - Can cause kidney infection.
  - Symptoms include fever, flank pain, chills; dysuria (painful or burning urination), discolored urine; and lower abdominal pain (especially during urination).
- Pyelonephritis.
  - Kidney infection/inflammation
  - Often from infection ascending from bladder
  - Most common in women
  - Patients typically febrile, with lower back or flank pain, chills, possible urinary burning
- Acute renal failure—Rapid deterioration of kidney function, potentially reversible.
  - Causes
    - — Reduced renal blood flow due to shock, dehydration, vasopressor agents.
    - — Kidney injury from trauma, nephrotoxic drugs, infection.
    - — Urine flow obstruction due to enlarged prostate or tumor.
    - — Metabolic waste products accumulate.
    - — Uremia is present.
- Chronic renal failure—Long-standing failure associated with loss of nephron mass, usually irreversible.
  - Complications
    - — Elevated potassium levels
    - — Uremic pericarditis and encephalopathy
    - — Pericardial tamponade
    - — Subject to drug toxicity—Failure to eliminate medications
    - — Fluid overload and noncardiac pulmonary edema
- Presentation with severe renal failure includes severe dyspnea, jugular vein distention (JVD), ascites, and rales at lung bases.
- Presentation with chronic renal failure includes wasted appearance, pasty yellow skin, thin extremities; frostlike appearance of skin in later stages, edema, jaundice, and oliguria.

REPRODUCTIVE SYSTEM EMERGENCIES—FEMALE

- Pelvic inflammatory disease (PID)
  - Infection of the female reproductive organs.
  - Presentation includes lower abdominal pain, pain during movement, vaginal discharge, fever, and chills.
- Ovarian cyst
  - Fluid-filled sac which forms on the ovaries; can rupture causing pain and tenderness.
  - Often presents with lower abdominal pain—Sudden or gradual onset.

- Mittelschmerz
  - Abdominal pain accompanying ovulation.
  - Associated with release of ovum from ovary.
  - Can cause severe pain.
- Ectopic pregnancy
  - Implantation of a developing fetus outside of the uterus, most commonly in the fallopian tube.
  - If tube ruptures, significant bleeding can follow.
  - History of missed menses or irregular periods.
  - Presents with low abdominal pain on either side, associated with vaginal bleeding and often pallor and weak pulse.
  - Pre-hospital treatment includes supplemental oxygen, prevention of shock, and rapid transport.

REPRODUCTIVE SYSTEM EMERGENCIES—MALE

- Testicular torsion
  - Part of a blood vessel becomes twisted or rotated stopping blood flow to testicle.
  - More common in younger males and children.
  - Presents with severe testicular pain, possibly associated lower abdominal pain and swollen, tender testicle.
- Epididymitis
  - Inflammation of the epididymis.
  - Secondary to gonorrhea, syphilis, TB, mumps, prostatitis, urethritis, or following prolonged use of indwelling catheter.
  - Presents with chills, fever, inguinal pain, and swollen epididymis.
- Prostatitis
  - Infection of the prostate.
  - Presents with urinary frequency, burning pain with ejaculation, occasional pain with defecation, fever and chills, nausea, and vomiting.

ASSESSMENT OF THE ACUTE ABDOMEN DIALYSIS PATIENT

- Hemodialysis
  - Waste products removed by machine.
  - Renal failure patients (two-three times per week).
  - Many patients have home dialysis units.
  - Osmotic mechanism.
  - Patient's blood comes in contact with dialysate which normalizes electrolytes and eliminates wastes.
- Peritoneal dialysis
  - Uses lining of the peritoneal cavity for dialysis.
  - Dialysate is introduced into the peritoneum.
  - Remains there for 1 to 2 hours before removal.
  - Major complication is peritonitis.
- Complications of dialysis
  - Hypotension from dehydration, blood loss, and sepsis

- Chest pain/dysrhythmias from hyperkalemia or ischemia
- Disequilibrium syndrome from rapid electrolyte and osmotic changes
- Air embolism from tube opening
- Clotting of shunt or fistula
- Hemorrhage from rupture of fistula or shunt
- Management of dialysis patient
  - Use arm opposite shunt for blood pressure.
  - Treat medical emergencies.
  - Remove patient from dialysis machine by:
    — Turning off dialysis machine
    — Clamping shunt tubing ends
    — Controlling shunt hemorrhage

? CHAPTER QUESTIONS

4. Abdominal pain is considered serious and a high priority when:

    a. there is a sudden, severe onset

    b. it is accompanied by syncope and hypotension

    c. it has lasted for more than an hour

    d. it is accompanied by fever and vomiting

5. A 59-year-old woman describes a sudden onset of severe, constant abdominal pain that radiates to her lower back. The pain is described as "tearing." On physical examination, you note a pulsating abdominal mass upon palpation of the area. You suspect:

    a. esophageal varices

    b. intestinal obstruction

    c. abdominal aortic aneurysm

    d. ulcer

Chapter 16
Infectious Diseases and Personal Protection

SCENE SAFETY

Body Substance Isolation (Bio-Hazard)

EMT and Patient Safety Takes Priority!

- Hand washing before and after an assignment is the number-one way to prevent transmission of infection or disease.
- Any infectious waste should be disposed of in a bio-hazard container (Fig. 16-1A).
- Eye protection (Fig. 16-1B).
  - Eye protection must be worn when there is a chance for an eye injury to occur (ie, broken glass in a motor vehicle collision).
  - If prescription eyeglasses are worn, removable side shields can be applied to them.
  - Goggles are not required, but should be worn when bodily fluids are present.
- Gloves (Fig. 16-1C).
  - Gloves (vinyl or latex) should be worn on every assignment to reduce the risk of exposure.
  - Gloves must be worn when there is any contact with blood or body fluids.
  - Gloves should be changed in between contact with different patients.
  - Gloves (utility).
- Gowns (Fig. 16-1D) are needed for large splash situations such as with field delivery and major trauma.
- Masks (Fig. 16-1E).
  - Surgical type for possible blood splatter (worn by care provider).
  - High-efficiency particulate air (HEPA) respirator if patient is suspected for or diagnosed with tuberculosis (worn by care provider).
  - Airborne disease—surgical type mask (worn by patient).

Clinical Significance

Universal precautions involve the use of protective barriers such as gloves, gowns, aprons, masks, or protective eyewear, which can reduce the risk of exposure of the health-care worker's skin or mucous membranes to potentially infective materials. In addition, under universal precautions, it is recommended that all health-care workers take precautions to prevent injuries caused by needles, scalpels, and other sharp instruments or devices.

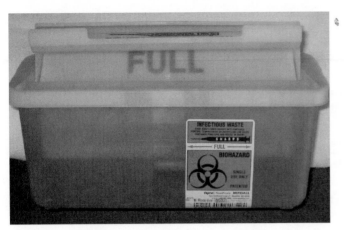

Figure 16-1A   Sharps container. *(Used with permission of Peter DiPrima)*

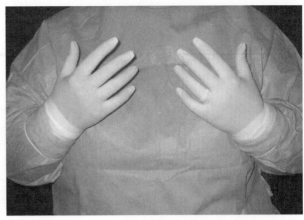

Figure 16-1C   Gloves. *(Used with permission of Peter DiPrima)*

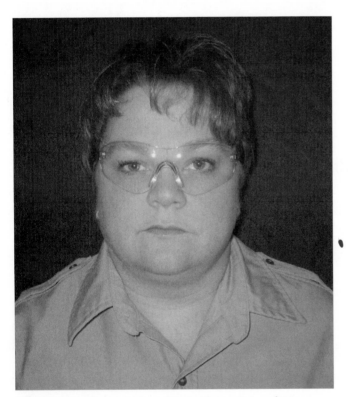

Figure 16-1B   Eye protection. *(Used with permission of Peter DiPrima)*

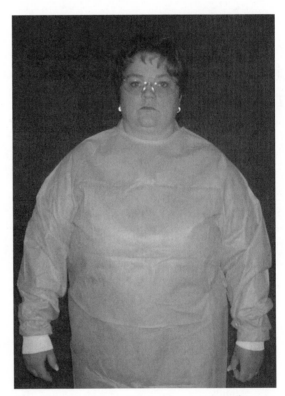

Figure 16-1D   Gown. *(Used with permission of Peter DiPrima)*

- Requirements and availability of specialty training.
  - Hazardous Waste Operations and Emergency Response standard (HAZWOPER) training.
  - Review Occupational Safety and Health Administration (OSHA)/state regulations regarding body substance isolation (BSI).
  - Review local notification and testing in an exposure incident.

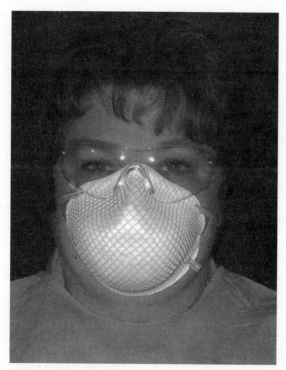

Figure 16-1E Mask. *(Used with permission of Peter DiPrima)*

PERSONAL PROTECTION AT HAZARDOUS MATERIAL INCIDENTS

- Identify possible hazards from a distance.
- Carrying binoculars on the ambulance is good for assessing a scene at a distance.
- Placards located on buildings or trucks aid in the identification of substances (Fig. 16-2).
- Carry the most updated version of the *Emergency Response Guidebook*, published by the US Department of Transportation (Fig. 16-3).[1]

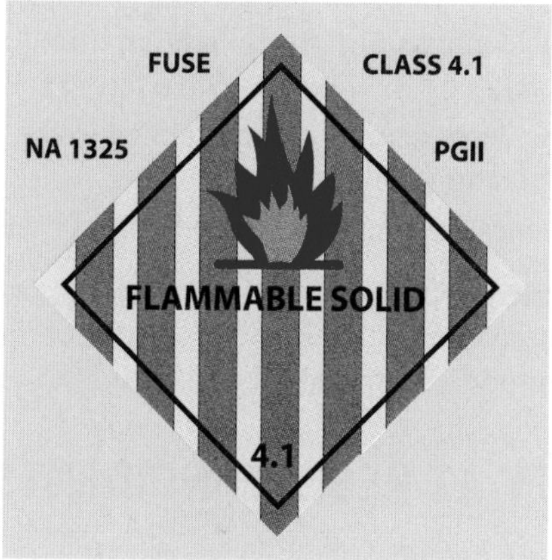

Figure 16-2 Placard example. *(Used with permission of Peter DiPrima)*

> **Clinical Significance**
>
> Vinyl gloves/nitrile gloves should be utilized if the emergency medical technician (EMT) has a latex allergy. Latex precautions should also be observed when confronted with a patient with latex allergies.

FUSE
CLASS 4.1
NA 1325
PGII
FLAMMABLE SOLID
4.1

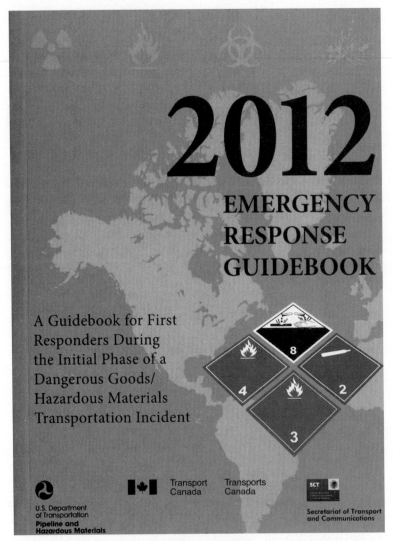

Figure 16-3   *Emergency Response Guidebook. (Reproduced with permission from http://hazmat.dot.gov/pubs/ erg/gydebook.htm)*

PROTECTIVE CLOTHING FOR HAZMAT INCIDENTS

- HAZMAT incidents require specialized hazardous material (HAZMAT) suits.
- HAZMAT incidents require special training in the use of self-contained breathing apparatus (SCBA).
- HAZMAT scenes are controlled by specialized HAZMAT teams.

EMTs provide emergency care only after the scene is safe and patient contamination has been eliminated. EMS personnel not operating in the capacity of a HAZMAT response team should operate in the "cold zone."

RESPONSIBILITY AT RESCUE INCIDENTS

Identify and reduce potential life threats, such as:

- Downed electrical lines
- Fire

- Explosion
- HAZMAT

EMTs should request assistance from trained personnel early in an incident.
EMTs should wear proper protective clothing such as:

- Turnout gear
- Puncture-proof gloves
- Helmet
- Eyewear

OPERATIONS AT THE SCENE OF A VICTIM OF VIOLENCE ASSIGNMENT

Scene security should always be controlled by law enforcement before the EMT provides patient care. Violence toward EMS personnel can occur when:

- Perpetrator of the crime is still on the scene.
- Bystanders interfere with patient care.
- Family members interfere with patient care.

Behavior at a crime scene includes:

- Do not disturb the scene unless required for medical care.
- Maintain the chain of evidence.
- When in doubt, request assistance from law enforcement.

PROTECTION FROM COMMUNICABLE DISEASES

Routes of transmission for communicable diseases are:

- Direct contact
- Indirect contact—Spread by inanimate objects
- Vector-borne—Carried by insects

Diseases of Concern for Pre-Hospital Personnel

- Herpes simplex
- Syphilis
- Human immunodeficiency virus (HIV)
- Hepatitis B and C virus
- Meningitis
- Tuberculosis

Potentially Infectious Bodily Fluids

- Blood, semen, vaginal secretions
- Cerebrospinal fluids
- Pleural, synovial fluids
- Peritoneal and amniotic fluids
- Saliva
- Fixed tissue or organ
- All other body fluids that may be contaminated, such as:
  - Urine
  - Vomitus

- o   Saliva
- o   Sweat
- o   Feces
- o   Sputum
- o   Tears
- o   Nasal secretions

Prevention

- OSHA establishes guidelines in reducing risk in the workplace.
- OSHA requires all EMTs to be trained to handle blood-borne pathogens.
- Washing hands and body areas exposed to blood or body fluids immediately after contact is an important means of preventing infection.
- Gloves should be worn when it is likely there will be contact with blood or other fluids.

Suggested immunizations EMTs should have are:

1. Tetanus prophylaxis
2. Hepatitis B vaccine
3. Verification of immune status with respect to commonly transmitted contagious diseases such as varicella, mumps, measles, and rubella
4. Access or availability of immunizations in the community (influenza)
5. Annual tuberculin purified protein derivative (PPD) testing

? CHAPTER QUESTIONS

1. An EMT should wear specific BSI clothing to avoid being exposed to infectious diseases. An example of BSI would be:

   a. leather gloves

   b. a helmet

   c. turnout gear

   d. latex/nitrile gloves

2. The number-one way an EMT can prevent infection is to vigorously wash their hands after every assignment.

   a. True

   b. False

Reference

1. US Department of Transportation, Transport Canada, and the Secretariat of Communications and Transportation of Mexico (SCT). *Emergency Response Guidebook*. Washington, DC: US Department of Transportation; 2004.

Chapter 17
Altered Mental Status and Diabetic Emergencies

A call comes into the local emergency medical services (EMS) system for an adult male diabetic emergency at 2144 Motorcycle Parkway. This address is known by both police and EMS for a diabetic patient who has uncontrolled diabetes. When he becomes hypoglycemic, he becomes very belligerent and violent. EMS and police arrive at this location to find the patient's son on the front lawn yelling into the front door of the premises. His son tells the police that his dad is hypoglycemic, violent, and is "tearing the house apart."

Police secures the scene and EMS is allowed to enter the premises. The 55-year-old man is found handcuffed on the floor, flailing around making incomprehensible noises. He is pale, cool, diaphoretic, and has an obviously altered mental status (AMS). You ask EMS dispatch to have an advanced life support (ALS) unit respond, and you begin to evaluate the patient. High-concentration oxygen is administered via a non-rebreather. The patient's vital signs are as follows: blood pressure 158/72; pulse rate 102, strong/bounding; respiratory rate 16; equal/full; skin pale, cool, and diaphoretic. You begin to package the patient and determine the patient has an intact gag reflex. Your partner hands you the Insta-glucose, and you administer the gel buccally (between the cheek and gums).

What is your next treatment modality, and is the treatment rendered *so* far correct?

ANATOMY AND PHYSIOLOGY OF THE ENDOCRINE SYSTEM

What Is a Hormone?

- A substance secreted by an endocrine gland that has effects upon other glands or systems of the body (Fig. 17-1).
- Greatly influenced by stress.

Pituitary Gland

- Located at the base of the brain (Fig. 17-2).
- Has two endocrine glands (regulatory).
- Master gland of the body.
- Regulates function of most other endocrine glands by hormone secretion.

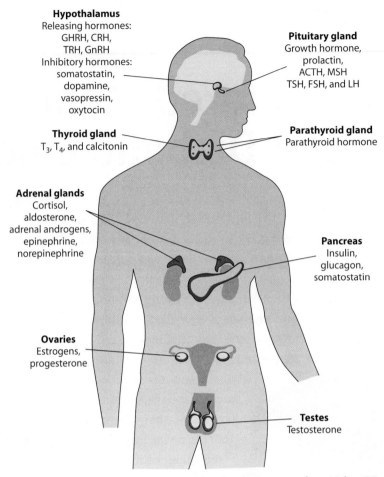

Figure 17-1   Endocrine system. *(Reproduced with permission from Molina PE. Endocrine Physiology. 2nd ed. New York: McGraw-Hill; 2006)*

Thyroid Gland

- Located in the neck.
- Anterior and lateral to the trachea.
- Below the larynx.
- Secretes thyroid hormones which regulate metabolic rate.

Parathyroid Gland

- Four small pea-sized glands on the posterior surface of the thyroid glands.
- Controls metabolism of calcium and phosphorus.

Adrenal Gland

- Located on top of the kidneys.
- Two glands that function as separate endocrine glands.

Adrenal Cortex

- Secretes glucocorticoids, mineralocorticoids, and small amounts of sex hormones.

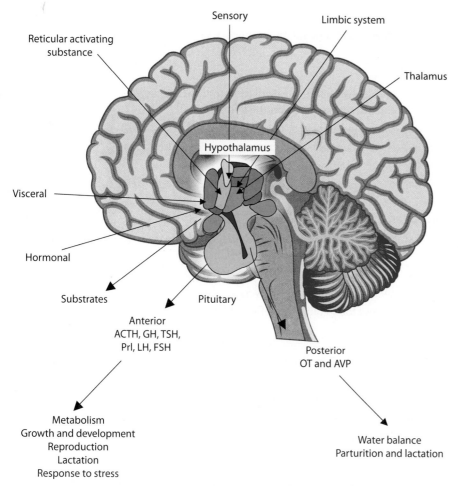

Figure 17-2 Effects of specific endocrine hormones secreted from the anterior and posterior pituitary gland. *(Reproduced with permission from Molina PE. Endocrine Physiology. 2nd ed. New York: McGraw-Hill; 2006)*

Adrenal Medulla

- Produces epinephrine and norepinephrine

Ovaries

- Paired in the pelvic cavity
- Reproduction

Estrogen

- Promotes monthly formation of inner uterine lining
- Promotes breast development during adolescence

Progesterone

- Aids in promotion of monthly formation of inner uterine lining
- Causes sodium/water retention

Testes

- Located in the scrotum
- Secretes testosterone

- Promotes growth.
- Develops and maintains secondary sexual characteristics.

Pancreas

- Located retroperitoneal adjacent to the duodenum on the right and extends to the spleen on the left.
- Endocrine and exocrine gland.
- Islets of Langerhans secrete two regulating hormones:
  - Insulin from beta cells (decreases blood sugar)
  - Glucagon from alpha cells (increases blood sugar)

Glucagon

- Fasting for a few hours, or a moderate decrease in blood glucose level, stimulates alpha cells to secrete glucagon.
- Increases liver glycogenolysis.
- Increases blood glucose levels.
- Allows for stabilization of sugar levels.

Insulin

- Secretion of insulin from the beta cells is stimulated by high blood sugar.
- Increases glucose transport into the cells.
- Increases glucose metabolism by cells; increases liver glycogenesis.
- Decreases blood glucose concentration toward normal levels (60-120 mg/dL).

PATHOPHYSIOLOGY OF DIABETES

Diabetes mellitus is defined as the inability of the pancreas to secrete insulin or the inability to produce enough insulin to control blood glucose levels.

- Diabetes mellitus, type I—Insulin dependent (1 in 10 diabetics)
  - Occurs after birth.
  - Juvenile may suffer more severe consequences/effects.
- Diabetes mellitus, type II—Noninsulin dependent
  - Obesity predisposes this form of diabetes.
  - Normally occurs in adults.
  - May be controlled with diet.
  - Some insulin may be produced but is ineffective in controlling blood sugar.

EFFECTS OF DIABETES

Osmotic Diuresis

- Glucose is filtered in the kidneys causing increased levels of glucose to be spilled into the urine.
- Secretion of glucose molecules in the urine eventually causes dehydration.

Ketone Body Formation (Body Begins to Go Into Starvation Mode)

- Fat breakdown increases to provide alternate energy.
- Fat breakdown products are called ketoacids/ketone bodies.

Renal Secretion of Ketoacids

- When more ketoacids are produced than the kidneys can excrete, they accumulate and produce metabolic acidosis (ketoacidosis).

Long-Term Effects

- Kidney disease in 10% of diabetics
- Blindness in about 5000 diabetics each year
- Peripheral neuropathy
- Heart disease—two to four times more likely than nondiabetics
- Stroke—two to six times more likely than nondiabetics

Signs/Symptoms of Diabetes

- Polydipsia—Abnormal thirst
- Polyphagia—Excessive hunger
- Polyuria—Excessive urination

HYPOGLYCEMIA

Pathophysiology

- Insulin lowers serum glucose by enhancing transfer into cells and by stimulating deposits of glycogen.
- Epinephrine tends to cause hypoglycemia by stimulating the breakdown of glycogen, by interfering with the utilization of glucose at the cell level.
- Glucose cannot enter muscle and fat cells.
- Glucose accumulates in blood, which increases blood osmotic pressure.
- Kidneys increase urine output.

Precipitating Factors

- Fasting or decreased food intake
- Chronic alcoholism—Alcohol depletes liver glycogen stores
- Tumor of the pancreas—Cancer
- Unusual physical activity
- Emotional stress
- Too much insulin or oral hypoglycemic medication
- Sepsis
- Administration of beta blockers
- Overdose of salicylates
- Malnutrition
- Liver disease
- Adrenal gland dysfunction

Onset of Hypoglycemia/Signs/Symptoms

- Rapid development
- Weak rapid pulse
- Cold, clammy skin
- Weakness and uncoordinated movements
- Headache
- Irritable, bizarre behavior (may appear intoxicated)
- Seizures and coma in severe cases
- Normal or shallow breathing

HYPOGLYCEMIA VERSUS HYPERGLYCEMIA

Pathophysiology of Diabetic Ketoacidosis

- Blood sugar is too high.
- Insulin dose is too small.
- Patient has not taken insulin:
  - When insulin levels are low, glucose cannot enter the cell and accumulates in the blood.
  - May be triggered by significant emotional stress, infection, excess alcohol, pregnancy, or trauma.
- Onset of hyperglycemia progresses slowly, 12 to 24 hours.

Signs/Symptoms

- Polyuria, polydipsia, polyphagia
- Nausea/vomiting
- Tachycardia, deep rapid respiration
- Warm, dry skin, fruity odor breath
- Fever, abdominal pain, and decreased consciousness

Compensatory Mechanism

- Deep rapid respiration in an attempt to blow off excess acids by CO_2 elimination (Kussmaul breathing)

Emergency Management of the Diabetic Patient

- Monitor and maintain the airway.
- Oral glucose (if the patient has an intact gag reflex).
- Call for ALS.
- Monitor vital signs.
- Transport.

COMA

Pathophysiology

- An abnormally deep state of unconsciousness from which the patient cannot be aroused by external stimuli.

Possible Causes of Coma (AEIOU-TIPS)

- *A*cidosis, alcohol
- *E*pilepsy
- *I*nfection
- *O*verdose
- *U*remia
- *T*rauma
- *I*nsulin related
- *P*sychosis
- *S*troke

Assessment of the coma patient includes eliciting specific information:

- Length of coma
- Onset—Sudden or gradual
- History of recent head trauma
- Under medical care
- Alcohol or drug abuse
- Complaints or symptoms prior to coma state
- Medic alert tag present

GLASGOW COMA SCALE

- The Glasgow Coma Scale (GCS) (Table 17-1) is used to determine a patient's level of consciousness. The patient is rated using a scale from 3 to 15. Specific evaluations of neurological function include eye opening, verbal response, and motor response. A score of 3 is the lowest score and a score of 15 is a normal score. This scale is used specifically to evaluate a patient's neurological function and is used in evaluating trauma, stroke, and AMS patients.

TABLE 17-1: **Glasgow Coma Scale**

Eye opening	Spontaneously	4
	To speech	3
	To pain	2
	None	1
Verbal response	Oriented	5
	Confused	4
	Inappropriate	3
	Incomprehensible	2
	None	1
Motor response	Obeys command	6
	Localizes pain	5
	Withdraws from pain	4
	Flexion to pain	3
	Extension to pain	2
	None	1
Maximum score		15

? CHAPTER QUESTIONS

1. A change in a patient's mental status is an indication that the central nervous system has been affected in some manner. Causes may include:

   a. brain injury due to trauma

   b. alteration in the patient's blood oxygen level

   c. alteration in the patient's blood sugar level

   d. any of the above

2. During your assessment of a patient with altered mental status, you note lacerations to the tongue. You should become suspicious of:

   a. a physical attack on the patient

   b. seizure activity

   c. loose dentures and possible airway compromise

   d. a suicide attempt

3. A high level of glucose in the blood is caused by:

   a. a lack of insulin to take glucose into the cells

   b. an adequate amount of insulin, but too much glucose in the blood

   c. too much glucose entering the cells of the body

   d. too much insulin leaving too much glucose in the blood

4. Contraindications to the use of glucose in a patient with altered mental status and a history of medication-controlled diabetes include:

   a. if it is unknown if the patient has taken insulin today

   b. the patient taking insulin today, but not eating

   c. a history of type II diabetes

   d. the patient being unable to swallow

Chapter 18
Psychiatric Emergencies

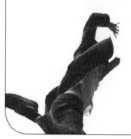 You and your partner are dispatched to the scene of major highway overpass where a 30-year-old man has just jumped from the bridge. He is lying supine on the ground below the bridge. The fall is approximately 50 ft. The patient appears to be conscious and is attempting to move. What is your next step in evaluating the scene?

Behavior is a manner in which a person acts or performs any or all activities including physical and mental activity.

BEHAVIORAL EMERGENCY

A situation where the patient exhibits abnormal behavior within a given situation that is unacceptable or intolerable to the patient, family, or community. This behavior can be due to extremes of emotion leading to violence or other inappropriate behavior or due to a psychological or physical condition such as lack of oxygen or low blood sugar in diabetics.

BEHAVIORAL CHANGE

General factors that may alter a patient's behavior—The number of factors which may alter a patient's behavior include situational stresses, medical illnesses, psychiatric problems, and alcohol or drugs. Below is a list of common causes for behavior alteration:

- Low blood sugar
- Lack of oxygen
- Inadequate blood flow to the brain
- Head trauma
- Mind-altering substances
- Psychogenic—resulting in psychotic thinking, depression, or panic
- Excessive cold
- Excessive heat

PSYCHOLOGICAL CRISES

- Panic
- Agitation
- Bizarre thinking and behavior
- Danger to self—Self-destructive behavior, suicide
- Danger to others—Threatening behavior, violence

ASSESSMENT FOR SUICIDE RISK

Depression

- Sad, tearful
- Thoughts of death or taking one's life

Suicidal Gestures

- The emergency medical technician (EMT) must recognize and intervene in self-destructive behavior before the patient commits the act of suicide. Risk factors may include:
  - Individuals over 40 years; single, widowed, or divorced; alcoholic, depressed
  - A defined lethal plan of action which has been verbalized
  - Unusual gathering of articles which can cause death such as purchase of a gun, large volumes of pills, and the like
  - Previous history of self-destructive behavior
  - Recent diagnosis of serious illness
  - Recent loss of significant loved one
  - Arrest, imprisonment, loss of job

Assessment

- Patient in an unsafe environment or with unsafe objects in hands
- Display of self-destructive behavior during primary assessment or prior to emergency response
- Important questions to be considered:
  - How does the patient feel?
  - Are there suicidal tendencies?
  - Is patient a threat to self or others?
  - Is there an underlying medical problem?
  - Any interventions?

Emergency Management

- Scene size-up, personal safety.
- Patient assessment.
- Calm the patient—Do not leave the patient alone.
- Restrain if necessary. Consider need for law enforcement.
- Transport, if overdose is suspected, bring medications or drugs found to medical facility.

COMMON PSYCHIATRIC DISORDERS

Affective Disorders

Affective disorders are a group of mental disorders characterized by mood disturbances such as depression, bipolar, and dysrhythmic disorders.

Alcohol Intoxication

Patients with emergencies related to alcohol are common. An intoxicated patient often gives an inaccurate medical history, abnormal response to physical problems, and has the potential for violent and disruptive behavior.

Amnesic Psychogenic Dissociative Disorder

An amnesic psychogenic dissociative disorder is an inability to remember personal information after a severe psychological stress. The patient is usually calm and other memories are intact.

Conversion Disorder

A conversion disorder is the loss of a physical function with no physical cause. The cause of a conversion disorder is often found to be a psychological conflict, such as a need to avoid an unpleasant task or a need to be removed from an unpleasant situation. The conversion places the patient in a situation where he can receive support. Symptoms are a loss of some bodily function.

Depersonalization

Depersonalization is an altered perception of the body or a sense of being outside of the body, characterized by feelings that one's actions and speech cannot be controlled. Depersonalization is usually a protecting mechanism to protect the self.

Drug Intoxication

In most instances, patients with acute drug intoxication present with physical symptoms or are brought in unresponsive by friends.

Dystonia

Haldol, Thorazine, and Compazine may cause dystonia, which is a reaction to medications that causes muscle spasm or contractions that usually involve the tongue, neck, and jaw. Treatment is Cogentin (benztropine mesylate).

Fugue Disorder

A fugue disorder is an abrupt, massive amnesic event with alteration of consciousness that presents as a new personality. A fugue disorder is often precipitated by extreme stress and is associated with drug and alcohol abuse.

Hypochondriasis

Hypochondriasis is a condition where the person has an abnormal preoccupation with the belief that they have a serious illness.

Panic Attacks

Panic attacks are acute, recurrent attacks of panic having no tangible cause. Symptoms include shortness of breath, chest pain, tachycardia, sweating, nausea, vomiting, diarrhea, and a feeling of approaching death.

Phobias

A phobia is a persistent and irrational fear of a specific activity or object that results in a compelling desire to avoid the situation. Phobias are classified into three types:

- Agoraphobias (a variety of everyday situations)
- Social phobias (embarrassment in public)
- Simple phobias (specific situations, eg, tunnels, flying, elevators)

Symptoms may include fear, shortness of breath, chest pain, tachycardia, sweating, nausea, vomiting, diarrhea, and a feeling that something terrible is about to happen.

Posttraumatic Stress Disorder

Posttraumatic stress disorder (PTSD) is a condition where a patient experiences recurrent dreams or thoughts about a traumatic event with feelings of detachment and estrangement from the environment. The disorder is associated with sleep disorders, hyperalertness, difficulty concentrating, and memory impairment.

The cause of PTSD is commonly military combat, rape, or a disaster. Symptoms may include fear, shortness of breath, chest pain, tachycardia, sweating, nausea, vomiting, diarrhea, and a feeling that something terrible is about to happen.

Organic Disorders

Organic disorders encompass a large group of acute and chronic mental disorders associated with brain damage or cerebral dysfunction. The patient may present with impaired consciousness, orientation, intellect, judgment, thought processing, or with hallucination and mood changes.

Paranoid Disorder

Paranoid disorder is a condition where the patient shows persistent delusions of persecution. Behavior can be consistent with the delusion, or bizarre and incoherent. The disorder usually occurs in mid or late adult life and may include anger that leads to violent behavior.

Schizophrenia

Schizophrenia is a group of mental disorders with disordered thinking and bizarre behaviors. Clinically, patients show disturbances of thought with delusions. Speech may be coherent but unassociated with the situation, mute, completely incoherent, or catatonic. Effect may be flat or inappropriate. Perception is disordered with visual and auditory hallucinations.

SOMATOFORM DISORDERS

Somatoform disorders are physical symptoms with no detectable organic physical cause; they are not under conscious control of the patient.

Somatization

Somatization is a condition where a person has multiple somatic complaints with 15 or more symptoms lasting over several years. The cause of somatization is unknown. Symptoms include multiple physical complaints, numerous surgeries, and many medical consults. The condition is frequently associated with alcohol abuse.

- 18 months to 3 years—Autonomy versus shame and doubt, self-control without loss of self-esteem, the ability to cooperate and express oneself.

- 3 to 5 years—Initiative versus guilt, realistic sense of purpose and ability to evaluate one's own behavior versus self-denial and self-restriction.

- 6 to 12 years—Industry versus inferiority, realization of competence, preservation, versus feeling that one will never be "any good" and withdrawal from school and peers.
- 12 to 20 years—Identity versus role diffusion, coherent sense of self; plans to actualize one's abilities versus feelings of confusion, indecisiveness, and the possibility of antisocial behavior.
- 18 to 25 years—Intimacy versus isolation, capacity for love as mutual devotion, commitment to work and relationships versus impersonal relationships and prejudice.
- 25 to 65 years—Generativity versus stagnation, creativity, production, concern for others versus self-indulgence, and impoverishment of self.
- 65 years to death—Integrity versus despair, acceptance of the worth and uniqueness of one's life versus a sense of loss and contempt for others.

PHYSICAL CHANGES DURING STRESS

Alarm Stage

The alarm stage is a condition where an increase in epinephrine and norepinephrine release occurs. The fight-or-flight reaction is activated. Blood pressure, pulse, respiratory rate, blood sugar, and alertness are increased.

Resistance Stage

The resistance stage is a stage where hormonal levels adjust and the patient uses coping and defensive behavior.

Exhaustion

When exhaustion occurs, the immune response decreases, the defense mechanisms are exaggerated, thinking is disorganized, sensory input is misperceived (auditory and visual illusions), reality concepts are distorted, and violent behavior can occur. Physical system failure and death can occur.

SUICIDOLOGY

The science of suicide includes causes, prediction of susceptibility, and prevention. In the United States, over 31,000 people intentionally kill themselves annually, which is equivalent to 1 in every 20 minutes. In recent years, suicides have doubled in children aged 10 through 19 years. Suicide is the ninth leading cause of death in the United States. More people die from suicide (11.9 per 100,000) than from homicide (8.5 per 100,000). Nearly 60% of all suicides are caused from firearms. Most suicide victims have consulted a physician within 6 months of the suicide and 10% have seen a physician within 1 week of the suicide. Health-care workers can prevent a suicide if they recognize the individual is at risk and intervene.

Warning Signs of Suicidal Ideation

- Specific lethal plan that does not include the possibility for rescue
- Depression (65% of suicides have a history of depression)
- History of suicide attempts (65% of suicides have a history of attempts)
- Limited psychological and social resources
- Taking actions to put their lives in order
- Giving away possessions

- Failure at work or school
- Recent loss and dealing with grief
- Poor work or school performance
- History of alcohol abuse
- History of drug abuse

Medical/Legal Considerations

- An emotionally disturbed patient who consents to care and transport significantly reduces legal problems.
- How to handle the patient who resists treatment:
  - Emotionally disturbed patient will often resist treatment.
  - May threaten EMTs and other responders.
  - To provide care against patient's will, you must show a reasonable belief that the patient would harm himself or others.
  - If a threat to self or others, the patient may be transported without consent after contacting medical direction. This action is performed by law enforcement.
- Avoiding unreasonable force:
  - Reasonable force depends on what force was necessary to keep patient from injuring himself or others.
  - Reasonable force is determined by looking at all circumstances involved.
    — Patient's size and strength
    — Type of abnormal behavior
    — Sex of patient
    — Mental state of patient and method of restraint
  - Be aware; after a period of combativeness and aggression, some calm patients may cause unexpected and sudden injury to self and others.
  - Avoid acts or physical force that may cause injury to the patient.
  - Emergency medical services (EMS) personnel may use reasonable force to defend against an attack by emotionally disturbed patients.

Police and Medical Direction Involvement

- Seek medical direction when you consider restraining a patient.
- Ask for police assistance, if during scene size-up the patient appears or acts aggressive, or combative.

Protection Against False Accusations

- Documentation of abnormal behavior exhibited by the patient is very important.
- Have witnesses in attendance especially during transport, if possible.
- Accusing EMTs of sexual misconduct is common by emotionally disturbed patients—Have help, same-sex attendants, and third-party witnesses.

PRINCIPLES FOR ASSESSING BEHAVIORAL EMERGENCY PATIENTS

- Identify yourself and let the person know you are there to help.
- Inform him/her of what you are doing.

- Ask questions in a calm, reassuring voice.
- Allow the patient to tell what happened without being judgmental.
- Show you are listening by rephrasing or repeating part of what is said.
- Acknowledge the patient's feelings.
- Assess the patient's mental status.
  - Appearance
  - Activity
  - Speech
  - Orientation for time, person, and place

ASSESSMENT OF POTENTIAL VIOLENCE

- Scene size-up.
- History—The EMT should check with family and bystanders to determine if the patient has a known history of aggression or combativeness.
- Posture—Stands or sits in a position which threatens self or others. May have fists clenched or lethal objects in hands.
- Vocal activity—Yells or verbally threatens harm to self or others.
- Physical activity—Moves toward caregiver, carries heavy or threatening objects, has quick irregular movements, muscles tense.

METHODS TO CALM BEHAVIORAL EMERGENCY PATIENTS

- Acknowledge that the person seems upset, and restate that you are there to help.
- Inform him of what you are doing.
- Ask questions in a calm, reassuring voice.
- Maintain a comfortable distance.
- Encourage the patient to state what is troubling him.
- Do not make quick moves.
- Respond honestly to patient's questions.
- Do not threaten, challenge, or argue with disturbed patients.
- Tell the truth; do not lie to the patient.
- Do not "play along" with visual or auditory disturbances of the patient.
- Involve trusted family members or friends.
- Be prepared to stay at the scene for a long time. Always remain with the patient.
- Avoid unnecessary physical contact. Call additional help, if needed.
- Use good eye contact.

Restraining Patients

Restraint should be avoided unless patient is a danger to self and others. When using restraints, have police present, if possible, and get approval from medical direction. If restraints must be used, do the following:

- Be sure to have adequate help.
- Plan your activities.
- Use only the force necessary for restraint.

- Estimate range of motion of patient's arms and legs and stay beyond range until ready.
- Once decision has been made—Act quickly.
- Have one EMT talk to patient throughout restraining.
- Approach with four persons, one assigned to each limb all at the same time.
- Secure limbs together with equipment approved by medical direction.
- Turn patient face down on stretcher.
- Secure to stretcher with multiple straps.
- Cover face with surgical mask if patient is spitting on EMTs.
- Reassess circulation frequently.
- Document indication for restraining patients and technique of restraint.
- Avoid unnecessary force.

MANAGING OTHER BEHAVIORAL ISSUES

- Always try to talk to the patient into cooperation.
- Do not belittle or threaten patients.
- Be calm and patient in your attitude.
- Do not agree with disturbed thinking.
- Be reassuring and avoid arguing with irrational patients.
- Suggest appropriate steps to take.
- Lower distressing stimuli.
- Avoid restraints unless necessary.
- Treat with respect.

? CHAPTER QUESTIONS

5. Which of the following is most likely at low risk for suicide?

   a. Older man without a spouse, unemployed, and in poor health
   b. People who are depressed
   c. Persons with a serious debilitating illness
   d. Married men, living spouse, and/or employed

Chapter 19
Genitourinary and Renal Emergencies

A 16-year-old adolescent boy comes to the emergency department (ED) complaining of severe right flank and scrotal pain beginning several hours ago, awakening him from sleep. He denies genitourinary (GU) trauma, fever, chills, sexual activity, dysuria, hematuria, urinary discharge, frequency, nocturia. On physical examination he appears in moderate pain. His blood pressure (BP) = 130/88, pulse (P) = 100, respiratory (R) = 20, temperature (T) = 37°C.

What is your differential diagnosis for acute scrotal pain, and what is this patient's "worst possible" diagnosis?

ACUTE RENAL FAILURE

Acute renal failure (ARF) or acute kidney injury is a rapid loss of kidney function.

Causes/Classifications

Prerenal

ARF secondary to hypoperfusion of the kidneys

- Excessive fluid loss: dehydration, hemorrhage, severe burns, polyuria, persistent vomiting/diarrhea/diaphoresis
- Decreased cardiac output: myocardial infarction, congestive heart failure (CHF), shock states (hypovolemic, cardiogenic, obstructive)

Intrinsic

ARF secondary to damage to renal parenchymal

- Acute tubular necrosis
- Nephritis: glomerulonephritis, interstitial nephritis, pyelonephritis, lupus nephritis
- Rhabdomyolysis
- Drug-related nephrotoxicity

Postrenal

ARF secondary to an obstruction of the outflow of urine

- Renal stones, blood clots, tumors, prostatic hypertrophy, urethral strictures

URINARY TRACT INFECTIONS

Infectious process located in the urinary tract.

Causes/Classifications

- Poor hygiene.
- *Sexual activity:* Not voiding after sexual activity increases risk of urinary tract infection (UTI) (especially in females).
- *Urinary catheterization:* Indwelling catheterization poses a greater risk than straight catheterization.
- *Stagnant urine:* Secondary to renal stones or enlarged prostate.
- *Incomplete bladder emptying:* Often seen with patients having spinal cord injuries.

Pyelonephritis is an infection of the renal pelvis.

Causes/Classifications

- *Ascending UTI:* Infection which has begun in the urinary tract has ascended to the renal pelvis.

URINARY CALCULI

A mineral deposit located in the urinary tract.

Causes/Classifications

- *Supersaturation of the urine:* The urine solution contains more solutes than can be dissolved and excreted. This may lead to the formation of crystalline structures (usually composed of calcium or uric acid).
- *Deficiency of chelating agents:* The urine solution contains chemical agents that prevent the formation of crystalline structures. If there is a deficiency of these agents the chance of calculi formation increases.
- *Contributing factors:* Dietary (excessive intake of refined sugars, animal proteins, sodium, cola drinks), persistent dehydration, calcium and vitamin C supplements, hyperparathyroidism, Crohn disease, diabetes mellitus (DM), excessive alcohol consumption.
- *Nephrolithiasis:* Calculi formation lodged in the kidney.
- *Ureterolithiasis:* Calculi formation lodged in the ureter.
- *Cystolithiasis:* Calculi formation lodged in the bladder.

TESTICULAR TORSION

Ischemia of the testicles and surrounding structures within the scrotum secondary to twisting of the spermatic cord.

Causes/Risk Factors

- *Bell clapper deformity:* A condition where the testis and epididymis fail to anchor to the tunica vaginalis. The deformity predisposes the testis to swing and rotate within the scrotum, increasing risk of torsion.
- Other risk factors or possible causes include:
  - Most common ages from 12 to 16 years
  - Cold temperatures
  - Physical activities
  - Trauma to scrotum

EPIDIDYMITIS

Inflammation of the epididymis (a coiled structure, posterior to the testicle where sperm is stored and matures).

Causes/Risk Factors

Infectious Epididymitis

- Sexually transmitted infections (particularly gonorrhea and chlamydia)
- Urinary tract infections (bacteria in the urethra travels through the urinary and reproductive structures to the epididymis)

Noninfectious Epididymitis

- Sterile urine backflows from the urethra to the epididymis (may be secondary to heavy lifting, straining, sexual intercourse with a full bladder, prostatitis).
- Amiodarone (antiarrhythmic drug) has been associated with inflammation of the epididymitis.

PROSTATITIS

An inflammation of the prostate gland.

Classifications

- *Acute bacterial prostatitis:* Sudden bacterial infection marked by inflammation of the prostate. Usually associated with severe symptoms requiring emergent attention.
- *Chronic bacterial prostatitis:* Develops gradually and continues for an extended time.
- *Chronic prostatitis without infection:* Also referred to as chronic pelvic pain syndrome. Inflammation without infection. Etiology unclear.
- *Asymptomatic inflammatory prostatitis:* Inflammation without symptoms. Etiology unclear.

Causes/Risk Factors of Acute Bacterial Prostatitis

- Intraprostatic ductal reflux (urinary backflow to the prostate)
- Pharoses (foreskin cannot be fully retracted)
- Spreading rectal infection
- Urinary tract infections
- Acute epididymitis
- Indwelling Foley catheter
- Transurethral surgery

PRIAPISM

A persistent, often painful, erection (without sexual stimulation) that occurs for more than 4 hours.

Causes/Classifications/Risks

- *Low flow:* Low-flow priapism is usually due to persistent venous occlusion, resulting in venous stasis and deoxygenated blood pooling within the penis tissue. Pain is usually associated.

Risk Factors

- Sickle cell disease.
- Leukemia.
- Malaria.
- Medication side effects.
- *High flow:* High-flow priapism usually is secondary to a rupture of a local artery and unregulated flow into the penis. Pain less likely to be associated or severe.
- Injury/trauma to the penis or the perineum
- Spinal cord injury (parasympathetic response)

A foreign body lodged (intentionally or unintentionally) somewhere in the genitourinary tract

- Often sexual or erotic in nature.
- Endoscopic and minimal invasive techniques of removal should be used whenever possible.
- Surgical retrieval of a foreign body may be required, particularly when there is a severe associated inflammatory reaction.

Special Considerations

- Very common complaint.
- Must take *all* complaints of abdominal pain seriously.
- History, assessment, and cooperation needed.
- Privacy is essential.
- Watch facial expression during examination.

ASSESSMENT

History of Present Illness and Review of Systems

General

The following characteristics of each symptom should be elicited and explored:

- Onset (sudden or gradual)
- Location
- Duration, chronology
- Characteristics/quality of symptom
- Associated symptoms
- Precipitating and aggravating factors
- Relieving factors
- Timing, frequency, and duration
- Current situation (same, improving, or deteriorating)
- Previous diagnosis of similar episodes
- Previous treatments and efficacy
- Effects on daily activities

Cardinal Signs and Symptoms

In addition to the general characteristics outlined previously, the following additional characteristics of specific symptoms should be elicited:

Abdominal Pain

- Quality—Sharp, burning, cramping
- Quantity—Constant, intermittent
- Radiation—Localized, generalized
- Timing—Related to eating or movement
- Severity

Consider GU indicators—Flank, suprapubic, genital, groin or low back pain, and ± tenderness

Nausea and Vomiting

- Frequency, amount
- Presence of bile
- Hematemesis
- Force
- Color
- Relationship to food intake

Dysphagia

- Solids or liquids.
- Site where food gets stuck.
- Food is regurgitated.

Bowel Habits

- Last bowel movement
- Frequency, color, and consistency of stool
- Presence of blood or melena
- Pain before, during, or after defecation
- Sense of incomplete emptying after bowel movement
- Use of laxatives—Type and frequency
- Tenesmus
- Hemorrhoids
- Belching, bloating, and flatulence
- Change in bowel habits

Urinary Symptoms

- Frequency, urgency, quantity
- Dysuria and its timing during voiding (at beginning or end, throughout)
- Difficulty in starting or stopping urinary stream
- Change in color and odor of urine
- Hematuria
- Incontinence (including urge and stress)
- Presence of stones or sediment in the urine
- Nocturia (new onset or increase in usual pattern)
- Urinary retention
- For men—Postvoid dribbling and/or feeling that bladder is incompletely empty

Jaundice

- Scleral icterus
- Tea-colored urine
- Clay-colored bowel movements
- Pruritis (itching)
- History of hepatitis A, hepatitis B, or hepatitis C

GU—Female

Where appropriate for females to rule out ectopic, pelvic inflammatory disease (PID), or pregnancy as the cause of symptoms:

- Any changes in the date of last menstrual period (LMP)?
- Dyspareunia or postcoital bleeding
- Lesions on external genitalia
- Itching
- Urethral or vaginal discharge
- Sense of pelvic relaxation (pelvic organs feel as though they are falling down or out)

GU—Male

- Testicular pain or swelling
- Discharge from penis, itching
- Lesions on external genitalia

Other Associated Symptoms

- Change in appetite
- Fever
- Malaise
- Headache
- Dehydration
- Meal pattern
- Recent weight loss or gain that is not deliberate
- Enlarged, painful nodes (axilla, groin)
- Skin—Dry, rash, itchy

History Specific to GI/GU Systems

- Allergies (seasonal as well as reactions)
- Past and current use of medications (prescription and over-the-counter [OTC], eg, aspirin [ASA], antacids, triple therapy for peptic ulcer disease, acetaminophen, antibiotics, laxatives, estrogen, progesterone [including birth control], anticholinergics, antihypertensives, antipsychotics, thiazide diuretics, immunosuppressants, digoxin, codeine)
- Herbal preparations and traditional therapies
- Immunizations

Diseases—GI

- Hiatus hernia, esophageal cancer
- Documented *Helicobacter pylori* or gastroesophageal reflux disease (GERD)

- Presence of hernia, masses
- Chronic constipation
- Irritable bowel syndrome (IBS), inflammatory bowel disease (IBD)
- Peptic ulcer disease (PUD)
- Diverticulosis
- Liver disease (hepatitis A, hepatitis B, hepatitis C, or cirrhosis), gallbladder disease
- Pancreatitis
- Diabetes mellitus

Diseases—GU

- Human papilloma virus, sexually transmitted infections (STIs), including human immunodeficiency virus (HIV)
- Renal disease, pyelonephritis, recurrent cystitis, renal stones
- Congenital structural abnormalities of GU tract

Male

- Hydrocele, epididymitis, prostatism, varicocele, hernia, undescended testis, spermatocele, erectile dysfunction, testicular torsion, vasectomy

Female

- Menstrual history—Menarche, LMP, interval, regularity, duration, and amount of flow
- Premenstrual syndrome (PMS) symptoms, dysmenorrhea, menopause, postmenopausal bleeding, PID
- Obstetrical history—Gravida, term, para, abortion, live (GTPAL), stillbirths, complications during pregnancies, deliveries, infertility

Other

- Abdominal surgery or examinations, including GU such as catheterization, vasectomy, gynecological procedures
- Blood transfusion
- Immunocompromised

Family History Specific to GI/GU Systems

- Household contact with hepatitis A or hepatitis B
- Household contact with recent gastrointestinal (GI) infections
- Food poisoning
- GERD, PUD
- Gallbladder disease
- Gastric or colon cancer
- Polyps
- Pancreatitis
- Metabolic disease (ie, diabetes mellitus, porphyria)
- Cardiac disease
- Renal disease (eg, renal cancer, polycystic kidneys, renal stones)
- Urinary tract infections

Personal and Social History Specific to GI/GU Systems

- Substance use—Alcohol, smoking, caffeine, street drugs, including injection drugs, steroids
- Dietary recall including foods avoided (and reasons for), fat intake, nitrate intake (eg, smoked foods)
- Obesity, anorexia, bulimia, or other eating disorder
- Travel to area where infectious GI conditions are endemic
- Body piercing or tattoos
- Stress at work, home, or school
- Quality of drinking water—Exposure to pollutants
- Sanitation problems at home or in the community
- Personal hygiene, toileting habits, use of bubble bath, douches, tight-fitting underwear or other clothing
- Sexual history and practices, including risk behaviors (unprotected oral, anal, or vaginal intercourse, multiple partners, sexual orientation) and contraceptives
- Symptomatic sexual partner
- Sexual or physical assault or spousal abuse
- Fear, embarrassment, anxiety
- Missing work, school or social functions because of GU symptoms (eg, incontinence)

PHYSICAL ASSESSMENT

Vital Signs

- Temperature
- Pulse
- Respiratory rate
- SpO_2
- Blood pressure

General

- Apparent state of health
- Appearance of comfort or distress
- Color
- Nutritional status
- State of hydration
- Match between appearance and stated age

Abdominal Inspection

- Abdominal contour, symmetry, scars, dilatation of veins
- Movement of abdominal wall with respiration
- Visible masses, hernias, pulsations, peristalsis
- Guarding and positioning for comfort
- Ability to mobilize and gait

Auscultation

- Auscultation should be performed *before* percussion and palpation so as not to alter bowel sounds.
- Presence, character, and frequency of bowel sounds.
- Presence of bruits (renal, iliac, or abdominal aortic).

Abdominal Examination: Peripheral Areas

- Jaundice, spider nevi on face, neck or upper trunk, palmar erythema, Dupuytren contracture, clubbing of fingers

The following GU signs and symptoms require immediate transport:

- Bleeding from the urethra, male or female
- Urinary retention
- Urethral discharge
- Severe GU pain (consider PID or ectopic pregnancy)
- Scrotal swelling
- Erectile dysfunction
- Systemic symptoms (sepsis)
- Incontinence (new onset)
- Recent urological/renal surgery

? CHAPTER QUESTIONS

1. Acute renal failure is the rapid loss of kidney function.

   a. True
   b. False

2. A persistent, often painful, erection (without sexual stimulation) that occurs for more than 4 hours is called:

   a. priapism
   b. tenesmus
   c. mittelschmerz
   d. dysuria

Chapter 20
Gynecological Emergencies

A 16-year-old G1P1, last menstrual period (LMP) 1 week ago, presents with a 1-week history of severe lower abdominal pain. Pain is constant, bilateral, and accompanied by fever and chills. She has had some nausea and several episodes of vomiting. She has been sexually active for 3 years and has had unprotected intercourse with several partners. She denies irregular bleeding, dysmenorrhea, or dyspareunia. Past medical history is negative except for childhood illness. Past surgical history is remarkable for tonsillectomy as a child and an uncomplicated vaginal delivery 1 year ago.

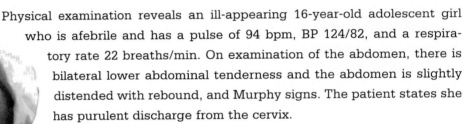

Physical examination reveals an ill-appearing 16-year-old adolescent girl who is afebrile and has a pulse of 94 bpm, BP 124/82, and a respiratory rate 22 breaths/min. On examination of the abdomen, there is bilateral lower abdominal tenderness and the abdomen is slightly distended with rebound, and Murphy signs. The patient states she has purulent discharge from the cervix.

What would be your treatment and diagnosis?

Goals in treating and interviewing the gynecological emergent patient include:

- Gathering a history requires attention to privacy and confidentiality.
- Obtain a full menstrual, contraceptive, and sexual history.
- Interview in the absence of family members.
- Consider pregnancy!

PHASES OF THE MENSTRUAL CYCLE

- The proliferative phase
- The secretory phase
- The ischemic phase
- The menopausal phase

Proliferation Phase

- This is the first 2 weeks of the menstrual cycle.
- Estrogen causes the uterine lining to thicken and became engorged with blood.
- Secretion of luteinising hormone (LH) day 14: Ovulation takes place.
- If the egg is not fertilized, menstruation takes place.

- If the egg is fertilized, the corpus luteum produces progesterone until the placenta takes over.
- Cilia sweep the egg toward the uterus.
- A fertilized egg normally implants in the lining of the uterus.
- If the egg is not fertilized, it is expelled from the uterine cavity.

Secretory Phase

- The secretory phase is referred to as ovulation.
- Progesterone increases and estrogen drops if the egg is not fertilized.
- The uterus becomes more vascular in preparation for implantation of a fertilized egg.

Ischemic Phase

- Estrogen and progesterone levels fall without fertilization.
- The endometrium breaks down.

Menopausal Phase

- *Menopause* is cessation of menstruation.
- Onset
  - Usually 50 to 51 years
    - If less than 40 years premature menopause
    - If less than 35 years premature ovarian failure (idiopathic, send genetic studies)
- Symptoms
  - Irregular menses
  - Hot flashes secondary to decreased estrogen
  - Mood changes
  - Depression
  - Lower urinary tract atrophy
  - Genital changes
  - Osteoporosis

Consequences of Decreased Estrogen

- Unfavorable lipid profile that could result in stroke and myocardial infarction (MI).
- Increased bone reabsorption because estrogen decreases osteoclast activity predisposing to hip fracture.
- Atrophy of skin and muscle tone.

PREMENSTRUAL SYNDROME

Second-half of cycle

Probable causes: Abnormal estrogen/progesterone balance, increased prostaglandin (PG) production, decreased endogenous endorphins; disturbance in renin-angiotensin-aldosterone system

Signs and Symptoms

- Decreased mood

- Anxiety
- Affective liability
- Decreased interest
- Irritability
- Concentration difficulty
- Decreased energy
- Change in appetite
- Overwhelmed
- Edema
- Weight gain
- Breast tenderness

Dysmenorrhea

Pain and cramping during menstruation that interfere with the acts of daily living

- Primary—Presents in less than 20 years because of increased PG occurs with ovulatory cycles
- Secondary—Endometriosis, adenomyosis, fibroids, cervical stenosis (congenital, trauma, surgery, infection), adhesions (history of infection pelvic inflammatory disease [PID], tuboovarian abscess [TOA])

Menorrhagia

- Heavy prolonged menstrual bleeding; over 80 cc/cycle.
- Average 35 mL of blood loss.
- More than 24 pads per day.
- Estrogen increases endometrial thickness.
- Progesterone matures endometrium and withdrawal of progesterone leads to secretion.
- Menstruation at regular intervals usually indicates ovulation.

ABNORMAL UTERINE BLEEDING

Abnormal uterine bleeding aka irregular periods indicates anovulation. Causes: Fibroids, adenomyosis, endometrial hyperplasia, endometrial polyps, cancer (CA), pregnancy complication

Metrorrhagia

- Intermenstrual bleeding
- Thick endometrial polyps
- Endometrial/cervical cancer
- Pregnancy complication

Polymenorrhea

- Cycles fewer than 21 days between periods, that is, anovulation

Oligomenorrhea

- More than 35 days apart—Disruption of pit/gonadal axis, pregnancy

POSTMENOPAUSAL BLEEDING

- More than 12 months after menopause
- Lower/upper genital tract

Mechanism

- Exogenous hormones
- Nongynecological causes: Rectal bleeding, prolapse, fissures, tumors, vaginal atrophy, CA (endometrial and cervical), endometrial hyperplasia, polyps

Fibroids

- Fibroids: Estrogen-dependent local proliferation of smooth muscle cells, usually occur in women of childbearing age and regress at menopause; African Americans are at higher risk; have a pseudocapsule of compressed muscle cells; are found in 20% to 30% American women at age 30.

Signs and Symptoms

- Menorrhagia
- Metrorrhagia
- Pressure (from pressing against bladder)
- Infertility
- About 50% are asymptomatic.
- Parasitic fibroids: Get their blood supply from the omentum.

Surgical Treatment

- Momectomy (only for fertility purposes)
- Hysterectomy indicated when anemic from bleeding
- Severe pain
- Size more than 12 weeks
- Urinary frequency
- Growth after menopause
- New role for embolization by interventional radiology

ENDOMETRIOSIS

Adenomyosis

Endometrium in myometrium

- Usually a 30-year-old multiparous woman with *heavy painful periods*, enlarged tender uterus described either as boggy/soft or woody/firm and pelvic heaviness.
- Treatment: Hysterectomy/analgesics.
- The tissue does not undergo proliferation phase of cell cycle.

TYPES OF SEXUALLY TRANSMITTED DISEASES

- Chlamydia
- Gonorrhea
  - Usually transfers more from male to female than female to male.
- Syphilis: *Treponema pallidum*

- Herpes simplex virus (HPV)
  - Types 6/11—Genital warts
  - Types: 16,18,31—Cervical cancer
- Chancroid: Caused by *Haemophilus ducreyi* and is a painful soft ulcer with inguinal lymphadenopathy
- Lymphogranuloma venerum: Primary = papules/shallow ulcer; secondary = painful inflammation of inguinal nodes with fever, headache, malaise, anorexia
- *Phthirus pubis/Sarcoptes scabiei*: Lice and scabies, respectively

Vaginitis

- *Candida*
  - Signs and symptoms: Burning, itching, vulvitis, cottage cheese discharge, dyspareunia
- *Trichomonas*: Unicellular flagellated protozoan
  - Signs and symptoms: Itching, including discharge (yellow/gray/green), frothy
- Bacterial vaginosis: *Gardnerella vaginalis*
  - Signs and symptoms: Odorous discharge, (not a sexually transmitted disease [STD]).

PID

- Organisms: *Neisseria, Chlamydia, Mycoplasma, Ureaplasma, Bacteroides*
- Signs and symptoms: Diffuse lower abdominal pain, vaginal discharge, bleeding, dysuria, dyspareunia, adnexal tenderness, gastrointestinal (GI) discomfort

Tuboovarian Abscess

- Persistent PID progresses to TOA in 3% to 16% of the time.
- Adnexal mass/fullness.

ENDOMETRITIS

- Usually after some type of instrument disruption of the uterus: C-section, vaginal delivery, D & E/C, intrauterine device [IUD])

TOXIC SHOCK SYNDROME

- Vaginal infection that is not associated with menstruation. Can be associated with delivery, C-sections, postpartum endometritis.
- *Staphylococcus aureus* produces epidermal TSS T-1 that produces fever, erythema rash desquamation of palmer surfaces, and hypotension. You may also see GI disturbances, amylase, mucus membrane hyperemia, change in mental status.

INCONTINENCE

- Urge incontinence: Aka detrusor instability
- Signs and symptoms: Urgency, often cannot make it to the bathroom
- Causes: Foreign body, urinary tract infection (UTI), stones, CA, diverticulitis

Stress Incontinence

- Symptoms: Involuntary loss of urine when there is an increased abdominal pressure mostly from sneezing, coughing, laughing which transmits pressure to the urethra
- Mechanism: Intrinsic sphincter defect, hypermobile bladder neck, pelvic relaxation
- Causes: Trauma, neurological dysfunction, associated with multiparity

Polycystic Ovarian Syndrome

This is a syndrome which can include numerous ovarian cysts, but really is more than that. It includes:

- Insulin resistance: Diagnosed by fasting glucose/insulin ratio less than 4.5 Tx: *metformin.*
- Hirsutism: From hyperandrogenemia.
- Anovulation: Irregular, heavy periods; if desires fertility treat with *metformin and Clomid.*
- Follicle-stimulating hormone (FSH): LH ratio is over 2.5:1.

Infertility

Inability to achieve pregnancy after 12 months of unprotected intercourse, 20% of population

- Idiopathic—10%
- Male and female—-10%
- Female causes—40%
  - Ovulatory—Anovulation, endocrine, polycystic ovary (PCO), premature ovarian failure

VAGINAL CA

- Women in their 50s
- Diethylstilbestrol (DES) exposure in utero resulting in clear cell adenocarcinoma
  - DES is a man-made (synthetic) form of estrogen, a female hormone.
- Asymptomatic for the most part but may have discontinued, bleeding, purities

CERVICAL CANCER

- Signs and symptoms: Vaginal bleeding, discontinue, pelvic pain, growth on cervix.
- Classic presentation: Postcoital bleeding, pelvic pain/pressure, abnormal vaginal bleeding rectal/bladder
- Types: Squamous large cell, keratinizing, nonkeratinizing, small cell (worse prognosis)
  - Adenocarcinoma
  - Mixed carcinoma
  - Glassy cell—occurs in pregnant women, usually fatal

Cervical Cancer Staging

O—Carcinoma

I—Contained to cervix

II—Carcinoma beyond cervix, no sidewall

II—Pelvic sidewall, hydronephrosis

IV—Extends beyond pelvis

OVARIAN TUMORS

- Family history, uninterrupted ovulation, low fertility, delayed childbearing, late-onset menopause
- Signs and symptoms: Asymptomatic until advanced stages, urinary frequency, dysuria, pelvic pressure, ascites

Ovarian Cancer Staging

I—Growth to one/both ovaries

II—With extension to pelvic structures

III—Peritoneum

IV—Distant metastatic CA

CA OF FALLOPIAN TUBES

- Adenocarcinoma from mucosa
- Disease progresses like ovarian CA
- Peritoneal spread
- Ascites
- Bilateral in 10% to 20% results often from metastatic CA
- Primary in very rare cases
- Asymptomatic but may have vague lower abdominal pain and discharge

? CHAPTER QUESTIONS

1. Signs and symptoms of pelvic inflammatory disease include all of the following *except*:

   a. diffuse lower abdominal pain

   b. vaginal discharge

   c. bleeding

   d. diarrhea

2. The first 2 weeks of the menstrual cycle is called:

   a. the proliferative phase

   b. the secretory phase

   c. the ischemic phase

   d. the menopausal phase

Section 6

Shock

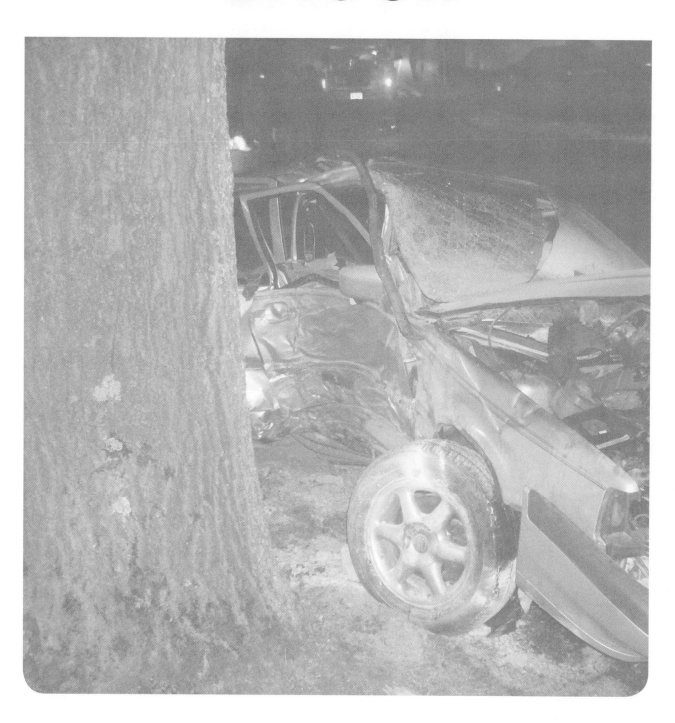

Chapter 21

Bleeding and Shock

Your unit is dispatched to University Avenue and West 190th Street for a victim of a stabbing. Upon arriving at the scene, you notice police frantically waving you down in front of the local bodega. The scene is safe to operate. As you survey the scene, you notice a very large pool of blood surrounding what appears to be a female patient. The patient is found lying prone in front of the location, unconscious and unresponsive. As you log roll the patient using C-spine precautions, your partner notices a very large knife impaled in the patient's sternum. You estimate blood loss to be significant and the patient is pale, cool, and diaphoretic. The patient has agonal breathing, and rescue breathing is started by another responder on-scene. Your partner tells you she cannot palpate a radial or femoral pulse, but has a weak and thready carotid pulse.

With this assessment, what type of shock is this patient presenting?

PATHOPHYSIOLOGY OF SHOCK

- Shock is defined as "inadequate tissue perfusion."
- Shock can result from trauma, fluid loss, heart attack, infection, spinal cord injury, and the like.
- Occurs first at the cellular level, and if allowed, can progress to organ failure and death.

PHYSIOLOGY OF PERFUSION

- Cells of the body require a constant supply of oxygen and nutrients (glucose) along with the elimination of carbon dioxide and waste products.
- The needs of the cells are fulfilled by the circulatory system in conjunction with our respiratory and gastrointestinal systems.
- Perfusion is dependent on three components of the circulatory system:
  ○ Pump (heart) (rate)
  ○ Fluid volume (blood)
  ○ Container (blood vessels)

Any derangement of any of these components can affect perfusion.

- The following organs require the most oxygen, and in the pecking order during decreased perfusion receive oxygenated blood over other organs and tissues:
  ○ The heart (circulatory system)
  ○ The brain (nervous system)

- ○ The lungs (respiratory system)
- ○ The kidneys

THE PUMP "HEART"

- The pump of the circulatory system receives blood from venous system.
- Pumps blood to the lungs to receive oxygen.
- Pumps blood to the peripheral tissues.

Stroke Volume

Defined as the amount of blood pumped by the heart in one contraction (average amount is 70 mL). Stroke volume is affected by preload, contractile force, and afterload.

Preload

- The amount of blood delivered to the heart during diastole.
- It is dependent on venous return.
- Variable venous capacitance can increase or reduce blood return to the heart.
- Increased preload = increased stroke volume.

Contractile Force

The force generated by the heart during each contraction.

Frank-Starling Mechanism

- The greater the preload, the more the ventricles are stretched.
- The greater the stretch, the greater the contractile force.

Afterload

- Resistance against which the heart must pump.
- When resistance is overcome, blood can be ejected.
- Determined by the degree of arterial peripheral vasoconstriction.
- Vasoconstriction = increased resistance = increased afterload = decreased stroke volume.

Cardiac Output

- Amount of blood pumped by the heart in 1 minute or stroke volume × heart rate = cardiac output.
- Expressed in liters per minute.
- An increase in stroke volume or heart rate = increased cardiac output
- A decrease in stroke volume or heart rate = decreased cardiac output

Cardiac output = (stroke volume) × (heart rate)

Blood Pressure

It is defined as, cardiac output × peripheral vascular resistance (afterload).

- Increased afterload = increased blood pressure
- Decreased afterload = decreased blood pressure

Baroreceptors

- Sensory fibers located in the aortic and carotid bodies.
- They monitor changes in blood pressure.
- If blood pressure increases, baroreceptors tell the brain to decrease heart rate, preload, and afterload.
- If blood pressure falls, baroreceptors signal the brain to activate the sympathetic nervous system to increase heart rate, preload, contractile force, afterload, and cardiac output.

THE FLUID "BLOOD"

- Blood is the fluid of the cardiovascular system.
- Blood is more viscous, thicker, and more adhesive than water.
- Because the cardiovascular system is closed, an adequate volume of blood must be present to fill the system.
- Blood transports oxygen, carbon dioxide, nutrients, hormones, metabolic waste products, and heat.

THE CONTAINER "BLOOD VESSELS"

- The blood vessels serve as the container of the cardiovascular system.
- They are a continuous, closed, pressurized pipeline that moves blood throughout the cardiovascular system.
- The blood vessels of the body include arteries, arterioles, capillaries, venules, and veins.
- Under the control of the autonomic nervous system, they regulate blood flow to different areas of the body by adjusting their size and rerouting blood flow through microcirculation.

Microcirculation

- Responsive to local tissue needs.
- Capillary beds can adjust size to supply undernourished tissue and bypass tissue with no immediate need.
- Precapillary sphincters and postcapillary sphincters open and close to feed or bypass tissues.

Blood Flow

- Occurs because of peripheral resistance and pressure within the system.
- Peripheral resistance is dependent on inner diameter and length of the vessel, and blood viscosity.
- Very little resistance in the aorta and arteries.
- Significant changes are seen in arterioles, which can change size fivefold.

System Pressures

- Contraction of the venous side increases preload and stroke volume.
- Contraction of the arteriole side increases afterload and blood pressure.

Oxygen Transport

- In addition to perfusion, oxygenation of peripheral tissues is essential.
- Oxygen diffuses across the alveolar-capillary membrane.

- Oxygen binds to the hemoglobin molecule of the red blood cells.
- Ideally, 97% to 100% of hemoglobin is saturated with oxygen.

Fick Principle

- Conditions for effective movement and utilization of oxygen in the body
- Adequate FiO_2 (concentration of O_2 in inspired air)
- Appropriate oxygen diffusion from alveoli into bloodstream
- Adequate number of red blood cells
- Proper tissue perfusion
- Efficient off-loading at the tissue level

Tissue Perfusion

- Tissue perfusion is dependent on the circulatory system and oxygenation by the respiratory system.
- Inadequate tissue perfusion can be caused by:
  - Inadequate pumping
  - Inadequate preload
  - Inadequate cardiac contractile strength
- Excessive afterload can be caused by:
  - Inadequate heart rate
  - Inadequate fluid volume
  - Hypovolemia
  - Inadequate container
  - Excessive dilation without change in fluid volume
  - Excessive systemic vascular resistance

PHYSIOLOGICAL RESPONSE TO SHOCK

- Normally the body can compensate for decreased tissue perfusion through a variety of mechanisms.
- When composition fails, shock develops, and if uncorrected becomes irreversible.
- Systemic response occurs when:
  - Progressive vasoconstriction
  - Increased blood flow to major organs
  - Shunted from skin, gastrointestinal (GI), and the like
  - Increased cardiac output
  - increased respiratory rate and volume
  - Decreased urine output
  - Decreased gastric activity

SHOCK AT THE CELLULAR LEVEL

Metabolism in Normal Conditions (Aerobic)

- Cell energy comes from glucose broken down through glycolysis into pyruvic acid.
- Pyruvic acid is further broken down in the Krebs cycle into CO_2, water, and energy.

Metabolism Poor Perfusion States (Anaerobic)

- Glucose breaks down into pyruvic acid, but not enough oxygen is present to enter into the Krebs cycle.
- Pyruvic acid accumulates, degrades into lactic acid, which also accumulates along with other metabolic acids.
- Cells die; tissues die; organs fail; organ systems fail; death ultimately ensues.
- Not enough O_2 in the cell for aerobic metabolism.
- Shifts to anaerobic metabolism using glycogen and fat (until stores depleted).
- Increased cell permeability.
- Na^+ and H_2O enter cell causing cellular swelling.
- K^+ leaks out of cell.
- Then Ca^{2+} enters cell.
- Buildup of lactic acid and CO_2 in cell.
- Cell eventually ruptures.

STAGES OF SHOCK

Compensated Shock

The body's defense mechanism in an attempt to preserve major organs.

- Precapillary sphincters close, blood is shunted to the core organs.
- Increased heart rate and strength of contractions.
- Increased respiratory function, bronchodilation.
- Will continue until problem is solved or shock progresses to next stage.
- Can be difficult to detect with subtle indicators.
- Tachycardia.
- Decreased skin perfusion.
- Alterations in mental status.
- Some medications such as propranolol can hide signs and symptoms (beta blockers).

Decompensated Shock

- Precapillary sphincters open, blood pressure falls.
- *Cardiac output falls.*
- Blood surges into tissue beds, blood flow stagnates.
- Red cells stack up in rouleaux.
- Easier to detect than compensated shock.
- Prolonged capillary refill time.
- Marked increase in heart rate.
- Rapid, thready pulse.
- Agitation, restlessness, confusion.
- *Decreased BP.*

Irreversible Shock

- Compensatory mechanisms fail, cell death begins, vital organs falter.
- Cannot be differentiated in the field.

- Patient may be resuscitated but will die later (acute respiratory distress syndrome [ARDS], renal and liver failure, sepsis).
- Organs have been deprived of O_2 for too long and cells have died causing organ failure.
- Brain, lungs, heart, kidneys.
- Development of disseminating intravascular coagulopathy (DIC).

Disseminating Intravascular Coagulopathy

- Presence of injured or lysed cells results in the release of phospholipids into the blood, triggering the intrinsic pathway.
- Prolonged states of low CO result in injury to the vascular endothelium, which also triggers the intrinsic pathway.
- Systemic coagulation.
- Diffuse fibrin formation.
- Clotting factors are exhausted.
- Activation of coagulation causes activation of fibrinolytic system.

TYPES OF SHOCK

Hypovolemic Shock

- Shock due to loss of intravascular fluid volume.

Possible Causes

- Internal or external hemorrhage
- Traumatic hemorrhage
- Long bone or open fractures
- Severe dehydration from GI losses
- Plasma losses from burns
- Diabetic ketoacidosis
- Excessive sweating
- Can result from internal third-space loss, possible causes include:
  - Bowel obstruction
  - Peritonitis
  - Pancreatitis
  - Liver failure resulting in ascites

Internal Bleeding

- Hematemesis—Blood in vomit
- Melena—Black, tarry stool
- Hemoptysis—coughing up blood
- Pain, tenderness, bruising, or swelling
- Broken ribs, bruises over the chest, distended abdomen

Characteristics of Bleeding

- Arterial—Blood is bright red and spurts.
- Venous—Blood is dark red and does not spurt.
- Capillary—Blood oozes out and is controlled easily.

External Bleeding

- Hemorrhage = bleeding.
- Body cannot tolerate greater than 20% blood loss.
- The average adult male has approximately 6 L of blood.
- Blood loss of 1 L can be dangerous in adults; in pediatrics, loss of 100 to 200 mL is serious.
- Hypovolemic shock is a volume problem.

What signs and symptoms would you expect to see and how would you treat the patient in the opening scenario in this chapter?

Controlling External Bleeding

DIRECT PRESSURE AND ELEVATION

- Direct pressure is the most common and effective way to control bleeding.
- Elevation controls bleeding.
- Wrap a pressure dressing around the wound once bleeding is controlled.
- If bleeding continues, apply additional dressings on top.

Pressure Points

- If bleeding continues, apply pressure on pressure point.
- Pressure at *proximal* pulse point greatly slows down circulation to extremity.
- The brachial artery and femoral artery are the two most common pressure points used.

Applying a Tourniquet

- Fold a triangular bandage into four in cravat.
- Wrap the bandage.
- Use a stick as a handle to twist and secure.
- Write "TK" on the patient's forehead, time it was placed, and what location on the body.

> **Clinical Significance**
>
> Stages of hypovolemia
> Stage 1: 10%-15% blood loss
> Stage 2: 15%-30% blood loss
> Stage 3: 30%-45% blood loss
> Stage 4: >45% blood loss

Cardiogenic Shock

- Inability to pump enough blood to supply all body parts.
- Primary cause is severe left ventricular failure (acute myocardial infarction [AMI], congestive heart failure [CHF]).
- Accompanying hypotension decreases coronary artery perfusion, worsening the situation.
- Other compensatory mechanisms—Increased peripheral resistance, increased myocardial O_2 demand (both worsen the situation).

Other Causes

- Chronic progressive heart disease.
- Rupture of papillary heart muscles or intraventricular septum.
- End-stage valvular disease.
- Patients may be normovolemic or hypovolemic.
- Usually have pulmonary edema.
- Pump failure (cardiogenic shock).
- Inadequate function of the heart.
- The heart muscle can no longer generate enough pressure to circulate blood to all organs.
- Causes a backup of blood into the lungs.
- Results in pulmonary edema.

A major difference between cardiogenic shock and other types of shock is the presence of pulmonary edema and dyspnea. Cardiogenic shock is a pump failure problem!

- What signs and symptoms would you expect to see?
- How would you manage a patient exhibiting signs and symptoms of cardiogenic shock?

Neurogenic Shock

- Shock resulting from inadequate peripheral resistance due to widespread vasodilatation (hypotension associated with C-spine or a high thoracic spinal cord injury).

Common Causes

- Spinal cord injury
- Central nervous system injuries

Neurogenic shock is a loss of vasomotor tone below the injury.

- What signs and symptoms would you expect to see?
  ○ Skin warm and dry below injury
  ○ Loss of sympathetic tone to the heart (bradycardia)
- How would you treat a neurogenic shock patient?

Septic Shock

- Shock resulting from systemic vasodilatation.
- Systemic increased vascular permeability.
- Usually a result of gram (–) bacterial infection.
- Development of bacteremia septic shock.
- Vessel and content failure.
- Caused by severe bacterial infections, *toxins,* or infected tissues.
- Toxins damage vessel walls, causing them to *leak* and become unable to contract well.
- Leads to *dilation* of vessels and loss of plasma, causing shock.
- How do you want to treat a septic shock patient?

Anaphylactic Shock

Anaphylactic shock is defined as a widespread hypersensitivity reaction to a specific antigen resulting in vasodilatation, peripheral pooling, relative hypovolemia leading to decreased perfusion, and impaired cellular metabolism.

- Provokes an extensive immune and inflammatory response
- Vasodilation
- Increased permeability
- Peripheral pooling
- Tissue edema
- Sudden onset and death can occur in minutes
- Anxiety
- Difficulty breathing
- GI cramps
- Edema
- Urticaria
- Pruritis
- Allergic reactions
- Vasodilation = produces drop in *BP*
- Bronchoconstriction = dyspnea

How would you treat a patient in anaphylactic shock?

- Psychogenic shock is caused by a sudden reaction of the nervous system that produces a temporary, generalized, vascular dilation.
- Commonly referred to as fainting or syncope.
- Causes range from fear or bad news to unpleasant sights.

EVALUATION OF THE SHOCK PATIENT

- Initial approach, approach with caution.
- What is the patient's mental status?
- Respiratory effort?
- Skin color?

Primary Assessment

- Check for airway patency; correct problems as needed.
- Assess breathing rate, quality; correct any life-threatening problems by administering high-concentration oxygen.
- Correct any obvious external bleeding.
- Location of palpable pulse as indicator of circulatory status.
  - Radial pulse—BP at least 80 mm Hg
  - Femoral pulse—BP at least 70 mm Hg
  - Carotid pulse—BP at least 60 mm Hg
- Assess skin color, temperature, and moisture.
  - Pale = decreased diffusion
  - Cyanotic = inadequate oxygenation

- - Mottled = late sign of shock
  - Cool = indicates vasoconstriction
- Assess capillary refill time in pediatric patients (<2 seconds is a normal finding).
- Level of consciousness is very early sign of impending circulatory collapse.
- Manifestations of reduction in cerebral flow include:
  - Agitation
  - Disorientation
  - Confusion
  - Inappropriateness of response
  - Unresponsiveness
- While altered mental status may result from drug/alcohol intake, assume the cause is decreased cerebral perfusion.

Secondary Assessment

- Rapid transport for life-threatening conditions.
- Ideally, expose the head, neck, chest, and abdomen.
- Reassess vital signs.
- Gather a patient history when appropriate.

GENERAL SHOCK MANAGEMENT

- *Ensure patent airway.*
- Maintain cervical spine support.
- Maintain airflow through the use of airway adjuncts or intubation, preferred in unresponsive shock patients.
- Provide suctioning as necessary.
- *Maintain adequate respiratory function.*
- Assist ventilations with bag-valve-mask (BVM) or other appropriate adjunct.
- Perform other interventions as needed to correct shock-related conditions leading to respiratory compromise.
- *Control major bleeding and treat hypotension.*
- Positioning of patient (supine with legs elevated 10-12 in).
- Upright if cardiogenic shock with pulmonary edema (check respirations and assist as needed).

? CHAPTER QUESTIONS

3. Which of the following forms of shock is most commonly seen in the trauma patient?

   a. Hypovolemic shock

   b. Cardiogenic shock

   c. Septic shock

   d. None of the above

4. A patient has lost 15% to 30% of their total blood volume, what class of shock would they be in?

   a. Class I
   b. Class II
   c. Class III
   d. Class IV

5. What is the most common cause of cardiogenic shock?

   a. Dysrhythmias
   b. Myocardial infarction
   c. Chest trauma
   d. Congenital valve disorders

Chapter 22
Mechanism of Injury, Kinematics of Trauma

Your volunteer ambulance company is toned out for a forthwith pedestrian auto accident with the patient still pinned under the motor vehicle. The first responder arrives on-scene and confirms the incident. She states the patient is an 8-year-old girl pinned under a sport-utility vehicle (SUV); she is alert to voice, and is complaining of severe abdominal pain. You arrive moments after that report; the fire department is operating on-scene removing the patient from under the vehicle with air bags to lift the vehicle off the patient. You approach the scene, determine scene safety, and establish there is one patient, and the firefighters are removing the victim as you arrive at the vehicle's side.

Your primary assessment reveals an 8-year-old girl with multiple grotesque deformities to both upper and lower extremities, no obvious life-threatening hemorrhaging, and obvious abrasion to the right upper quadrant of her abdomen.

Does this patient have a significant mechanism of injury (MOI)?

Figure 22-1 shows the interior of a vehicle following a high-speed lateral impact motor vehicle collision. Notice the seat and steering column displacement. This car struck a tree on the driver's side at a high rate of speed. What type of injuries would you expect to see with this MOI?

KINEMATICS OF TRAUMA

- Trauma is the leading cause of death and disability in the United States among children and young adults (1-44 years old).
- Trauma is the third leading cause of death in all age groups.
- Annually, one in four Americans is injured severely enough to seek medical attention. An estimated 23 to 28 million people are treated in the emergency department (ED) annually for injury, of which 90% are not admitted to the hospital.
- Traumatic injury occurs to the body when the body tissues are exposed to energy levels beyond their tolerance. Work is defined as force acting over a distance. Forces that bend, pull, or compress tissues beyond their inherent limits result in the work that causes injury.

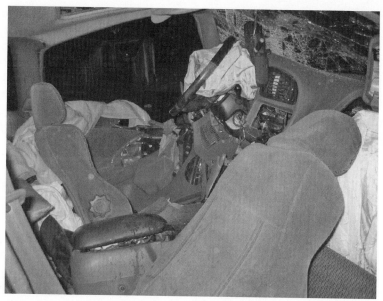

Figure 22-1   High-speed lateral impact motor vehicle collision. *(Used with permission of Peter DiPrima)*

- Kinetic energy (KE) is the energy of a moving object (motion).
  - The formula for determining kinetic energy is:

$$KE = \frac{mass\ (weight) \times velocity\ (speed)^2}{2}$$

- In the case of a motor vehicle crash (MVC), the kinetic energy of the speeding car is converted into the work of stopping the car (crushing the car). Similarly, the passengers have kinetic energy, and this is converted to the work of stopping them (injury).
- The energy that is available to cause injury doubles when an object's weight doubles, but quadruples when its speed doubles.
- Velocity has a greater influence than mass.
- Increasing a car's speed from 50 to 70 mph doubles the energy that is available to cause injury.
- Potential energy—The product of mass (weight), force of gravity, and height.
- A child in a tree has potential energy. When the child falls, the potential energy is converted into kinetic energy. As the child hits the ground, the kinetic energy is converted into work, that is, the work of bringing the child's body to a stop and thereby damaging tissues, bones, and so on.

BLUNT TRAUMA: "LEADING CAUSE OF TRAUMATIC DEATH IN THE UNITED STATES"

- Motor vehicle crashes—One of the most common sources of blunt trauma.
  - Each MVC typically consists of three collisions:
    - First—Vehicle against a hard object—MOI
    - Second—Passenger against the interior of the car
    - Third—Passenger's internal organs against the solid structures of the body

With new automotive technology (ie, air bags, energy-absorbing structural components, restraint systems), the severity of injuries to passengers in a motor vehicle collision is reduced. Air bags, which were introduced in the automotive community in the 80s and 90s, deploy very aggressively at speeds of 140 to 200 mph. This rapid deployment increased the potential of significant injury to unrestrained passengers, as well as children under 12 years old.

It is important to understand the effects of seating position, restraint type, restraint use, and vehicle type in assessing a patient from an MVC.

- Types of crashes (Figs. 22-2 through 22-7) include:
  - Frontal collisions—Is there intrusion into patient compartment? Were restraints used? Did the air bag deploy?
  - Rear-end collisions—High potential for whiplash injuries. Were restraints used?
  - Lateral collisions—T-bone, were restraints used? Twenty-five percent of severe aortic injuries result from lateral MVCs.
  - Rollover collisions—Ejection or partial ejection. Were restraints used?
  - Rotational impacts.

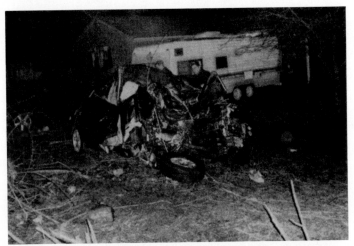

Figure 22-2   Significant mechanism of injury, car versus tree. (*Used with permission of Peter DiPrima*)

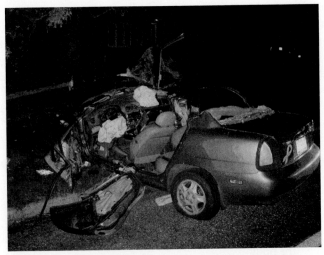

Figure 22-3   High-speed motor vehicle collision. (*Used with permission of Peter DiPrima*)

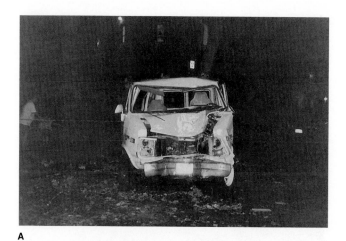

A

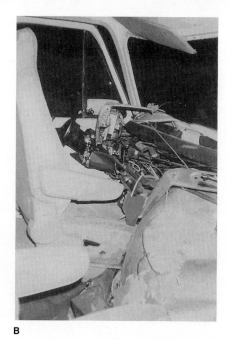

B

Figure 22-4 A. Van versus tree. B. Photo of inside the van. Notice the seat displacement and steering column displacement. *(Used with permission of Peter DiPrima)*

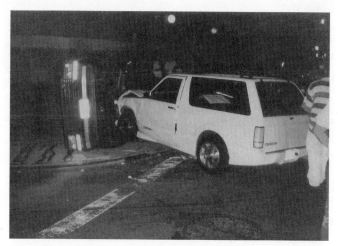

Figure 22-5 Lateral impact motor vehicle collision with a rollover. *(Used with permission of Peter DiPrima)*

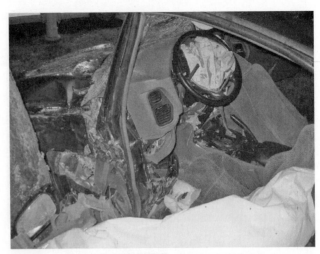

Figure 22-6 Lateral impact car versus tree. *(Used with permission of Peter DiPrima)*

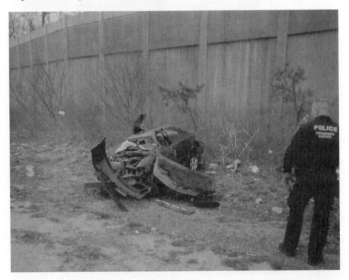

A

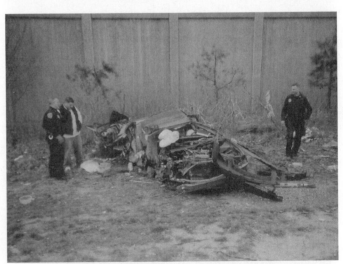

B

Figure 22-7 High-speed rollover motor vehicle collision with passenger ejection. *(Used with permission of Captain Richard Mancuso, Station 2, Lakeland FD)*

PENETRATING TRAUMA

- Second largest cause of traumatic death in the United States.
- Low-velocity penetrating injuries, that is, knives, ice picks, and the like. Injury closely follows path of penetrating object.
- Medium-velocity and high-velocity penetrating injuries—Bullet, pressure waves emanating from path of bullet can cause remote damage (cavitation). If the mass of a bullet is doubled, the energy that can cause injury is doubled. If the velocity (speed) of the bullet is doubled, the energy that can cause damage is quadrupled.

FALLS

- Considered to be the most common cause of trauma.
- The severity of an injury from a fall is directly related to the height of the fall and the surface the patient lands on.
- A fall from more than 12 to 15 ft, or three times the victim's height, is considered to be a significant mechanism of injury.
- Always consider internal injuries in a patient who has fallen from a significant height.
- Factors involving mechanism of injury from a fall include:
  o Height of the fall
  o Type of surface struck
  o The part of body that hit first
- Always consider syncope or other underlying medical causes of the fall.

BLAST INJURIES

- Three mechanisms of injury involving a blast injury:
  o Primary phase—Injuries occur from the pressure wave of the blast. (Injuries are seen to gas-containing or hollow organs.)
  o Secondary phase—Injuries occur by flying debris.
  o Tertiary phase—Injuries occur when the victim is thrown against an object.

TRAUMA PATIENT ASSESSMENT

- Three key decision points in trauma assessment process are:
  o MOI determination
  o General impression of the patient
  o Priority determination—At end of the primary assessment, is this a load-and-go situation?

Secondary Assessment

- Rapid trauma examination is quick and covers key areas of body with patients who have a significant MOI.
- Focused examination on patients without a significant MOI focuses only on an injured area.
- Rapid examination is quick and looks for "major" life-threatening injuries.
- Detailed examination is slower, more complete, and checks the "nooks and crannies." It is performed en route to hospital in most cases.

General Idea

- Care for serious patients occurs at hospitals/operating rooms.
- Trauma care for serious patients is a balance of care for life-threatening injuries and transport.
- Early identification of serious patients is the key!

MOI determination is as important in initial assessment decisions as actual patient care.

? CHAPTER QUESTIONS

1. The type of crash predicts the injury pattern associated with vehicular trauma.

   a. True
   b. False

2. MVCs cause three points of impact that produce injury. They include collision with the object, body impact with the vehicle, and:

   a. organ impact on the body
   b. side impact crashes
   c. both a and b
   d. none of the above

Chapter 23
Soft Tissue Injuries

Upon arrival at the scene, you find a huge crowd standing around a patient who is lying on the floor. As you approach, a police officer tells you that witnesses state that the patient was at the bar about 1 hour ago and had a couple of drinks before a woman, who said she was his ex-girlfriend, walked into the bar and shot him. He is now supine on the street corner with an obvious gunshot wound to the chest. His mental status is alert, and he is sweating profusely.

What is your first step in assessing this patient?

FUNCTION OF THE SKIN

- Skin protects the body.
- Skin is watertight and not penetrable by bacteria.
- Skin regulates body temperature. Water evaporates from the skin surface in hot weather, and surface blood vessels constrict in cold weather.

LAYERS OF THE SKIN

(Fig. 23-1)

- Epidermis—Outermost layer consists of dead cells constantly being rubbed off and replaced.
  - Deeper part of the epidermis contains cells which contain some pigment granules.
- Dermis—Contains many special structures of the skin:
  - Sweat glands
  - Sebaceous glands
  - Hair follicles
  - Blood vessels
  - Specialized nerve endings
- Subcutaneous tissue—Beneath the skin is a layer composed largely of fat that serves as a body insulator.

TYPES OF SOFT TISSUE INJURIES

Closed Soft Tissue Injuries

Contusion (Bruise)

- Epidermis remains intact.
- Cells are damaged and blood vessels torn in the dermis.

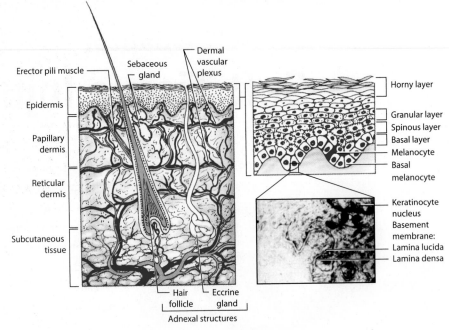

Figure 23-1 Layers of the skin. *(Reproduced with permission from Bruncardi FC, Andersen DK, Billiar TR, et al. (eds). Schwartz's Principles of Surgery. 8th ed. New York: McGraw-Hill; 2005)*

- Swelling and pain are typically present.
- Blood accumulation causes discoloration.

Hematoma

- Collection of blood beneath the skin.
- Larger amount of tissue damage as compared to contusion.
- Larger vessels are damaged.
- May lose one or more liters of blood.

Crush Injuries

- Crushing force applied to the body.
- Can cause internal organ rupture.
- Internal bleeding may be severe with shock (hypoperfusion).

Emergency Management

- Body substance isolation (BSI)
- Proper airway/artificial ventilation/oxygenation
- If shock (hypoperfusion) or internal bleeding is suspected:
  - Treat for shock (hypoperfusion).
  - Splint a painful, swollen, deformed extremity.
  - Transport.
  - Complete the pre-hospital care report. Document all pertinent findings of the patient assessment, treatment, and transport decisions.

Open Soft Tissue Injuries

Abrasion

- Outermost layer of skin is damaged by shearing forces.
- Painful injury, even though superficial.
- Very little or no oozing of blood.

Laceration

- Break in skin of varying depth.
- May be linear (regular) or stellate (irregular) and occur in isolation or together with other types of soft tissue injury.
- Caused by forceful impact with sharp object.
- Bleeding may be severe.

Avulsion

Flaps of skin or tissue are torn loose or pulled completely off.

Penetration/Puncture

- Caused by sharp pointed object.
- May be no external bleeding.
- Internal bleeding may be severe.
- Exit wound may be present.
- Examples are:
  - Gunshot wound
  - Stab wound

Amputations

- Involves the extremities and other body parts.
- Massive bleeding may be present or bleeding may be limited.

Crush Injuries

- Damage to soft tissue and internal organs.
- May cause painful, swollen, deformed extremities.
- External bleeding may be minimal or absent.
- Internal bleeding may be severe.

Emergency Management

- Body substance isolation.
- Maintain proper airway/artificial ventilation/oxygenation.
- Management of open soft tissue injuries.
- Expose the wound.
- Control the bleeding.
- Prevent further contamination.
- Apply dry sterile dressing to the wound and bandage securely in place.
- Keep the patient calm and quiet.
- Treat for shock (hypoperfusion), if signs and symptoms are present.

Special Considerations

- *Chest injuries*—Occlusive dressing to open wound
  - Administer high-concentration oxygen.
  - Position of comfort, if no spinal injury suspected.
- *Abdominal injuries*—Evisceration (organs protruding through the wound)
  - Do not touch or try to replace the exposed organ.
  - Cover exposed organs and wound with a sterile dressing, moistened with sterile water or saline, and secure in place.
  - Flex the patient's hips and knees, if uninjured.

- *Impaled objects*—Do not remove the impaled object, unless it is through the cheek and obstructing the airway, if it would interfere with chest compressions, or if interferes with transport.
  - Manually secure the object.
  - Expose the wound area.
  - Control bleeding.
  - Utilize a bulky dressing to help stabilize the object.
- *Amputations*—Concerns for reattachment
  - Wrap the amputated part in a sterile dressing.
  - Wrap or bag the amputated part in plastic and keep cool.
  - Transport the amputated part with the patient.
  - Do not complete partial amputations.
  - Immobilize to prevent further injury.
- *Open neck injury*
  - May cause air embolism.
  - Cover with an occlusive dressing.

? CHAPTER QUESTIONS

1. A wound under the skin that involves a blood vessel, characterized by a large lump with bluish discoloration is called a:

   a. crush injury

   b. concussion

   c. hematoma

   d. contusion

2. When performing the primary assessment and history and secondary assessment on a trauma patient, which of the following should be kept in mind?

   a. Severe bleeding should be treated as soon as your primary assessment is completed.

   b. BSI precautions should be taken if there is any external bleeding.

   c. DCAP-BTLS (*d*eformities, *c*ontusions/*c*repitation, *a*brasions, *p*unctures/*p*enetrations, *b*urns, *t*enderness, *l*acerations, *s*welling) during your rapid trauma assessment.

   d. SAMPLE (*s*igns/*s*ymptoms, *a*llergies, *m*edications, *p*ast medical problems, *l*ast oral intake, *e*vents) history should be obtained prior to your physical examination.

3. When providing emergency medical care for a closed soft tissue injury, remember that:

   a. large contusions, hematomas, and crush injuries usually heal themselves without treatment

   b. modern protective gloves have made hand washing unnecessary

   c. splinting painful, swollen, deformed extremities reduce the patient's pain

   d. high-concentration oxygen is usually not appropriate for soft tissue injuries

4. All the types of open wounds have one thing in common. That is:

   a. they all involve underlying soft tissue that is torn loose or pulled completely off.

   b. the patient is at risk for contamination with dirt, bacteria, and infection.

   c. they are all more serious internally than they appear externally.

   d. the wounds are all linear.

5. Scraping, rubbing, or shearing away of the outermost layer of the skin is called a/an:

   a. contusion

   b. laceration

   c. abrasion

   d. avulsion

6. Which of the following statements is true regarding punctures and penetrations?

   a. Powder burns around a gunshot wound are indicative of a small-caliber bullet.

   b. They are often more serious internally than they appear externally.

   c. The entrance wound of a gunshot is larger than the exit wound when shot at close range.

   d. Stab wounds are always easily detected due to the external bleeding.

7. When caring for a patient with a large, open neck injury, remember:

   a. dark, oozing blood indicates the carotid artery has been damaged

   b. to apply a pressure dressing circumferentially around the neck to control bleeding

   c. to cover the wound with an occlusive dressing, taped on three sides

   d. to immediately place a gloved hand over the wound to prevent air embolism

Chapter 24

Head, Face, Neck, and Spine Injuries

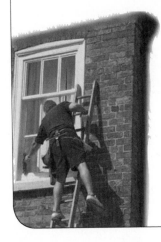

A 911 call is received, and your ambulance is dispatched for a man with a head injury which occurred from a fall from a ladder. Upon arrival you find a 30-year-old man lying in a fetal position with what appears to be a head laceration.

As you approach and determine scene safety, you find the patient to be exhibiting what appears to be seizure activity.

What is your next step?

INJURIES TO THE BRAIN AND SKULL

- Traumatic brain injuries (TBIs) are the leading cause of death and disability for children and adults ages 1 to 45 years of age.
- About 1.6 million head injuries occur each year in the United States.
- Approximately 52,000 people die each year from TBI.
- About 70,000 to 90,000 people are left with neurological disabilities.

THE IMPORTANCE OF AIRWAY, BREATHING, CIRCULATION

- Airway
  - Is the airway open?
    - Use the modified jaw thrust maneuver for opening the airway of a suspected C-spine injury.
  - Is the airway patent?
- Breathing
  - Is the patient breathing?
  - Is the breathing pattern irregular?
  - Don't be shy; be aggressive with managing the breathing of a head-injured patient.
  - Rescue breathing (hyperventilation) should be limited to 20 breaths/min.
- Circulation
  - Check for a radial, brachial, femoral, or carotid pulse.

- No pulse, begin cardiopulmonary resuscitation (CPR) according to American Heart Association (AHA) guidelines.
- Treat for shock.
- Is bleeding controlled?

HEAD INJURIES

- Injuries to the scalp (Fig. 24-1)
  - Very vascular, may bleed more than expected.
  - Control bleeding with direct pressure.
  - Injuries to the brain—Injury of brain tissue or bleeding into the skull will cause an increase of pressure in the skull.

Related Nontraumatic Conditions

- Nontraumatic injuries to the brain may occur due to clots or hemorrhaging.
- Nontraumatic brain injuries can be a cause of altered mental status.
- Signs and symptoms parallel that of traumatic injuries with the exception of evidence of trauma and a lack of mechanism of injury (MOI).

Skull Injury—Signs and Symptoms

- Mechanism of injury
- Contusions, lacerations, hematomas to the scalp

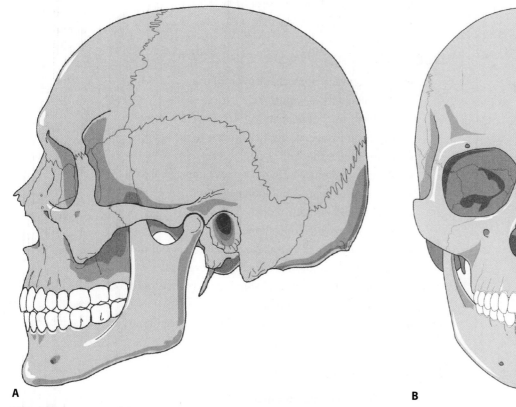

A   B

Figure 24-1 Image of the skull. A. Side view. B. Frontal view. (*©Unlisted images / Fotosearch.com*)

- Deformity to the skull
- Blood or fluid (cerebrospinal fluid [CSF]) leakage from the ears or nose
- Bruising (discoloration) around the eyes
- Bruising (discoloration) behind the ears (mastoid process)

Traumatic Brain Injury—Signs and Symptoms

- Altered or decreasing mental status is the best indicator of a brain injury (Glasgow Coma Scale [GCS] <9).
  - Confusion, disorientation, or repetitive questioning
  - Conscious—Deteriorating mental status
  - Unresponsive
- Irregular breathing pattern.
- Consideration of mechanism of injury.
  - Deformity of windshield
  - Deformity of helmet
- Contusions, lacerations, hematomas to the scalp.
- Deformity to the skull.
- Blood or fluid (CSF) leakage from the ears and nose.
- Bruising (discoloration) around the eyes (raccoon eyes).
- Bruising (discoloration) behind the ears (mastoid process) (Battle sign).
- Neurological disability.
- Nausea and/or vomiting.
- Unequal pupil size with altered mental status.
- Systolic blood pressure.
- Seizure activity may be seen.
- Oxygen saturation less than 90%.

Open Head Injury—Signs and Symptoms

- Consideration of mechanism of injury.
  - Deformity of windshield
  - Deformity of helmet
- Contusions, lacerations, hematomas to the scalp.
- Deformity to the skull.
- Penetrating injury—Do not remove impaled objects in the skull.
- Soft area or depression upon palpation.
- Exposed brain tissue if open.
- Bleeding from the open bone injury.
- Blood or fluid (CSF) leakage from the ears and nose.
- Bruising (discoloration) around the eyes.
- Bruising (discoloration) behind the ears (mastoid process).
- Nausea and/or vomiting.
- Possible signs and symptoms of a closed head injury may exist if brain injury has occurred.

Signs of Cerebral Herniation

- Unconscious and unresponsive
- Dilated pupils with no reaction to light

- Asymmetric pupils
- Nonresponsive to painful stimulus
- Posturing
  - Decorticate
  - Decerebrate
- Cushing reflex
  - ↑ in blood pressure, ↓ in pulse, and an irregular respiratory pattern

Emergency Management

- Body substance isolation (BSI).
- Maintain airway/artificial ventilation/oxygenation. Maintain an oxygen saturation of greater than 90%.
- Primary assessment should be done on-scene with a complete secondary physical examination en route hospital.
- With any head injury, the emergency medical technician (EMT) must minimize spinal movement.
- Closely monitor the airway, breathing, pulse, and mental status for deterioration.
- Control bleeding.
- Do not apply pressure to an open or depressed skull injury.
- Dress and bandage open wound as indicated in the treatment of soft tissue injuries.
- If a medical injury or nontraumatic injury exists, place patient on the left side.
- Be prepared for changes in patient condition.
- Immediately transport the patient.

Injuries to the Spine

Your unit is dispatched to the scene of a motor vehicle collision. The scene is safe to operate and you approach the vehicle. You note major damage to the driver's side of the car with major intrusion into the passenger compartment. The driver of vehicle is unconscious and appears to be the only patient.

How are you going to treat this patient?

SPINAL CORD INJURIES

- Mismanagement of spinal injuries can result in paralysis.
- Approximately 20,000 people suffer spinal cord injuries each year.
- The most common age group for spinal cord injuries is 16 to 35 years.
- Most common cause of spinal injuries is motor vehicle collisions.

THE NERVOUS SYSTEM REVIEW

Spinal Cord

- Consists of 31 segments; each gives rise to a pair of spinal nerves.
- Provides conduction pathways to and from the brain.
- Functions as a center for reflex action.

Peripheral Nervous System

- Cranial nerves—12 pairs are numbered according to order in which they arise; conducts impulses between brain and structures in head, neck, thoracic, and abdominal cavities.
- Spinal nerves—31 pairs; each nerve consists of a dorsal (sensory) root and a ventral (motor) root.

Autonomic Nervous System

- Involves involuntary or autonomic function.
- Impulses are conveyed to smooth muscle, cardiac muscle, and glandular epithelium.
- Center is located in the hypothalamus.
- Two parts—Sympathetic and parasympathetic.

Function of the Sympathetic Nervous System

- Increases cardiovascular response
- Pupil dilation
- Decreases peristalsis
- Regulates temperature
- Increases blood sugar
- Increases secretion of sweat glands
- Adrenal medulla—Epinephrine

Function of the Parasympathetic Nervous System

- Third, seventh, and tenth cranial nerves
- Pupillary constriction
- Decreases heart rate
- Stimulates watery secretions
- Relaxes bladder and rectal sphincters

Function of the Skeletal System in Relation to the Spine

The skeletal system provides protection and support to the spinal cord. Components of the skeletal system in relation to the spine include:

- Skull (Fig. 24-2)
- Spinal column (Fig. 24-3)
  - Thirty-three bones
  - Surrounds and protects the spinal cord

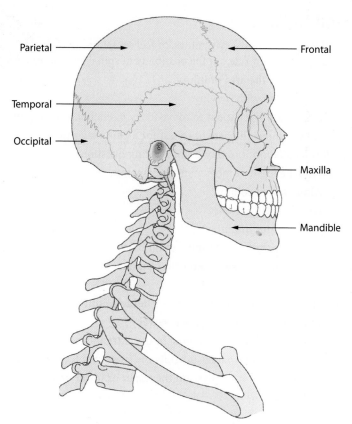

Figure 24-2 Skeletal system of the skull. (*©Unlisted images / Fotosearch.com*)

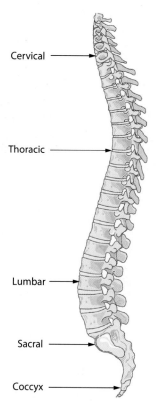

Figure 24-3 Skeletal system of the spine. (*©Unlisted images / Fotosearch.com*)

INJURIES TO THE SPINE—MECHANISM OF INJURY

- Compression injuries can occur from falls, diving accidents, or motor vehicle accidents.
- Excessive flexion, extension, rotation can cause serious injury to the spine.
- Lateral bending can cause serious injury to the spine.
- Distraction injuries occur from:
  ○ Pulling apart the spine
  ○ Hangings

The EMT must maintain a high index of suspicion for the following mechanisms of injury:

- Motor vehicle crashes
- Pedestrian/vehicle collisions
- Falls
- Blunt trauma
- Penetrating trauma to head, neck, or torso
- Motorcycle crashes
- Hangings
- Diving accidents
- Any unknown mechanism of injury that involves an unconscious trauma victim

Signs and Symptoms

- Ability to walk, move extremities, or feel sensation (or lack of pain to spinal column) does not rule out the possibility of spinal column or cord damage.
- Tenderness in the area of injury.
- Pain associated with moving.
  - Do not ask the patient to move to try to elicit a pain response.
  - Do not move the patient to test for a pain response.
- Tell the patient not to move while asking questions.
- Pain independent of movement or palpation.
  - Along spinal column
  - Lower legs
  - May be intermittent
- Obvious deformity of the spine upon palpation.
- Soft tissue injuries associated with trauma.
  - Head and neck to cervical spine
  - Shoulders, back, or abdomen—Thoracic, lumbar
  - Lower extremities—Lumbar, sacral
- Numbness, weakness, or tingling in the extremities.
- Loss of sensation or paralysis below the suspected level of injury.
- Loss of sensation or paralysis in the upper or lower extremities.
- Incontinence.

Assessing the Potential Responsive Spine Injury Patient

- What is the mechanism of injury?
- Questions to ask:
  - Does your neck or back hurt?
  - What happened?
  - Where does it hurt?
  - Can you move your hands and feet?
  - Can you feel me touching your fingers?
  - Can you feel me touching your toes?
- Inspect for contusions, deformities, lacerations, punctures, penetrations, swelling.
- Palpate for areas of tenderness or deformity.
- Assess equality of strength of extremities:
  - Hand grip
  - Gently push feet against hands

Unresponsive Patient

- Mechanism of injury.
- Primary assessment.
- Inspect for:
  - DCAP-BTLS
- Palpate for areas of tenderness or deformity.
- Obtain information from others at the scene to determine information relevant to mechanism of injury or patient's mental status prior to the EMT's arrival.

Complications of Spinal Injuries

- Inadequate breathing effort
- Paralysis

Emergency Management

- Body substance isolation.
- The patient should be placed in a properly fit cervical collar and spinal movement should be minimized.
- Perform primary assessment.
- Airway control must be done with in-line stabilization.
- Artificial ventilation must be done with in-line stabilization.
- Assess pulse, motor, and sensory, in all extremities.
- Assess the cervical region and neck.
- Apply a rigid, cervical immobilization device.
- Properly size the cervical immobilization device.
- An improperly fit immobilization device will do more harm than good.
- Quickly assess posterior body if not already done in the secondary physical examination.
- Reassess pulses, motor, and sensory, and record.
- If the patient is critically injured, perform a rapid extrication The patient should be placed in a properly fit cervical collar and spinal movement should be minimized.
- Transport the patient immediately.

SPINAL IMMOBILIZATION

Indications for Use of Cervical Spine Immobilization Devices

- Any suspected injury to the spine based on mechanism of injury, history, or signs and symptoms.

Sizing

- Various types of rigid cervical spine immobilization devices (CSIDs) exist; therefore, sizing is based on the specific design of the device.
- An improperly sized immobilization device has a potential for further injury.
- Do not obstruct the airway with the placement of a cervical immobilization device.
- If it doesn't fit, use a rolled towel and tape to the board and manually support the head. An improperly fitting device will do more harm than good.

Special Considerations

Indications for Rapid Extrication

- Unsafe scene.
- Unstable patient condition warrants immediate movement and transport.
- Patient blocks the EMTs' access to another, more seriously injured, patient.
- Rapid extrication is based on time and the patient, and not the preference of the EMTs.

Helmet Removal

Special assessment needs for patients wearing helmets:

- The helmet is removed to assure a properly maintained airway, or to adequately suction the patient, or to facilitate bag-valve-mask ventilation when necessary.

Indications for Leaving the Helmet in Place

- Good fit with little or no movement of the patient's head within the helmet.
- No impending airway or breathing problems.
- Removal would cause further injury to the patient.
- Proper spinal immobilization could be performed with helmet in place.
- No interference with the EMTs' ability to assess and reassess airway and breathing.

Indications for Removing the Helmet

- Inability to assess and/or reassess airway and breathing.
- Restriction of adequate management of the airway or breathing.
- Improperly fitted helmet allowing for excessive patient head movement within the helmet.
- Proper spinal immobilization cannot be performed due to helmet.
- Cardiac arrest.

Infants and Children

- Immobilize the infant or child on a rigid board appropriate for size (short, long, or padded splint), according to the procedure outlined in the "Spinal Immobilization" section.

Special considerations include:

- Pad from the shoulders to the heels of the infant or child, if necessary, to maintain neutral immobilization.
- Properly size the cervical immobilization device. If it doesn't fit, use a rolled towel and tape to the board and manually support head. An improperly fitted immobilization device will do more harm than good.

Injuries to the Eyes, Face, and Neck

It is after midnight on a summer night and you have been dispatched to the scene of a motor vehicle collision (MVC). Upon arrival, you establish the scene as being safe. You notice the patient walking around at the scene and he appears to be in his mid-twenties. You note the patient's car struck a light pole and there is significant damage to the front end of the car.

The patient appears upset as you approach him. His right eye is swollen and you notice he has a laceration above both of his eyes. He states, "I had too much to drink!" He is concerned about the damage he did to his mother's car, and is complaining of neck pain.

How would you manage this patient?

Eye, face, and neck injuries are significant because of the associated loss of function that occur secondary to the injury. The EMT must not only deal with the seriousness of the injury, but also the emotional distress the patient may have when fearing loss of vision, scarring, or even significant hemorrhage.

THE EYE

(Fig. 24-4)

- The eyeball is a sphere about 1 in in diameter.
- Its outer covering is the sclera (white portion).
- The cornea is the transparent region overlying the center.
- The pupil is the dark center, which is surrounded by the colored iris.

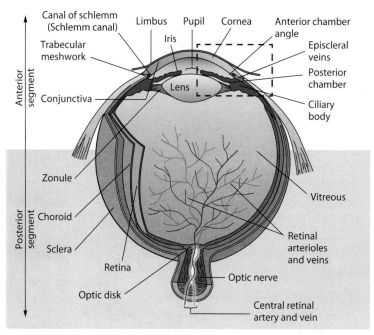

Figure 24-4A   Anatomy of the eye.

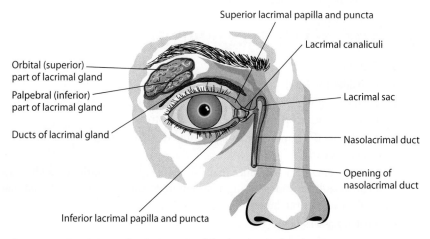

Figure 24-4B   Surrounding structures of the eye. (*Reproduced with permission from Brunton LL, Lazo JS, Parker KL. Goodman & Gilman's The Pharmacological Basis of Therapeutics. 11th ed. New York: McGraw-Hill; 2006*)

- The lens of the eye allows for the focusing of images on the retina, which is located to the back of the eye.
- Another structure of the eye is the conjunctiva, which lines the inner surface of the eyelids.
- Each side of the lens is a chamber. The anterior chamber contains aqueous humor, and posterior to the lens is the vitreous body that houses vitreous humor (gives the eye its shape).
- The eye is housed in the orbit socket of the skull.

THE FACE

- The face has 14 bones, 13 of which are immovable, with the only moveable one being the mandible.
- The face is also extremely vascular, and bleeds readily to even minor trauma. Trauma to the face can not only distort these bony structures, but it may also cause hemorrhage and airway occlusion.
- Any trauma of sufficient force to injure the face can easily result in head or neck trauma as well.

THE NECK

- The neck contains major structures of the body:
  - Carotid arteries
  - Jugular veins
  - Larynx and trachea
- Damage to these vascular and airway structures can cause life-threatening bleeding and airway compromise.
- Injuries to the neck can easily cause life-threatening conditions.
- While injuries to these locations can vary, they do create some common findings:
  - They all tend to hemorrhage profusely.
  - Many times, these types of injuries are the result of an assault.
  - You may deal with not only physical trauma, but emotional trauma also.
  - These types of injuries should not be taken lightly by the EMT-B, as they can rapidly deteriorate as well.

ASSESSMENT: EYE, FACE, AND NECK INJURIES

- Scene size-up.
- Consider the MOI.
- It may be difficult to gather information from the patient because often they are in extreme pain and emotional distress.
- Determine the number of patients injured and the need for additional resources early.
- Finally, remember that since many of these types of injuries come by way of an assault, consider having a law enforcement officer there, should that be the cause of the injury.
- Primary assessment.
- Be aware of the alteration in the patient's mental status.
- Establish in-line manual stabilization of the head.

- Open the airway with a jaw-thrust maneuver if needed and suction out any blood or vomitus.
- Determine quality and adequacy of breathing.
- Typically bleeding is profuse and easy to assess. Be sure, however, that you are properly managing bleeds to the head.
- Determine the priority status of the patient.

Primary Assessment Findings That Demonstrate a Critical or High-Priority Patient

- Chemical burns to the eye
- Impaled object in the eye
- An extruded eyeball
- Respiratory distress
- Severe injuries to the face and neck
- Major bleeding
- Alteration in mental status

Secondary Assessment

- Consistent with other traumatically injured patients, your completion of the physical examination, vitals, and SAMPLE (*s*igns/symptoms, *a*llergies, *m*edications, *p*ast medical problems, *l*ast oral intake, *e*vents) history are determined by your priority status.
- Often, injuries to the eye, face, and neck are critical, so commonly you'll complete a rapid trauma assessment followed by vitals and the SAMPLE history.
- Use the OPQRST (*o*nset, *p*rovokes, *q*uality, *r*adiates, *s*everity, *t*ime) mnemonic to assess any other complaints of pain.
- If the patient is critical, deliver only necessary treatment and initiate transport following the history and physical examination.

Secondary Assessment And Reassessment

- Secondary assessment will be completed when the patient's condition is stable.
- If the patient is unstable, or if you are too close to the hospital, then skip the detailed examination and start the ongoing assessment.
- Repeat the ongoing assessment for the unstable patient every 5 minutes, and every 15 minutes for the stable patient.
- Notify the receiving facility of the patient's condition, response to your treatment, and estimated time of arrival.

ASSESSING THE EYE-INJURED PATIENT

- Asses the orbits for bruising, swelling, lacerations, or tenderness.
- Assess the lids for bruising, swelling, and lacerations.
- Assess the conjunctiva for redness, pus, and foreign bodies.
- Assess the globes for redness, abnormal coloring, and lacerations.
- Assess the pupils for size, shape, equality, and reactivity.
- Evaluate eye muscle movement in all directions.
- Assess the eye for any abnormality.

- Assess motor function of the eyes by having the patient follow your finger movement in a large "H" pattern.
- If the eye is swollen shut, avoid excessive manipulation.
- Do not force eyelid open unless you're flushing it.
- Consult medical direction prior to irrigating the eye.
- Do not add medicine to the eye.
- Sponge or wipe blood away that exits the eye; do not remove blood from the eye itself.
- Keep patient supine and quiet.
- Give the patient nothing by mouth.
- If you're going to cover the injured eye, just cover both at the same time to limit motion.

Foreign Object in the Eye

Methods in removing a foreign object include:

- Flushing foreign particle from the eye.
- Inverting the eyelid and removing the object.
- Removing object from the upper lid.
- Grasping eyelid and telling the patient to look down.
- Placing applicator swab along center of upper eyelid.
- Pulling eyelid up and over applicator swab.
- Once you expose the undersurface of the eye, the foreign material can be removed.

Orbit Injury

- Management includes placing a dressing and a cold pack over the eye to reduce swelling.
- Do not, however, use a cold pack if you suspect a globe injury.

Lid Injury

- Stop any bleeding with light pressure.
- Preserve any avulsed tissue.
- Cover with a moist sterile dressing.
- Also cover opposite eye.

Globe Injury

- Due to the various injuries possible, it is best to just apply patches lightly to both eyes.
- Apply a shield to the injured eye to avoid any pressure being exerted on it.

Chemical Burn Injury

- The burning mechanism can cause rapid and permanent injury.
- Start irrigation with large amounts of water immediately.

Extruded Eyeball

- Cover the eye carefully so that no additional pressure is applied to the eyeball.
- Cover the other eye as well to limit motion and rapidly transport.

Impaled Object in the Eye

- Like an extruded eyeball, care should be taken to rapidly treat it and provide transport.
- Place padding around the object.
- Impaled object in the eye.
- Stabilize the impaled object with a cup.
- Bandage the cup in place and provide transport.

Removing Contact Lenses

- Eye injuries may be further complicated by the presence of contact lenses.
- Examine with a penlight to assess for shadowing over the outer portion of the eye (soft lens), or shadowing over the iris (hard lens).
- Some people only wear one contact lens, so don't dismiss them until you look in both eyes.
- Seek medical direction for permission to remove the lens.
- The type of lens typically determines how it should be removed.

INJURIES TO THE FACE

- Injuries to the face occur often due to common mechanisms of injury (ie, MVC), and their location.
- About 75% of MVC victims sustain some type of facial trauma.
- Some injuries can be life threatening due to their imposition on airway maintenance.
- Don't forget to consider cervical injuries with any type of facial trauma.

Emergency Management

- Establish cervical stabilization.
- Carefully assess the oral cavity, and retrieve any broken-off teeth, torn-away tissue, or other foreign material.
- Suction blood from the mouth (may need to be constantly repeated).
- Provide oxygen via non-rebreather (NRB) or positive-pressure ventilation (PPV), depending on breathing.
- Control any severe bleeding.
- Treat any avulsed teeth by wrapping in saline gauze.
- Treat for hypoperfusion (shock), and transport.

Impaled Object to the Cheek

- Generally, pack each side if the patient is stable.
- If the impalement compromises the airway, remove it in the direction of entry and pack both sides.

INJURIES TO THE NOSE

- Never pack the internal nares; however, external bleeds should be controlled.
- Try not to position the patient supine as any bleeding may compromise the airway.
- Treat nasal fractures with cold compresses.

INJURIES TO THE EAR

- Apply direct pressure to external bleeding.
- Preserve any tissue avulsions.
- Never pack the ear, but rather allow a sterile dressing to collect the blood.

INJURIES TO THE NECK

- Can be caused by blunt or penetrating trauma.
- Basic care includes:
  - Immobilization
  - Control of the airway, oxygen, and ventilation as needed
  - Cover neck wounds with occlusive dressing
  - Rapid transport

Severed Blood Vessel in the Neck

- Use a gloved hand to cover the wound initially.
- Use digital pressure on carotid artery only as a last resort.
- Apply an occlusive dressing.
- Cover with a regular bulky dressing.
- Only apply enough pressure to control the bleeding.
- Once bleeding is controlled, secure with roller gauze bandaging that is anchored around the shoulder and axillary region.
- Transport the patient on their left side with the head tilted down.
- If the patient is immobilized, then simply tilt the spinal board to the left.
- Continue oxygen therapy and treatment for shock.

? CHAPTER QUESTIONS

1. A patient that sustained a traumatic injury to the face must also be assessed for:

   a. brain injury

   b. airway obstruction

   c. spinal injury

   d. all of the above

2. Double vision, a marked decrease in vision, or a loss of sensation above the eyebrow, over the cheek, or in the upper lip may be caused by:

   a. detached retina

   b. orbital fracture

   c. cervical spine injury

   d. temporal bone fracture

3. The 12 vertebrae that comprise the upper back are the:

   a. sacral spine

   b. coccyx

   c. lumbar spine

   d. thoracic spine

4. During the primary assessment of a trauma patient:

   a. initiate immediate manual in-line spinal stabilization based on mechanism of injury

   b. open the airway of the unconscious patient using the head-tilt-chin-lift method

   c. the patient's skin may be cool, pale, and moist below the site of spinal injury, and warm and dry above the site of injury

   d. inadequate breathing will result from spinal cord damage involving the lumbar spine

5. The three major complications of spinal injury include which of the following?

   a. Systemic vasodilatation, resulting in reduced tissue perfusion

   b. Paralysis of the respiratory muscles, occurring with injury to the lumbar spine

   c. Paralysis to only one side of the body that does not resolve

   d. Inadequate circulation indicated by tachycardia and cool, clammy skin

6. The outermost layer of the three meninges is called the:

   a. pia mater

   b. dura mater

   c. alma mater

   d. arachnoid

7. Signs and symptoms of a brain injury may include:

   a. discoloration behind the ears (Battle sign)

   b. a ketone odor to the breath, which indicates the presence of CSF

   c. neck vein distention

   d. total or partial paralysis

8. When assessing the vital signs of a head injury patient, keep in mind that:

   a. head injury alone will not result in signs and symptoms of shock

   b. sudden hypotension indicates increased intracranial pressure

   c. a rapid or rising pulse indicates rising intracranial pressure

   d. hypotension in a head injury patient is due to bleeding elsewhere

9. Cushing reflex is a sign of severe head injury, and causes:

   a. seizure-like activity and apnea

   b. increased BP, decreased pulse, and respiratory pattern changes

   c. decorticate posturing and abnormal breathing patterns

   d. unconsciousness, decerebrate posturing, and vomiting

Chapter 25
Chest Trauma

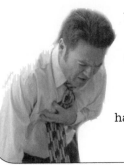

You are dispatched to the state police station for a man with chest pain. Upon arrival you learn the patient was struck in the chest with an object during an attempted robbery. The patient's vital signs are as follows:

BP 124/72, RR 28 labored, HR 100; skin is pale, cool, and dry.

With this mechanism of injury (MOI), what type of injuries may this patient have?

- Unlike trauma to the extremities, thoracic trauma rarely involves large visible injuries. In fact, an injury to these locations may be lethal, but have very minimal external signs of injury.
- Early recognition and treatment save lives.
- Thoracic injuries can interfere with normal breathing and gas exchange, and abdominal injuries may result in significant abdominal bleeding.

ANATOMY OF THE CHEST

- Surrounded by ribs, with the sternum on the anterior thorax, and the spine in the posterior.
- Inferior border is diaphragm.
- Contains lungs, heart, trachea, esophagus, and major blood vessels.
- Lungs are surrounded by the visceral and parietal pleura, which plays a role in certain types of thoracic injuries (Fig. 25-1).

TYPES OF CHEST INJURIES

- Open chest injuries result from some type of penetrating mechanism.
- These injuries can allow the pleural space to fill with air that gets entrained from outside causing the collapse of the lung.
- At times, the hole in the chest may cause air to get pulled in and create an audible "sucking" sound. This is referred to as a "sucking chest wound."
- Open chest wounds can also cause vascular damage to blood vessels in the chest causing the hemothorax to fill with blood (collapsing the lung and causing hypoperfusion).
- Even small injuries are sufficient to cause life-threatening air or blood accumulation in the pleural space.

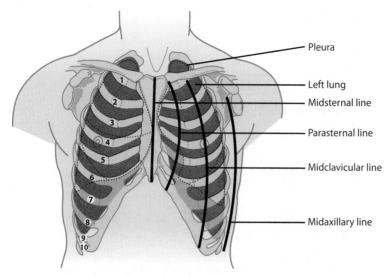

Figure 25-1 Anatomy of the chest. *(Reproduced with permission from Doherty GM, ed. Current Diagnosis & Treatment: Surgery, 13th ed. New York: McGraw-Hill; 2010)*

Pneumothorax

- A pneumothorax is a type of chest injury that can occur with an open or closed chest injury. As mentioned previously, a hole in the chest wall can allow air to be sucked in during inhalation. The problem is the air entering through the chest wound does not reach the alveoli for gas exchange. Rather, it accumulates in the "subatmospheric" space between the pleural linings until the lung collapses.
- The collapsing of the lung results in diminished ability to exchange oxygen and eliminate carbon dioxide.

Tension Pneumothorax

- This injury can progress from a pneumothorax when a large amount of air collects in the pleural cavity and causes significant disruption to the lungs.
- Another type of chest injury is referred to as a "closed" chest injury, and is the usual result of blunt forces applied to the chest wall.
- These injuries may be more challenging to discern because of the lack of external symptoms (other than some early signs of soft tissue trauma to the chest wall).
- Injuries that could result from closed chest wall injuries include both pneumothorax and tension pneumothorax, but also broken ribs, flail segments, and vascular trauma causing a hemothorax.

Signs and Symptoms

- Decreased or absent breath sounds on the affected side
- Jugular venous distension (late sign)
- Tracheal deviation toward unaffected side (late sign)
- Hyperresonance on percussion
- Unequal chest rise
- Dyspnea

- Tachypnea
- Tachycardia
- Hypotension
- Hypoxia
- Pale, cool, clammy skin
- Subcutaneous emphysema
- Cyanosis

Flail Segment

- A flail segment occurs when there are adjacent ribs that are fractured in numerous places.
- In effect, the flailed region becomes "detached" from the skeletal framework of the thoracic wall.
- As a result, the flailed segment moves opposite of the normal chest excursion during breathing because it is affected by the negative and positive pressure in the thorax created by breathing, rather than the muscular activity of the respiratory effort.
- This results in poor air exchange and hypoxemia.
- Paradoxical motion occurs when the flailed segment moves opposite of the normal chest wall.

Hemothorax

- A hemothorax could result from either a closed or open chest wall injury.
- The mechanism behind its occurrence is the hemorrhage of blood from a lacerated thoracic blood vessel, and the blood accumulates in the pleural space.
- As the blood accumulates, it forces the lung to collapse, which alters normal oxygenation, as well as promotes hypoperfusion as this is a type of internal bleeding which can make the patient hypovolemic.
- Hemothorax can result from either open or closed chest wall trauma. In either instance, its occurrence has a large effect on the patient's ability to oxygenate and maintain peripheral perfusion.

ASSESSMENT: CHEST INJURIES

- Scene size-up—As with other types of trauma, be certain that the scene is safe, making sure the injuries sustained are not from some type of violence or hazardous location.
- Take necessary body substance isolation (BSI); consider eye and face protection.
- Analyze the MOI, and try to determine if the patient may have an open or closed thoracic injury.
  - Sport accidents usually cause closed chest injuries.
  - Falls could cause closed or open chest injuries.
  - Was there a fight or shooting (common with open injuries)?
  - Crushing mechanism usually causes closed chest injuries.
  - An explosion could cause an open or closed chest injury.
- Remember to take in-line manual stabilization when needed.

Primary Assessment

- Determine your general impression. As you approach, does the patient seem to be in significant respiratory distress?
- Assess the airway for patency. Be certain there is no blood, vomitus, or secretions causing occlusion.
- Closely assess the respiratory effort. If you note inadequate breathing, immediately start artificial ventilation. You will determine the cause of the poor breathing during the rapid trauma assessment.
- During your assessment of the circulatory status, the presence of tachycardia, poor capillary refill, poor peripheral perfusion, and weak/absent peripheral pulses are all indications of hypoperfusion, possibly from an internal (or even external) bleeding.
- The patient should be considered a priority if any of the following is present:
  - Loss of function or impairment to the airway, breathing, or circulation
  - An acute change in mental status
  - Abnormal findings during focused history and physical examination
  - Indications of significant chest injury
  - Subtle clues or findings that may indicate chest wall injuries

Emergency Management

- When dealing with chest trauma, remember that the following conditions must be supported immediately:
  - Airway inadequacy (blood, vomitus, foreign bodies, etc)
  - Breathing insufficiency (per minute ventilation)
  - Circulatory compromise (hemorrhage, hypoperfusion)
- Maintain an open airway and establish cervical immobilization.
- Use a jaw-thrust maneuver if cervical spine injury suspected.
- Use an oral pharyngeal airway (OPA) or nasopharyngeal airway (NPA) if the airway is still difficult to control.
- Provide oral suctioning as needed.
- Provide oxygen therapy at 15 L/min.
- Evaluate/assure breathing adequacy.
- Provide artificial ventilation if needed; however, avoid forceful ventilations as this may aggravate chest injuries.
- Provide stabilization to any impaled object found in the chest.
  - If found, do not remove the impaled object.
- Occlude any open soft tissue injuries noted.
  - First with your gloved hand, then with an occlusive dressing
- Completely immobilize the patient.
  - As needed for spinal precautions
- Treat the patient for shock, and provide rapid transport to the hospital.
  - Warmth, positioning, oxygen therapy, and the like

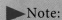Note:

The following injuries are considered immediate life threats and should be treated immediately:

- Open chest wound
- Flail segment
- Major hemorrhage

Specific Management of Chest Injuries

Open Chest Wound

- Place a nonporous dressing to the chest wall and tape it on three sides.
- This helps limit inward movement of air during breathing and relief of trapped air on exhalation.

Flail Segment

- Upon finding a flail segment, initially provide stabilization with your hand (to limit paradoxical motion). Continue stabilization by applying a bulky dressing or clean towel to the chest wall for splinting purposes.
- Secure the dressing. You can use the patient's arm to help splint the flail segment.

Secondary Assessment and Reassessment

- En route to the hospital, if time and the patient's condition permit, perform a secondary assessment to assess for any problems that may have been overlooked during the primary assessment.
- During the reassessment, reevaluate the effectiveness of your treatment and assess for further deterioration. Reassess and record the baseline vital signs.
- Contact the receiving hospital, and keep them advised of any further changes in the patient's status.

? CHAPTER QUESTIONS

1. Your patient has received an open chest wound from a screwdriver. Emergency management should include all the following *except*:

    a. high-concentration oxygen

    b. sealing the wound with an occlusive dressing

    c. placing in a position of comfort, if there is no spinal injury

    d. cleaning the wound with saline

Chapter 26
Abdominal and Genitourinary Trauma

A 25-year-old man presents with a stab wound to the right upper abdomen. Vital signs are BP 88/48, HR 122 weak and thread; RR 20; skin is pale, cool, and moist. The abdomen is not distended, soft, nontender. Bowel sounds are present.

How would you manage this patient?

ANATOMY OF THE ABDOMEN

- The abdomen contains major organs of the digestive, urinary, and endocrine systems.
- Organs are enveloped by a visceral and parietal peritoneum.
- Organs within the abdomen can be characterized as:
    - Hollow
    - Solid
    - Vascular

ABDOMINAL INJURIES

- Injuries to the abdomen could be caused by either blunt or penetrating trauma.
- Like chest injuries, abdominal injuries are considered to be either open or closed in nature.
- Because of the number of organs within the abdominal cavity (including highly vascular ones), trauma to the abdomen can cause significant disturbances in homeostasis, as well as acute hemorrhage and death should a vascular structure become damaged.

TRAUMA ASSESSMENT: ABDOMINAL INJURIES

- Scene size-up.
- The mechanism of injury (MOI) can give you clues as to the nature of the injury to the abdomen (blunt or penetrating injury).
- Ensure your own safety, and search the scene for clues such as guns, knives, sharp metal, etc.
- If the MOI was a motor vehicle collision (MVC) (which is the most common cause of blunt trauma), try to determine particularities of the crash (type of vehicle, speed of travel, points of impact, etc).

- Contact additional resources as necessary.
- Determine if any other victims (whether abdominally injured or not) are on-scene and in need of care.

Primary Assessment

- Form a general impression upon your approach to the patient.
- Note the position the patient is in; this may give you a clue as to the nature of the problem.
- Continue with your assessment of the patient's mental status by using the AVPU (*a*lert, *v*erbal, *p*ainful stimulus, *u*nresponsive) mnemonic.
- Ensure the patient's airway is open by assessing the oral cavity and listening for abnormal airway sounds.
- Breathing may be noted to be hypopneic as abdominal pain tends to make the patient's breathing shallow.
- Assess circulation by taking a core and peripheral pulse, evaluate the quality of peripheral perfusion, and determine the skin characteristics.
- Determine priority status of the patient.
- Focused history and physical examination are necessary.
- Consider the patient's complaints, MOI, and clinical status when determining whether to perform a trauma assessment.
- While performing a trauma assessment, be sure to use good assessment skills to detect any rigidity, guarding, soft tissue trauma, masses, tenderness, or other abnormal finding.
- Follow this with your assessment of baseline vitals and determination of the SAMPLE (*s*igns/*s*ymptoms, *a*llergies, *m*edications, *p*ast medical problems, *l*ast oral intake, *e*vents) history.
- Maintain an open airway and appropriate spinal protection.
- Provide high-flow oxygen at 15 L/min via an appropriate oxygenation adjunct.
- Reassess the breathing status; if found to be inadequate, then begin positive-pressure ventilation (PPV).
- Treat for shock (hypoperfusion) as appropriate.

Abdominal Evisceration

- This occurs when the trauma to the abdomen allows abdominal tissue to protrude out.
- Do not touch or replace the tissue.

Emergency Management: Abdominal Evisceration

- First, cut away any clothing.
- Place a premoistened dressing over the wound, and gently tape it in place.
- Do not try to replace intestines within the abdomen.
- Apply an occlusive dressing (such as plastic wrap) over the moistened dressing.
- Secure all the material in place with tape or other suitable material.

GENITALIA ANATOMY

Anatomy of both male and female (Figs. 26-1 and 26-2) is comprised largely of soft tissue.

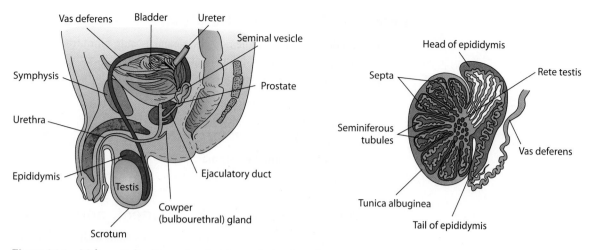

Figure 26-1 Male genitalia. *(Reproduced with permission from Ganong WF. Review of Medical Physiology. 22nd ed. McGraw-Hill; 2005)*

Injuries to the Male Genitalia

- Lacerations
- Abrasions
- Avulsions
- Penetrations
- Amputations
- Contusions
- Severe pain

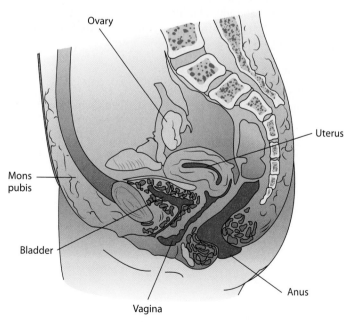

Figure 26-2 Female genitalia. *(Reproduced with permission from Benson RC. Handbook of Obstetrics & Gynecology. 8th ed. New York: McGraw-Hill; 1983)*

Injuries to the Female Genitalia

- Can occur from straddle injuries, sexual assault, blunt trauma, abortion attempts, traumatic childbirth, and foreign body insertion.
- Injury manifestation includes:
    - Soft tissue crush injuries
    - Amputation and avulsions
    - Lacerations
    - Contusions and hematoma
    - Severe pain

For Either Gender, Basic Assessment, and Treatment

- Essentially, the injury will be managed consistent with other soft tissue injuries.
- Apply direct pressure to stop any bleeding (never pack the female's vagina).
- Save and transport any avulsed or amputated tissue.
- Consider the application of a cold compress to help with pain management and swelling.
- Try to have a same gender emergency medical technician (EMT) provide the care, and be empathetic to the fright, pain, and anxiety that typically accompany these types of injuries.

? CHAPTER QUESTIONS

2. A 33-year-old male patient has been involved in a motor vehicle crash and has an open abdominal injury with a protruding bowel secondary to being partially ejected from the vehicle. Your treatment of the injury should include:

   a. replacing the exposed bowel
   b. keeping the patient's legs straight
   c. covering the exposed bowel with a sterile dressing moistened with saline
   d. covering the bowel with dry sterile gauze prior to transport

Chapter 27
Orthopedic Trauma

You are responding to a report of a patient pinned between a tractor trailer and a loading dock. Upon arrival, the bystanders have already removed the truck from the patient. The patient is conscious and alert and is complaining of severe pain to his pelvic region. You begin your assessment and determine the patient has a possible fractured pelvis.

How would you begin your treatment of this patient?

BONE AND JOINT INJURIES

Mechanisms of injury (MOI) resulting from:

- Direct force
- Indirect force
- Twisting force

Types of injuries are:

- Open—Break in the continuity of the skin
- Closed—No break in the continuity of the skin

Signs and Symptoms

- Deformity or angulation
- Pain and tenderness
- Grating (crepitus)
- Swelling
- Bruising (discoloration)
- Exposed bone ends
- Joint locked into position

Emergency Management

- Body substance isolation (BSI).
- Administer oxygen if not already done and indicated.
- After life-threatening injuries have been treated, splint injuries in preparation for transport.
- Elevate the extremity.

Splinting Rationale

- Prevent movement of bone fragments, bone ends, or angulated joints.
- Minimize complications and damage to muscles, nerves, or blood vessels caused by broken bones.

- Reduce the risk of a closed, painful, swollen, deformed extremity to an open, painful, swollen, deformed extremity.
- Minimize the reduction of blood flow as a result of bone ends compressing blood vessels.
- Reduce excessive bleeding due to tissue damage caused by bone ends.
- Decrease pain associated with movement of bone ends.
- Reduce the possibility of paralysis of extremities due to a damaged spine.

Rules of Splinting

- Assess pulse, motor, and sensation distal to the injury prior to and following splint application, and record findings.
- Immobilize the joint above and below the injury.
- Remove or cut away clothing.
- Cover open wounds with a sterile dressing.
- If there is a severe deformity or the distal extremity is cyanotic or lacks pulses, align with gentle traction before splinting.
- Do not intentionally replace the protruding bones.
- Pad each splint to prevent pressure and discomfort to the patient.
- Splint the patient before moving when feasible and no life threats.
- When in doubt, splint the injury when feasible and no life threats.
- If patient has signs of shock (hypoperfusion), align in normal anatomical position and transport.

Complications of Splinting

- Compression of nerves, tissues, and blood vessels from the splint.
- Delay in transport of a patient with life-threatening injury.
- Splint applied too tight on the extremity reducing distal circulation.
- Aggravation of the bone or joint injury.
- Cause or aggravate tissue, nerve, vessel, or muscle damage from excessive bone or joint movement.

Splinting a Joint Injury

- Body substance isolation.
- Apply manual stabilization.
- Assess pulse, motor, and sensory function.
- Align with gentle traction if distal extremity is cyanotic or lacks pulses and no resistance is met.
- Immobilize the site of injury.
- Immobilize bone above and below the site of injury.
- Reassess pulse, motor, and sensation after application of splint, and record.

Traction Splinting

Indications for use are a painful, swollen, deformed mid-thigh with no joint or lower leg injury (mid-shaft femur fracture).

Contraindications for the use of a Traction Splint

- Injury is close to the knee.
- Injury to the knee exists.

- Injury to the hip/pelvis.
- Partial amputation or avulsion with bone separation, distal limb is connected only by marginal tissue. Traction would risk separation.
- Lower leg or ankle injury.

Traction Splinting Procedure

- Assess pulse, motor, and sensation distal to the injury, and record.
- Body substance isolation.
- Perform manual stabilization of the injured leg.
- Apply manual traction—required when using a bipolar traction splint.
- Prepare/adjust splint to proper length.
- Position splint under injured leg.
- Apply proximal securing device (ischial strap).
- Apply distal securing device (ankle hitch).
- Apply mechanical traction.
- Position/secure support straps.
- Reevaluate proximal/distal securing devices.
- Reassess pulses, motor, sensation distal to the injury after application of the splint, and record.
- Secure torso to the long board to immobilize hip.
- Secure splint to the long board to prevent movement of splint.

? CHAPTER QUESTIONS

3. The three kinds of muscles found in the body, each with a specific function, are called:

   a. voluntary, involuntary, and cardiac muscles

   b. controlled, autonomic, and contracting muscles

   c. long, flat, and specialized muscles

   d. flat, striated, and walled muscles

4. Injuries to the musculoskeletal system include:

   a. a dislocation, which is the displacement of a bone

   b. a strain, which is damage to, or tearing of, ligaments

   c. a sprain, which is the overextending or stretching of a muscle and/or tendon

   d. a comminuted injury, which is the detachment of a muscle from a bone

5. Bone and joint injuries may exhibit crepitus, which is:

   a. deformity or angulation of the injured extremity

   b. swelling of the injury site

   c. the discoloration of the skin at and around the injury site

   d. the sound or feeling of broken bone fragments grinding against each other

6. Emergency medical care of bone and joint injuries should include:

    a. splinting any painful extremity
    b. applying a heat pack to the injury to alleviate pain
    c. determining the injury, such as a fracture, dislocation, and the like
    d. realigning deformed extremities prior to splinting

7. The basic reasons for splinting a bone or joint injury include:

    a. preventing further movement to reduce the chance of further injury
    b. replacing exposed bone ends back into the extremity
    c. setting the bone ends back into their proper position
    d. preventing swelling which might complicate the emergency-room (ER) physician's examination

8. When caring for an extremity injury, the emergency medical technician (EMT) should assess the distal pulse, motor function, and sensation:

    a. after application of a splint
    b. both before and after application of a splint
    c. prior to application of a splint
    d. every 5 minutes until arrival at the hospital

Chapter 28
Environmental Emergencies

It is the beginning of a very hot summer day. The temperature outside is 99°F, with a heat index of 110°F. An elderly woman is complaining of dizziness, nausea, vomiting, and an episode of syncope. Her husband determines she cannot withstand the extreme heat and summons emergency medical services (EMS). You arrive on-scene, determine the scene is safe, and enter the house. You establish the cause of the patient's complaints is from the house having no ventilation. You look on the wall to see a thermometer reading 112°F. The patient is pale, warm, and extremely diaphoretic. She denies chest discomfort and shortness of breath. She states, "I feel like I am going to pass out!"
What is your next course of action?

TEMPERATURE REGULATION

Regulation of temperature is based on heat loss versus heat gained.

When heat loss exceeds heat gained, the result is *hypothermia* (low body temperature). Heat loss occurs by:

- Radiation—Transfer of heat from the surface of one object to another without physical contact.
- Convection—Body heat is lost to surrounding air.
- Conduction—Body heat is lost to surrounding objects through direct physical contact.
- Evaporation—Body heat causes perspiration, which is lost from the surface of the body when changed from liquid to vapor.
- Respiration—Heat loss through the process of breathing.

Emergency technicians (EMTs) must be aware of methods of heat loss when treating patients with hypothermia to prevent further heat loss. When heat gained exceeds heat lost, the result is *hyperthermia* (high body core temperature).

Important questions to ask patients exposed to the environment are:

- What is the source?
- How is the environment the patient is in?
- Any loss of consciousness?
- Effects
  - General versus local injury or illness

EXPOSURE TO COLD

Figure 28-1 shows NOAA's National Weather Service wind-chill chart.

New windchill chart
Wind (mph)

Calm	5	10	15	20	25	30	35	40	45	50	55	60
40	36	34	32	30	29	28	28	27	26	26	25	25
35	31	27	25	24	23	22	21	20	19	19	18	17
30	25	21	19	17	16	15	14	13	12	12	11	10
25	19	15	13	11	9	8	7	6	5	4	4	3
20	13	9	6	4	3	1	0	−1	−2	−3	−3	−4
15	7	3	0	−2	−4	−5	−7	−8	−9	−10	−11	−11
10	1	−4	−7	−9	−11	−12	−14	−15	−16	−17	−18	−19
5	−5	−10	−13	−15	−17	−19	−21	−22	−23	−24	−25	−26
0	−11	−16	−19	−22	−24	−26	−27	−29	−30	−31	−32	−33
−5	−16	−22	−26	−29	−31	−33	−34	−36	−37	−38	−39	−40
−10	−22	−28	−32	−35	−37	−39	−41	−43	−44	−45	−46	−48
−15	−28	−35	−39	−42	−44	−46	−48	−50	−51	−52	−54	−55
−20	−34	−41	−45	−48	−51	−53	−55	−57	−58	−60	−61	−62
−25	−40	−47	−51	−55	−58	−60	−62	−64	−65	−67	−68	−69
−30	−46	−53	−58	−61	−64	−67	−69	−71	−72	−74	−75	−76
−35	−52	−59	−64	−68	−74	−73	−76	−78	−79	−81	−82	−84
−40	−57	−66	−71	−74	−78	−80	−82	−84	−86	−88	−89	−91
−45	−63	−72	−77	−81	−84	−87	−89	−91	−93	−95	−97	−98

Temperature (°F)

Frostbite occurs in 15 minutes or less

$$\text{Wind Chill (}^\circ\text{F)} = 35.74 + 0.6215T - 35.75(V^{0.16}) + 0.4275T(V^{0.16})$$

Where, T = Air temperature (°F)
V = Wind speed (mph)

Figure 28-1   NOAA's National Weather Service Wind Chill chart (effective 11/1/2001). *(Reproduced with permission from http://www.weather.gov/os /windchill/index.shtml)*

Generalized Cold Emergency—Generalized Hypothermia

Hypothermia occurs when the body loses more heat than it can produce!

- Predisposing risk factors include:
  - Cold environment
  - Immersion
  - Age (extreme ages)
    - Pediatric patients have a large surface area compared to their overall size.
    - Small muscle mass and the ability to shiver are not well developed in pediatric patients.
    - Children and infants have less body fat.
    - Younger children need help to protect themselves; they cannot put on or take off their clothes.
- Medical conditions that affect body temperature include:
  - Shock (hypoperfusion)
  - Head injury
  - Burns
  - Generalized infection

- Injuries to the spinal cord
- Diabetes and hypoglycemia
- Certain drugs/poisons
- Environmental conditions of cold exposure include:
  - Obvious exposure
  - Subtle exposure
  - Ethanol ingestion
  - Underlying illness
  - Overdose/poisoning
  - Major trauma
  - Outdoor resuscitation
  - Ambient temperature decreased (home of elderly patient)

Signs and Symptoms of Generalized Hypothermia

- Cool/cold skin temperature—The EMT should place the back of his hand between the clothing and the patient's abdomen to assess the general temperature of the patient. The patient experiencing a generalized cold emergency will present with cool abdominal skin temperature.
- Decreasing mental status or motor function—Correlates with the degree of hypothermia.
- Poor coordination.
- Memory disturbances.
- Reduced or loss of sensation to touch.
- Mood changes.
- Less communicative.
- Dizziness.
- Speech difficulty.
- Stiff or rigid posture.
- Muscular rigidity.
- Shivering may be present or absent.
- Breathing variations are:
  - Early—Rapid breathing
  - Late—Shallow, slow, or even absent breathing
- Slowly responding pupils (sluggish).
- Pulse:
  - Early—Rapid
  - Late—Slow and barely palpable and/or irregular, or completely absent
- Low-to-absent blood pressure.
- Poor judgment/poor coordination—Patient may actually remove clothing.
- Complaints of joint/muscle stiffness.
- Skin:
  - Red—Early
  - Pale
  - Cyanotic—Blue-gray
  - Stiff/hard

Emergency Management for Generalized Hypothermia

- Remove the patient from the environment and protect the patient from further heat loss.
- Remove wet clothing and cover with a dry warm blanket.
- Handle the patient gently. Avoid rough handling.
- Do not allow the patient to walk or exert him/herself.
- Administer oxygen if not already done as part of the primary assessment—Oxygen administered should be warm and humidified, if possible.
- Assess pulses for 45 to 60 seconds before starting cardiopulmonary resuscitation (CPR).
- If the patient is alert and responding appropriately, rewarm actively.
  - Warm blankets.
  - Apply heat packs or hot water bottles to the groin, axillary, and cervical regions.
  - Turn the heat up high in the patient compartment of the ambulance.
- If the patient is unresponsive or not responding appropriately, rewarm passively:
  - Warm blankets.
  - Turn the heat up high in the patient compartment of the ambulance.
  - Do not allow the patient to eat or drink stimulants.
  - Do not massage extremities.

Local Cold Injuries—Localized to Specific Area of Body

- Look for predisposing factors.
- Tend to occur on the distal end of extremities such as exposed ears, nose, and face.

Signs and Symptoms of Local Cold Injuries

- Local injury with clear demarcation of cold injury site.
- Early or superficial injury includes:
  - Blanching of the skin—Palpation of the skin in which normal color does not return.
  - Loss of feeling and sensation in the injured area.
  - Skin remains soft.
  - If rewarmed, tingling sensation.
- Late or deep injury include:
  - White, waxy skin.
  - Firm to frozen feeling upon palpation.
  - Swelling may be present.
  - Blisters may be present.
  - If thawed or partially thawed, the skin may appear flushed with areas of purple and blanching or mottled and cyanotic.

Emergency Management for Local Cold Injuries

- Remove the patient from the environment.
- Protect the cold injured extremity from further injury.
- Administer oxygen if not already done as part of the primary assessment.

Clinical Significance

Rough handling can cause the patient to go into ventricular fibrillation. *Remember—Move the patient with extreme care.*

- Remove wet or restrictive clothing.
- If early or superficial injury, splint and cover the extremity.
- Do not rub or massage.
- Do not reexpose to the cold.
- If late or deep cold injury, then:
  - Remove jewelry.
  - Cover with dry clothing or dressings.

Do Not

- Break blisters.
- Rub or massage area.
- Apply heat directly to the extremity.
- Allow the patient to walk on the affected extremity.

When an extremely long or delayed transport is inevitable, active rapid rewarming should be done.

- Immerse the affected part in a warm water bath (100°F-110°F).
- Monitor the water to ensure it does not cool from the frozen part.
- Continuously stir water.
- Continue until the body part is soft, and color and sensation return.
- Dress the area with dry sterile dressings. If hand or foot, place dry sterile dressings between fingers or toes.
- Protect against refreezing the warmed part.
- Expect the patient to complain of severe pain.

EXPOSURE TO HEAT

Figure 28-2 shows NOAA's National Weather Service heat index.

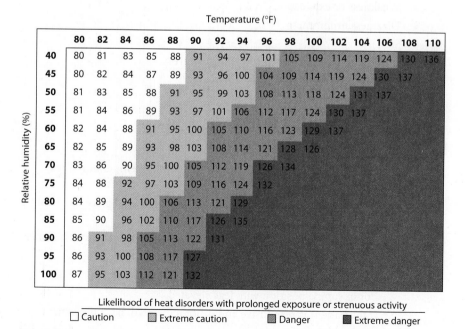

Temperature (°F)

Relative humidity (%)	80	82	84	86	88	90	92	94	96	98	100	102	104	106	108	110
40	80	81	83	85	88	91	94	97	101	105	109	114	119	124	130	136
45	80	82	84	87	89	93	96	100	104	109	114	119	124	130	137	
50	81	83	85	88	91	95	99	103	108	113	118	124	131	137		
55	81	84	86	89	93	97	101	106	112	117	124	130	137			
60	82	84	88	91	95	100	105	110	116	123	129	137				
65	82	85	89	93	98	103	108	114	121	128	126					
70	83	86	90	95	100	105	112	119	126	134						
75	84	88	92	97	103	109	116	124	132							
80	84	89	94	100	106	113	121	129								
85	85	90	96	102	110	117	126	135								
90	86	91	98	105	113	122	131									
95	86	93	100	108	117	127										
100	87	95	103	112	121	132										

Likelihood of heat disorders with prolonged exposure or strenuous activity

☐ Caution   ☐ Extreme caution   ☐ Danger   ☐ Extreme danger

Figure 28-2 NOAA's National Weather Service heat index. *(Reproduced with permission from http://www.weather.gov/om/heat/index.shtml (effective 11/1/2001))*

- Predisposing factors include:
  - Climate.
  - High ambient temperature reduces the body's ability to lose heat by radiation.
  - High relative humidity reduces the body's ability to lose heat through evaporation.
- Exercise and activity
  - Can lose more than 1 L of sweat per hour.
  - Loss of electrolytes (sodium, chloride, and fluid through sweat).
- Factors regarding age
  - Elderly
    — Poor thermoregulation.
    — Certain medications (beta blockers) affect ability to respond to heat.
    — Lack of mobility—Cannot escape hot environment.
  - Newborn/infants
    — Poor thermoregulation
    — Cannot remove own clothing
- Preexisting illness and/or conditions that may affect the patient who is experiencing a heat emergency:
  - Heart disease
  - Dehydration
  - Obesity
  - Fever
  - Fatigue
  - Diabetes
  - Drugs/medications

Signs and Symptoms

- Muscular cramps
- Weakness or exhaustion
- Dizziness or faintness
- Skin
  - Moist, pale; normal to cool temperature
  - Hot, dry, or moist—"True emergency"
- Rapid heart rate
- Altered mental status to unresponsive

Emergency Management of Heat Emergencies

- Patient with moist, pale skin; normal to cool skin temperature *(heat exhaustion)*
  - Remove the patient from the hot environment and place in a cool environment (back of air-conditioned ambulance).
  - Administer oxygen if not already done during the primary assessment.
  - Loosen or remove clothing.
  - Cool patient by fanning.
  - Put in supine position with legs elevated.
  - If the patient is responsive and is not nauseated, have the patient drink water.
  - If the patient is unresponsive or is vomiting, transport to the hospital with patient on his left side.

- Patient with hot, dry, or moist skin *(heat stroke)*
    - Remove the patient from the hot environment and place in a cool environment (back of air-conditioned ambulance with air conditioner running on high).
    - Remove clothing.
    - Administer oxygen if not already done during the primary assessment.
    - Apply cool packs to neck, groin, and armpits.
    - Keep the skin wet by applying water by sponge or wet towels.
    - Fan aggressively.
    - Transport immediately.

BITES AND STINGS

Humans can be injured by the bites or stings of many kinds of animals, including mammals such as dogs, cats, and fellow humans; arthropods such as spiders, bees, and wasps; snakes; and marine animals such as jellyfish and stingrays.

It is a very warm summer night. The streets are full of people celebrating a national holiday. The time is 8 PM when emergency medical services (EMS) is summoned to respond to a private address for a victim with an animal bite. As EMS arrives on-scene, the local police department has secured the site. The police officer approaches the ambulance and states, "You have one to go. She is in front of the location. Apparently the neighbor's bull mastiff attacked her when she entered the neighbor's backyard."

As you approach the patient, you witness bystanders upset about what has occurred. The patient, a young 25-year-old woman, conscious, is complaining of severe pain to her right forearm and left leg. You notice bright red blood on a towel the neighbor was using to control the bleeding. The patient has an obvious deformity to her right forearm, and bleeding appears to be controlled.

What steps should be performed while evaluating and treating this patient?

Mammals

Dogs

In the United States, where the dog population exceeds 50 million, dogs surpass all other mammals in the number of bites inflicted on humans. However, most dog-bite injuries are minor. Each year, about 10 to 20 Americans, mostly children under 10 years of age, are killed by dogs.

Dog bites result in an estimated 340,000 emergency-room visits annually throughout the United States. More than half of the bites seen by emergency departments occur at home. Children under 10 years old, especially boys between 5 and 9 years of age, are more likely than older people to visit an emergency room for bite treatment. Children under 10 years old are also much more liable to be bitten on the face, neck, and head. Nearly all of the injuries suffered by people seeking treatment in emergency rooms were of "low severity," and most were treated and released without being admitted to a hospital or sent to another facility. Many of the bites resulted from people attempting to break up fights between animals.

Cats

Although cats are found in nearly a third of US households, cat bites are far less common than dog bites. The tissue damage caused by cat bites is usually limited, but they carry a high risk of infection. Whereas the infection rate for dog-bite injuries is 15% to 20%, the infection rate for cat bites is 30% to 40%. A typical person who has been bitten, is a young girl playing with a pet.

Humans

Bites from mammals other than dogs and cats are uncommon, with one exception—human bites. There are approximately 70,000 human bites each year in the United States. Because the human mouth contains a multitude of potentially harmful microorganisms, human bites are more infectious than those of most other animals.

Arthropods

Arthropods are invertebrates belonging to the phylum Arthropoda, which includes insects, arachnids, crustaceans, and other subgroups. There are more than 700,000 species in all. The list of arthropods that bite or sting humans is extensive and includes lice, bedbugs, fleas, mosquitoes, black flies, ants, chiggers, ticks, centipedes, scorpions, and other species. Spiders, bees, and wasps are the three kinds of arthropod that most often bite people.

Spiders

In the United States, only two kinds of venomous spider are truly dangerous: black widow spiders and brown (violin or fiddle) recluse spiders. The black widow, which is found in every state but Alaska, is probably the most notorious spider. It prefers dark, dry places such as barns, garages, and outhouses, and also lives under rocks and logs. Disturbing a female black widow or its web may provoke a bite. Brown recluse spiders also prefer sheltered places, including clothing, and may bite if disturbed.

Bees and Wasps

Bees and wasps will sting to defend their nests or if they are disturbed. Species common to the United States include honeybees, bumblebees, yellow jackets, bald-faced hornets, brown hornets, and paper wasps. Of note also are Africanized bee species, also called "killer bees," that have been found in the United States since 1990. More than 50 Americans die each year after being stung by a bee, wasp, or ant. Almost all of those deaths are the result of allergic reactions, and not of exposure to the venom itself.

Snakes

There are 20 species of venomous snakes in the United States. These snakes are found in every state except Maine, Alaska, and Hawaii. Each year about 8000 Americans receive a venomous snakebite, but no more than about 15 die, mostly from rattlesnake bites.

The venomous snakes of the United States are divided into two families, the Crotalidae (pit vipers) and the Elapidae. Pit vipers, named after the small heat-sensing pit that lies between each eye and nostril, are responsible for about 99% of the venomous snakebites suffered by Americans. Rattlesnakes, copperheads, and cottonmouths (also called water moccasins) are pit vipers. This family of snakes delivers its venom through two long, hinged fangs in the upper jaw. Some pit vipers carry potent venom that can threaten the brain and spinal cord. The venom of others, such as the copperheads, is less harmful.

The Elapidae family includes two kinds of venomous coral snakes indigenous to the southern and western states. Because coral snakes are bashful creatures that come out only at night, they almost never bite humans, and are responsible for approximately 25 bites a year in the United States. Coral snakes also have short fangs and a small mouth, which lowers the risk of a bite actually forcing venom into a person's body. However, their venom is quite poisonous.

Marine Animals

Several varieties of marine animals may bite or sting. Jellyfish and stingrays are two kinds that pose a threat to people who live or vacation in coastal communities.

Signs and Symptoms

Dogs

A typical dog bite results in a laceration, tear, puncture, or crush injury. Bites from large, powerful dogs may even cause fractures and dangerous internal injuries. Also, dogs trained to attack may bite repeatedly during a single episode. Infected bites usually cause pain, cellulitis (inflammation of the connective tissues), and a pus-filled discharge at the wound site within 8 to 24 hours. Most infections are confined to the wound site, but many of the microorganisms in the mouths of dogs can cause systemic and possibly life-threatening infections. Examples are bacteremia and meningitis, especially severe in people diagnosed with acquired immunodeficiency syndrome (AIDS) or other health condition that increases their susceptibility to infection. Rabies is rare among pet dogs in the United States, most of which have been vaccinated against the disease. Tetanus is also rare but can be transmitted by a dog bite, if the victim is not immunized.

Cats

The mouths of cats and dogs contain many of the same microorganisms. Cat scratches and bites are also capable of transmitting the *Bartonella henselae* bacterium, which can lead to cat-scratch disease, an unpleasant but usually not life-threatening illness.

Cat bites are mostly found on the arms and hands. Sharp cat teeth typically leave behind a deep puncture wound that can reach muscles, tendons, and bones, which are vulnerable to infection because of their comparatively poor blood supply. This is why cat bites are much more likely to become infected than dog bites. Also, people are less inclined to view cat bites as dangerous and requiring immediate attention; the risk that infection has set in by the time a medical professional is consulted is thus greater.

Humans

Human bites result from fights, sexual activity, medical and dental treatment, and seizures. Bites also raise the possibility of spousal or child abuse. Children often bite other children, but those bites are hardly ever severe. Human bites are capable of transmitting a wide range of dangerous diseases, including hepatitis B, syphilis, and tuberculosis.

Human bites fall into two categories: occlusion (true) bites and clenched-fist injuries. The former presents a lower risk of infection. The latter, which are very infectious and can permanently damage the hand, usually result from a fist hitting teeth during a fight. People often wait before seeking treatment for a clenched-fist injury, with the result that about half of such injuries are infected by the time they are seen by a medical professional.

Spiders

As a rule, people rarely see a black widow bite, nor do they feel the bite as it occurs. The first (and possibly only) evidence that a person has been bitten may be a mild swelling of the injured area and two red puncture marks. Within a short time, however, some victims begin to experience severe muscle cramps and rigidity of the abdominal muscles. Other possible symptoms include excessive sweating, nausea, vomiting, headaches, and vertigo as well as breathing, vision, and speech problems.

A brown recluse spider's bite can lead to necrotic arachnidism, in which the tissue in an area of up to several inches around the bite becomes necrotic (dies), producing an open sore that can take months or years to disappear. In most cases, however, the bite simply produces a hard, painful, itchy, and discolored area that heals without treatment in 2 to 3 days. The bite may also be accompanied by a fever, chills, edema (an accumulation of excess tissue fluid), nausea and vomiting, dizziness, muscle and joint pain, and a rash.

Bees and Wasps

The familiar symptoms of bee and wasp stings include pain, redness, swelling, and itchiness in the area of the sting. Multiple stings can have much more severe consequences, such as anaphylaxis, a life-threatening allergic reaction that occurs in hypersensitive persons.

Snakes

Venomous pit viper bites usually begin to swell within 10 minutes and sometimes are painful. Other symptoms include skin blisters and discoloration, weakness, sweating, nausea, faintness, dizziness, bruising, and tender lymph nodes. Severe poisoning can also lead to tingling in the scalp, fingers, and toes; muscle contractions; an elevated heart rate; rapid breathing; large drops in body temperature and blood pressure; vomiting of blood; and coma.

Many pit viper and coral snakes (20%-60%) fail to poison (envenomate) their victim, or introduce only a small amount of venom into the victim's body. The wounds, however, can still become infected by the harmful microorganisms that snakes carry in their mouths.

Coral snake bites are painful but may be hard to see. One to seven hours after being bitten, a person begins to experience the effects of the venom, which include tingling at the wound site, weakness, nausea, vomiting, excessive salivation, and irrational behavior. Major nerves of the body can become paralyzed for 6 to 14 days, causing double vision, difficulty in swallowing and speaking, respiratory failure, and other problems. Six to eight weeks may be needed before normal muscular strength is regained.

Jellyfish

Jellyfish venom is delivered by barbs called nematocysts, which are located on the creature's tentacles and penetrate the skin of people who brush up against them. Instant painful and itchy red lesions usually result. The pain can continue up to 48 hours. Severe cases may lead to skin necrosis, muscle spasms and cramps, vomiting, nausea, diarrhea, headaches, excessive sweating, and other symptoms. In rare instances, cardio respiratory failure may also occur.

Sting Rays

Tail spines are the delivery mechanism for stingray venom. Deep puncture wounds result that can cause an infection, if pieces of spine become embedded in the wound. A typical stingray injury scenario involves a person who inadvertently steps on a resting stingray and is lashed in the ankle by its tail. Stingray venom produces immediate, excruciating pain that lasts several hours. Sometimes the victim suffers a severe reaction, including vomiting, diarrhea, hemorrhage (bleeding), a drop in blood pressure, and cardiac arrhythmia (disordered heart beat).

Emergency Management

- If stinger is present, remove it.
  - Scrape stinger out, that is, with the edge of a credit card.
  - Avoid using tweezers or forceps as these can squeeze venom from the venom sac into the wound.
- Wash area gently.
- Remove jewelry from injured area before swelling begins, if possible.
- Place injection site slightly below the level of the patient's heart.
- Do not apply cold to snakebites.
- Consult medical direction regarding constricting band for snakebite.
- Observe for development of signs and symptoms of an allergic reaction, treat as needed.

? CHAPTER QUESTIONS

1. Hypothermia occurs when:

   a. the body loses more heat than it produces

   b. cold food or drink is ingested

   c. the body produces more heat than it loses

   d. specific parts of the body are exposed to cold temperatures

2. Emergency care for local cold injuries includes:

   a. packing the affected area with snow or a cold pack

   b. encouraging the patient to walk on an injured extremity to restore circulation

   c. rubbing the affected area to restore circulation, as soon as possible

   d. immersing the affected area in warm (tepid) water, just above body temperature (100°F-110°F)

3. All of the following are heat-related emergencies *except*:

   a. heat cramps

   b. heat exhaustion

   c. heat stroke

   d. heat index

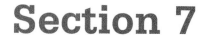

Section 7
Special Patient Populations

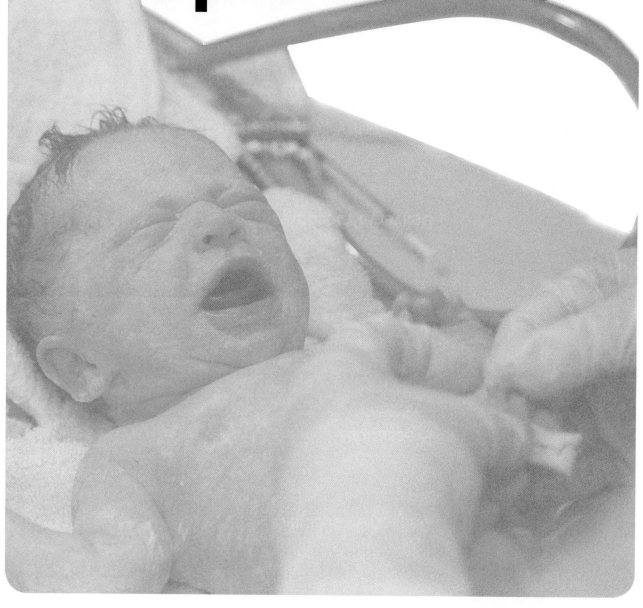

Section 7

Special Patient
Populations

Chapter 29
Obstetric and Neonatal Emergencies

You are the first arriving emergency medical services (EMS) unit on-scene. As you enter the apartment, you find a 27-year-old woman complaining of abdominal pain from contractions. She states she is 5 months pregnant, has 9 children, and her water has broken. As you approach, you notice the head of the baby crowning. As you begin your assessment and prepare for delivery, you notice intravenous (IV) drug track marks up both arms.

How should you begin to prepare for this imminent delivery?

REPRODUCTIVE ANATOMY AND PHYSIOLOGY

(Fig. 29-1)

- Fetus—Developing unborn baby
- Uterus—Organ in which a fetus grows, responsible for labor and expulsion of infant
- Birth canal—Vagina and lower part of the uterus
- Placenta—Fetal organ through which fetus exchanges nourishment and waste products during pregnancy
- Umbilical cord—Cord that is an extension of the placenta through which fetus receives nourishment while in the uterus
- Amniotic sac (bag of water)—The sac that surrounds the fetus inside the uterus
- Vagina—Lower part of the birth canal
- Perineum—Skin area between vagina and anus, commonly torn during delivery
- Crowning—The bulging-out of the vagina which is opening as the fetus' head or presenting part presses against it
- "Bloody show"—Mucus and blood that may come out of the vagina as labor begins
- Labor—The time and process (defined in three or four stages) beginning with the first uterine muscle contraction until delivery of the placenta
  - Delivery is imminent.
  - Crowning.
  - In the process of delivering.

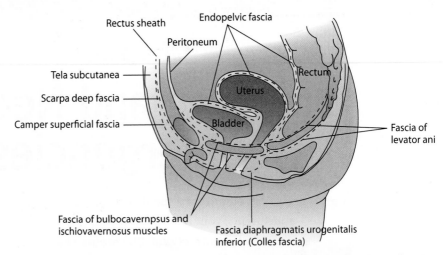

Figure 29-1   OB anatomy. *(Reproduced with permission from DeCherney AH, Nathan L. Current Diagnosis & Treatment Obstetrics and Gynecology. 10th ed. New York: McGraw-Hill; 2007)*

- Presenting part—The part of the infant/fetus that comes first (usually the head)
- Abortion/miscarriage—Delivery of products of conception early in pregnancy

ASSESSMENT OF THE PREGNANT PATIENT

- Your primary goal is to focus on whether you will need to deliver in the pre-hospital setting or you have time to transport.
- A complete assessment should include an extensive history. Questions to ask include:
  - What is the age of the patient?
  - Is there a possibility of the patient being pregnant?
  - Did the patient miss her period and when was the last menstrual period?
  - Any abdominal pain (location/quality)?
  - Any nausea or vomiting?
  - What is the EDC—Expected date of confinement (due date)?
  - Gravida—Number of pregnancies?
  - Para—Number of pregnancies that made it far enough that a fetus would have been expected to be viable?
  - Ab—Abortions, spontaneous or elective?
  - Prenatal care?
  - ROM—Any rupture of membranes?
  - Vaginal bleeding present?
  - Expulsion of the mucous plug?
  - Contractions, and what is the frequency?
  - Are there any preexisting medical conditions or illnesses that are a consequence of pregnancy?
  - Medications, including prenatal vitamins?
  - Last oral intake?

OBSTETRICAL EMERGENCIES

Ectopic Pregnancy

- Zygote implants in a location other than the uterine cavity.
- About 95% are in the fallopian tube.
- This is a life-threatening emergency!

Signs and Symptoms

- Abdominal pain may be absent.
- Some patients do not miss their period.
- Some patients have negative pregnancy tests.
- Lower abdominal pain or unexplained hypovolemia in a woman of child-bearing age is an ectopic pregnancy until proven otherwise!

Emergency Management

- High-concentration oxygen
- Treatment for hypovolemia
- Transport immediately

Spontaneous Abortion

- Miscarriage
- Pregnancy terminating before the 20th week
- Usually occurs in the first trimester

Signs and Symptoms

- Vaginal bleeding
- Cramping, lower abdominal pain, or pain in the back
- Passage of fetal tissue
- Complications include:
  - Incomplete abortion
  - Hypovolemia
  - Infection leading to sepsis

Emergency Management

- High-concentration oxygen
- Transport in the Trendelenburg position
- Transport any tissue to the hospital
- Provide emotional support

Preeclampsia

- Acute hypertension after the 24th week of gestation.
- About 5% to 7% of all pregnancies.
- Most often occurs with first pregnancies.
- Other risk factors include young mothers, no prenatal care, multiple gestations, lower socioeconomic status.
- Triad—Hypertension, proteinuria, edema.

Signs and Symptoms

- Hypertension
  - Systolic greater than 140 mm Hg

- ○ Diastolic greater than 90 mm Hg
- ○ Or either reading greater than 30 mm Hg above patient's normal blood pressure
- Edema, particularly of the hands and face is present early in the day.
- Rapid weight gain.
  - ○ About 3 lb/wk in the second trimester
  - ○ Greater than 1 lb/wk in the third trimester
- Decreased urine output.
- Headache and blurred vision.
- Nausea and vomiting.
- Epigastric pain.
- Pulmonary edema.
- Complications include:
  - ○ Eclampsia
  - ○ Premature separation of the placenta
  - ○ Cerebral hemorrhage
  - ○ Retinal damage
  - ○ Pulmonary edema
  - ○ Lower birth weight infants

Emergency Management

- High-concentration oxygen.
- Transport left lateral recumbent.
- Avoid excessive stimulation.
- Reduce light in patient compartment.

Eclampsia

- Most severe form of pregnancy-induced hypertension
- Occurs in less than 1% of all pregnancies

Signs and Symptoms

- Include signs and symptoms of preeclampsia
- Seizures
- Coma
- Complications include:
  - ○ About 10% maternal mortality rate
  - ○ About 25% fetal mortality rate

Emergency Management

- High-concentration oxygen, assist ventilations as needed.
- Transport left lateral recumbent.
- Reduce light.
- Transport immediately.
- Consider advanced life support (ALS) intercept.

Abruptio Placenta

- Premature separation of the placenta

- High-risk groups include:
  - Older patients
  - Hypertensive patients
  - Multigravidas

Signs and Symptoms

- Mild-to-moderate vaginal bleeding.
- Sharp abdominal pain.
- Rigid tender uterus.
- Hypovolemia.
- Remember: Third trimester abdominal pain equals abruptio placenta until proven otherwise.

Management

- High-concentration oxygen.
- Transport left lateral recumbent.
- Treat hypovolemia.
- Transport rapidly.

Placenta Previa

- Implantation of the placenta over the cervical opening

Signs and Symptoms

- Painless, bright red vaginal bleeding
- Soft nontender uterus
- Hypovolemia

Management

- High-concentration oxygen.
- Transport left lateral recumbent.
- Treat hypovolemia.
- Transport rapidly.

Uterine Rupture

- Blunt trauma to the pregnant uterus
- Prolonged labor against an obstruction
- Weaken uterine wall from old cesarean scar

Signs and Symptoms

- Tearing abdominal pain.
- Hypovolemic shock.
- Firm rigid abdomen.
- Vaginal bleeding may or may not be present.

Emergency Management

- High-concentration oxygen administration.
- Anticipate shock.
- Consider ALS intercept.

EMERGENCY CHILDBIRTH—NORMAL DELIVERY

- Predelivery considerations—*Remember* body substance isolation (BSI)/personal protective equipment (PPE)!
  - Have the obstetric (OB) kit open and begin setup.
  - Have oxygen and resuscitation equipment available for both mother and baby.
- It is best to transport an expecting mother, unless delivery is expected within a few minutes based on assessment of:
  - How long have you been pregnant?
  - Are there contractions or pain?
  - Any bleeding or discharge?
  - Is crowning occurring with contractions?
  - What is the frequency and duration of contractions?
  - Does she feel as if she is having a bowel movement with increasing pressure in the vaginal area?
  - Does she feel the need to push?
  - Rock hard abdomen?

Precautions

- Use body substance isolation.
- Do not touch vaginal areas except during delivery and when your partner is present.
- Do not let the mother go to bathroom.
- Do not hold mother's legs together.
- Recognize your own limitations and transport even if delivery must occur during transport.
- If delivery is eminent with crowning, contact medical direction for decision to commit to delivery on site. If delivery does not occur within 10 minutes, contact medical direction for permission to transport.

Delivery Procedures

(Fig. 29-2)

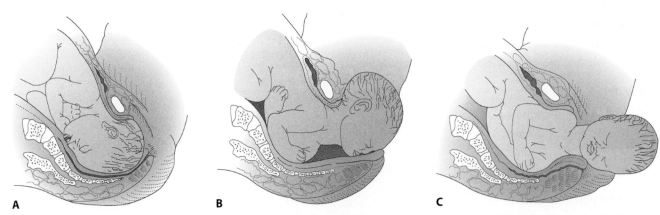

A   **B**   **C**

Figure 29-2   Delivery. A. Anterior rotation of the head. B. Extension of the head. C. External rotation of the head. *(Reproduced with permission from DeCherney AH, Nathan L. Current Diagnosis & Treatment Obstetrics and Gynecology. 10th ed. New York: McGraw-Hill; 2007)*

- Apply gloves, mask, gown, and eye protection for infection control precautions.
- Have mother lie with knees drawn up and spread apart.
- Elevate buttocks with blankets or pillow.
- Create sterile field around vaginal opening with sterile towels or paper barriers.
- When the infant's head appears during crowning, place fingers on bony part of skull (not fontanels or face) and exert very gentle pressure to prevent explosive delivery. Use caution to avoid fontanels.
- If the amniotic sac does not break, or has not broken, use a clamp to puncture the sac and push it away from the infant's head and mouth as they appear.
- As the infant's head is being born, determine if the umbilical cord is around the infant's neck; slip over the shoulder or clamp, cut and unwrap.
- After the infant's head is born, support the head; suction the mouth two or three times and the nostrils. Use caution to avoid contact with the back of the mouth.
- As the torso and full body are born, support the infant with both hands.
- As the feet are born, grasp the feet.
- Wipe blood and mucus from mouth and nose with sterile gauze, suction mouth and nose again.
- Wrap infant in a warm blanket and place on its side, head slightly lower than trunk.
- Keep infant level with vagina until the cord is cut.
- Assign partner to monitor infant and complete initial care of the newborn.
- Clamp, tie, and cut umbilical cord (between the clamps) as pulsations cease, approximately four fingers' width from infant.
- Observe for delivery of placenta while preparing mother and infant for transport.
- When delivered, wrap placenta in towel and put in plastic bag, transport placenta to hospital with mother.
- Place sterile pad over vaginal opening, lower mother's legs, help her hold them together.
- Record time of delivery and transport mother, infant, and placenta to hospital.

APGAR SCORING

The APGAR score is a quick way to assess a newborn infant (see Table 29-1). It is composed of five separate components. Each of the parts is assigned a score from 0 to 2. The composite score is computed at 1 and 5 minutes. Scores of 7 or above are considered normal. Scores of 4 to 6 are intermediate. Lower scores suggest the baby was subject to birth stress.

Vaginal bleeding following delivery—Up to 500 cc of blood loss is normal following delivery. A 500-cc blood loss is well tolerated by the mother following delivery. The emergency medical technician (EMT) must be aware of this loss so as not to cause undue psychological stress on him-/herself or the new mother.

With excessive blood loss, massage the uterus.

TABLE 29-1: APGAR Scoring Chart

Signs	0	1	2	1 Min	5 Min
Heart rate	Absent	<100	>100		
Respiratory effort	Absent	Slow, irregular	Good, crying		
Muscle tone	Limp	Some flexion	Active motion		
Reflex irritability	No response	Grimace	Cough, sneeze, cry		
Color	Blue, pale	Body pink	Completely pink		
	Blue	extremities blue			
			Total Score:		

- Hand with fingers fully extended.
- Place on lower abdomen above pubis.
- Massage (knead) over area.
- Bleeding continues—Check massage technique and transport immediately, providing oxygen and ongoing assessment.

Regardless of estimated blood loss, if mother appears in shock (hypoperfusion), treat as such and transport prior to uterine massage. Massage en route.

INITIAL CARE OF THE NEWBORN

(Figs. 29-3)

Abnormal Deliveries

Prolapsed Cord

- Condition where the cord presents through the birth canal before delivery of the head; presents a serious emergency which endangers the life of the unborn fetus.
  - Size-up.

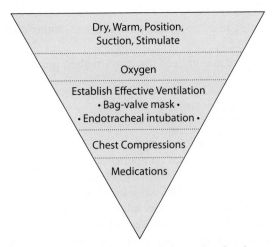

Figure 29-3   Inverted pyramid. *(Reproduced with permission from http://www.health.state.ny.us/nysdoh/ems/ppcctoc.htm)*

- Primary assessment.
- Mother should have high-flow oxygen.
- History and physical examination.
- Assess baseline vitals.
- Treatment based on signs and symptoms.
- Position mother with head down or buttocks raised using gravity to lessen pressure in birth canal.
- Insert sterile gloved hand into vagina pushing the presenting part of the fetus away from the pulsating cord.
- Transport rapidly, keeping pressure on presenting part and monitoring pulsations in the cord.

Breech Birth Presentation

- Breech presentation occurs when the buttocks or lower extremities are low in the uterus and will be the first part of the fetus delivered.
- Newborn at great risk for delivery trauma, prolapsed cord more common, transport immediately upon recognition of breech presentation.
- Delivery does not occur within 10 minutes.
- Emergency medical care.
- Immediate rapid transportation upon recognition.
- Place mother on oxygen.
- Place mother in head down position with pelvis elevated.

Limb Presentation

- Occurs when a limb of the infant protrudes from the birth canal. Is more commonly a foot when infant is in breech presentation.
  - Immediate rapid transportation upon recognition.
  - Place mother on oxygen.
  - Place mother in head down position with pelvis elevated.

Multiple Births

- Be prepared for more than one resuscitation.
- Call for additional assistance.

Meconium

Amniotic fluid that is greenish or brownish-yellow rather than clear is an indication of possible fetal distress during labor.

- Do not stimulate before suctioning oropharynx.
- Suction.
- Maintain airway.
- Transport as soon as possible.

Premature Birth

- Always at risk for hypothermia.
- Usually requires resuscitation, should be done unless physically impossible.

? CHAPTER QUESTIONS

1. Which of the following conditions indicates a predelivery emergency for a pregnant patient?

   a. Swelling of the face and/or extremities
   b. A fever
   c. Flu-like symptoms
   d. Nausea

2. Vaginal bleeding is discovered during your physical examination. Which of the following you should do?

   a. Place a sanitary napkin over the vaginal opening
   b. Massage the uterus to control internal bleeding
   c. Pack the vagina with sterile gauze or a dressing
   d. Apply direct pressure to the vaginal area until bleeding is controlled

3. Which of the following is true regarding trauma to a pregnant woman?

   a. Keep spine boards absolutely flat to facilitate blood flow to the fetus.
   b. Even minor trauma to the abdomen can cause serious fetal injuries.
   c. Early signs of shock are very obvious in pregnant women.
   d. If a pregnant woman dies as a result of an accident, cardiopulmonary resuscitation (CPR) may save the life of the unborn infant.

4. Expect delivery of the infant within a few minutes if:

   a. the patient's "water breaks"
   b. the patient's abdomen gets very soft
   c. the patient has the sensation of a bowel movement
   d. contractions are 5 minutes apart, and last 15 to 30 seconds

5. Emergency care of the patient in active labor for a normal delivery includes:

   a. immediately clamping and cutting the umbilical cord if wrapped around the infant's neck
   b. suctioning the infant's nose first, as newborns are obligate nose-breathers
   c. exerting gentle pressure against the infant's skull to prevent explosive delivery
   d. having the patient lay on her left side during the delivery

6. As your patient delivers the infant, your emergency medical care should include:

   a. holding the infant upside down by the feet to help drain fluid
   b. cutting, then clamping, the umbilical cord
   c. massaging the uterus to decrease vaginal bleeding after delivery
   d. yanking on the umbilical cord after delivery to assist with placental expulsion

7. Which of the following is not a correct treatment for a cord presentation?

   a. Cover the cord with a saline-moist, sterile towel.

   b. With a sterile gloved hand, place the cord back into the vagina.

   c. Position the mother with her head down in the "knee-chest" position.

   d. Insert a sterile gloved hand into the vagina and push the presenting part of the fetus back and away from the cord.

8. Meconium staining is:

   a. the passing of a bowel movement by the infant in the amniotic fluid

   b. urine expelled by the infant during delivery

   c. a yellowish bubbly fluid caused by the infant's lungs being compressed during delivery

   d. blood that has leaked out of the umbilical cord during delivery

9. Additional care that you should provide to a premature infant includes:

   a. not suctioning the infant's mouth, as you may cause trauma

   b. placing a surgical mask on the infant's face to prevent contamination

   c. drying the infant thoroughly and wrapping in warm blankets, covering the head

   d. applying high-concentration oxygen by a pediatric non-rebreather mask

10. The signs of a severely depressed newborn include:

    a. poor or absent skeletal muscle tone

    b. an APGAR score of under 6

    c. a heart rate over 140 or under 100 beats/min

    d. a respiratory rate under 60 beats/min

11. An abnormally low placenta may tear or separate from the uterus, causing painless hemorrhaging. This condition is known as:

    a. ectopic pregnancy

    b. ruptured uterus

    c. placenta previa

    d. abruptio placenta

12. Eclampsia most frequently occurs during the last trimester and most often affects women in their 20s who are pregnant for the first time. Signs and symptoms of toxemia, or eclampsia, include:

    a. vaginal bleeding without pain

    b. increased urinary output

    c. seizures

    d. history of severe allergic reactions

13. An ectopic pregnancy means:

    a. the egg has implanted outside the uterus

    b. a naturally aborted fetus due to any number of reasons

    c. a pregnancy that continues past the expected due date

    d. the fetus is developing in an abnormal position in the uterus

14. The fetus, or unborn infant, develops in the:

   a. vagina
   b. placenta
   c. cervix
   d. uterus

15. The organ through which the fetus receives oxygen and nourishment from the mother is the:

   a. placenta
   b. umbilical cord
   c. amniotic sac
   d. uterus

16. The fluid-filled bag in which the infant floats is called the:

   a. placenta
   b. uterus
   c. amniotic sac
   d. vagina

17. During the first stage of labor, which of the following occurs?

   a. The placenta separates from the uterine wall.
   b. The cervix becomes fully dilated.
   c. The infant's head appears at the opening of the birth canal.
   d. All of the above.

18. Indications that delivery is imminent include:

   a. the onset of contractions
   b. bulging of the perineum
   c. the "bloody show"
   d. the breaking of the amniotic sac

19. During the third stage of labor which of the following takes place?

   a. The infant is actually delivered.
   b. The amniotic sac ruptures.
   c. The placenta is expelled from the uterus.
   d. The head of the infant appears at the opening of the birth canal.

20. Questions that should be asked regarding due date include which of the following?

   a. How many previous pregnancies are there?
   b. How many children does the patient have?
   c. Has the patient had any prenatal care?
   d. All of the above.

Chapter 30
Infants and Children

Emergency medical services (EMS) is dispatched to a private house for an unconscious female child. Upon entering the house, from across the room you see a 2-year-old girl listless in her mother's arms. As you approach, the patient's father urgently summons you to "help his daughter." The mother states the patient "stopped breathing and turned blue." You ask the mother if you can take the baby from her arms, and immediately begin assessing the patient's airway. What is your next step during your assessment?

THE HUMAN BODY (INFANTS AND CHILDREN)

Developmental Differences

Newborns (Birth to 1 Month) and Infants (1-12 Months)
- Minimal stranger anxiety.
- Separation anxiety from parents.
- Do not want to be suffocated by an oxygen mask.
- Need to be kept warm—Make sure hands and stethoscope are warmed before touching the child.
- Breathing rate best obtained at a distance—Watch chest rise, note color, and level of activity.
- Examine heart and lungs first, head last. This is done to build confidence. It is best to obtain heart and lung sounds before the child becomes agitated.

Toddlers: 1 to 3 Years
- Do not like to be touched.
- Do not like being separated from parents.
- Do not like having clothing removed. Remove, examine, replace.
- Do not want to be suffocated by an oxygen mask.
- Assure the child that he was not bad. Children think their illness/injury is punishment.
- Afraid of needles.
- Fear of pain.
- Should be examined trunk-to-head approach. This is done to build confidence. It should be done before child becomes agitated.

Preschool: 3 to 6 Years

- Do not like to be touched.
- Do not like being separated from parents.
- Do not like having clothing removed. Remove, examine, replace.
- Do not want to be suffocated by an oxygen mask.
- Assure the child that he was not bad. Children think that the illness/injury is a punishment.
- Afraid of blood.
- Fear of pain.
- Fear of permanent injury.
- Modest.

School Age: 6 to 12 Years

- Afraid of blood.
- Fear of pain.
- Fear of permanent injury.
- Modest.
- Fear of disfigurement.

Adolescent: 12 to 18 Years

- Fear of permanent injury.
- Modest.
- Fear of disfigurement.
- Treat them as adults.
- These patients may desire to be assessed privately, away from parents or guardians.

Table 30-1 shows Pediatric Assessment Tools.

Anatomical and Physiological Concerns: The Pediatric Airway

- Small airways throughout the respiratory system are easily blocked by secretions and airway swelling.
- Tongue is large relative to small mandible and can block airway in an unconscious infant or child.
- Positioning the airway is different in infants and children, do not hyperextend the neck. Place the head in a neutral position.
- Infants are obligate nose breathers, so suctioning a secretion-filled nasopharynx can improve breathing problems in an infant.
- Children can compensate well for short periods of time.
  - Compensate by increasing breathing rate and increasing effort of breathing.
  - Compensation is followed rapidly by decompensation due to rapid respiratory muscle fatigue and general fatigue of the infant.

Airway

The most important component of pediatric care is airway, airway, airway!

- The pediatric airway is more anterior than the adult's.
- The diameter of the airway is smaller than the adult patient's.

TABLE 30-1: Pediatric Assessment Tools

Pediatric Pulse Rates

Age	Low	High
Infant (birth-1 y)	100	160
Toddler (1-3 y)	90	150
Preschooler (3-6 y)	80	140
School-age (6-12 y)	70	120
Adolescent (12-18 y)	60	100

Pediatric Respiratory Rates

Age	Rate (breaths/min)
Infant (birth-1 y)	30-60
Toddler (1-3 y)	24-40
Preschooler (3-6 y)	22-34
School-age (6-12 y)	18-30
Adolescent (12-18 y)	12-16

Low-Normal Pediatric Systolic Blood Pressure

Age*	Low Normal
Infant (birth-1 y)	>60*
Toddler (1-3 y)	>70*
Preschooler (3-6 y)	>75
School-age (6-12 y)	>80
Adolescent (12-18 y)	>90

*Normal vital sign ranges.

This curriculum was developed by the Fire Department of the City of New York under contract with the New York State Department of Health/Health Research Incorporated. Funding was provided through grant #6 H33 MC 00036 from the Emergency Medical Services for Children Program. The Emergency Medical Services for Children (EMSC) Program is administered by the Maternal and Child Health Bureau, Health Resources and Services Administration, Public Health Service, US Department of Health and Human Services in cooperation with the National Highway Traffic Safety Administration.

Health Research Incorporated (HRI) retains title and copyright of this curriculum. This curriculum should not be published or duplicated without prior written consent of HRI, except as required by law. Any references to this curriculum should include the New York State Department of Health and the State of New York. Authors: Ann M. Fitton, EMT-P, WilfredoSilvestry, EMT-P, John S. McFarland, EMT-P, Peter N. Andryuk, EMT-P, Contributors: Andres Rodriguez, EMT-P, John C. Clappin, Gustave Pappas, EMT-P.

- Large tongue in relation to the jaw.
- Infants favor breathing through the nose.

Breathing

- Pediatric patients are dependent on the contraction of their diaphragm to breathe.
- Bradycardia is a late sign of low oxygenation in the pediatric patient.
- Pediatric patients compensate for respiratory distress by increasing their rate, but fatigue easily.

Circulation

- Compensate in shock effectively, but decompensate rapidly.
- Mental status change is a good indicator of hypoperfusion.
- Blood pressure is an unreliable indicator of perfusion in the pediatric patient.
- Hypovolemia can result from vomiting and diarrhea in children.
- Compare strength of central pulses with those of peripheral pulses.

Oxygen Therapy

- High concentration via pediatric non-rebreather mask
- Blow-by techniques such as:
  - Holding oxygen tubing 2 in from the patient's face (and oxygen that is set at a liter flow of 1-6 L/min).
  - Insert tubing into a paper cup, and let the patient hold the cup by their face.

Artificial Ventilation

- Bag-valve-mask sizing is important.
- Mask seal
  - Two-hand method (preferred method)
  - One-hand method
- Mouth-to-mask artificial ventilations with supplemental oxygen attached.
- Use of the bag-valve-mask requires skill and practice!
  - Squeeze bag slowly and evenly enough to make chest rise adequately.
  - Rates for child and infant are 20 breaths/min.
  - Provide high-concentration oxygen by using an oxygen reservoir.

ASSESSMENT

General impression of a well versus sick child can be obtained from overall appearance. The emergency medical technician (EMT) should assess the following:

- Mental status
- Effort of breathing
- Color
- Quality of cry/speech
- Interaction with environment and parents
  - Normal behavior for child of this age.
  - Playing.
  - Moving around.
  - Attentive versus nonattentive.
  - Eye contact.
  - Recognizes parents.
  - Responds to parents' calling.
- Emotional state
- Response to the EMT
- Tone/body position

General Approach to the Pediatric Patient Should Begin From Across the Room

- Mechanism of injury
- Assessment of surroundings
- General impression of well versus sick
- Respiratory assessment
  - Note chest expansion/symmetry
  - Effort of breathing

  - Nasal flaring
  - Stridor, crowing, or noisy
  - Retractions
  - Grunting
  - Respiratory rate
- Perfusion assessment—Skin color

Hands-On Approach to Infant or Child Patient Assessment

- Assess breath sounds.
- Assess circulation.

Detailed Physical Examination

Begin with a trunk-to-head approach.

COMMON PROBLEMS ENCOUNTERED WITH PEDIATRIC PATIENTS

Airway Obstructions

Mild Airway Obstruction: Signs and Symptoms in the Pediatric Patient

- Good air exchange.
- Responsive and can forcefully cough.
- Wheezing may be present.

Severe Airway Obstruction: Signs and Symptoms in the Pediatric Patient

- Poor air exchange
- No air exchange
- High-pitched noise while inhaling (stridor)
- Increased difficulty breathing
- Cyanosis
- Unable to speak or cry
- May exhibit the "universal choking sign"
- Inability to move air

Emergency Management

1 YEAR TO ADOLESCENT (CONSCIOUS)

- Ask, "Are you choking?"
- Give abdominal thrusts/Heimlich maneuver.
- Repeat until foreign body is dislodged or the child goes unconscious.
- Summon advanced life support.

1 YEAR TO ADOLESCENT (UNCONSCIOUS)

- Begin cardiopulmonary resuscitation (CPR).
- Look into the mouth while opening the airway; use a finger sweep only if a foreign body is visible.
- Continue CPR for five cycles or 2 minutes, continue cycles until foreign object is dislodged and prepare for transport.

Less Than 1 Year of Age (Conscious)

- Confirm severe airway obstruction.
- Evaluate for sudden onset of severe difficulty breathing, ineffective or silent cough, weak or silent cry.
- Give five back slaps and five chest thrusts.
- Repeat until effective or the patient becomes unconscious.
- Summon advanced life support.

Less Than 1 Year of Age (Unconscious)

- Begin CPR.
- Look into the mouth while opening the airway; use a finger sweep only if a foreign body is visible.
- Continue CPR for five cycles or 2 minutes, continue cycles until foreign object is dislodged and prepare for transport.

Respiratory Emergencies

- Recognize the difference between upper airway obstruction and lower airway disease.
  - Upper airway obstruction—Stridor on inspiration
  - Lower airway disease
    - Wheezing and breathing effort on exhalation
    - Rapid breathing (tachypnea) without stridor

Recognize Signs of Increased Effort of Breathing

Respiratory distress is indicated by any of the following:

- Nasal flaring
- Intercostal retraction (neck muscles), supraclavicular, subcostal retractions
- Stridor
- Neck and abdominal muscles—Retractions
- Audible wheezing
- Grunting

Respiratory Failure

Respiratory failure presents with the same signs and symptoms of respiratory distress, and any of the following:

- Breathing rate less than 10/min
- Heart rate greater than 60
- Cyanosis
- Decreased muscle tone
- Severe use of accessory muscles
- Poor peripheral perfusion
- Altered mental status
- Grunting

Respiratory Arrest

- Apneic
- Limp muscle tone
- Unconscious

- Slower, absent heart rate
- Weak or absent distal pulses

Emergency Management

- Provide high-concentration oxygen to all children with respiratory emergencies.
- Provide high-concentration oxygen and assist ventilation for severe respiratory distress.
  - Respiratory distress and altered mental status
  - Presence of cyanosis with oxygen
  - Respiratory distress with poor muscle tone

Childhood Respiratory Disease

Croup is a group of respiratory diseases that often affect infants and children under the age of 6. It is characterized by a barking cough; a whistling, obstructive sound (stridor) as the child breathes in; and hoarseness due to obstruction in the region of the larynx. It may be mild, moderate, or severe, and severe cases, with breathing difficulty, can be fatal. Another type of croup is known as spasmodic croup. People with spasmodic croup first catch a cold, rarely with fever, and then the croupy cough begins. In some cases, spasmodic croup may begin suddenly without any preceding cold symptoms. Unlike viral croup, spasmodic croup usually recurs, and can occur in older children, and rarely even in adults. Spasmodic croup is thought to be related to allergies.

- A Westley score of less than or equal to 2 designates mild croup (Table 30-2). The characteristic barking cough and hoarseness may be present but without resting stridor.
- A score of 3 to 7 is classified as moderate croup, and typically there will be signs of increased respiratory effort, including accessory muscle recruitment and sternal recession.
- A score of greater than or equal to 8 indicates severe croup, and these children are at the greatest risk of respiratory failure. There is marked in drawing of the sternum, and the child may become fatigued and distressed.

One alarming feature is the reduction of stridor in a child previously demonstrating severe obstructive signs. With worsening airway obstruction, air movement is so limited that the characteristic sound is lost.

TABLE 30-2: **The Westley Score: Classification of Croup Severity**

Feature	Severity			
Chest wall retraction	None = 0	Mild = 1	Moderate = 2	Severe = 3
Stridor	None = 0	With agitation = 1	At rest = 2	
Cyanosis	None = 0	With agitation = 4		At rest = 5
Level of consciousness	Normal = 0 (including sleep)	Disoriented = 5		
Air entry	Normal = 0	Decreased = 1	Markedly decreased = 2	

Data from *Muñiz A, Molodow RE, Defendi GL. Croup. Available on: http://emedicine.medscape.com/article/962972-overview.*

Signs and Symptoms

Croup is characterized by a harsh "barking" cough and sneeze, inspiratory stridor (a high-pitched sound heard on inhalation), nausea/vomiting, and fever. Hoarseness is usually present. More severe cases will have respiratory distress.

The "barking" cough (often described as seal-like) of croup is diagnostic. Stridor will be provoked or worsened by agitation or crying. If stridor is also heard when the child is calm, critical narrowing of the airway may be imminent.

Epiglottitis

Epiglottitis is inflammation of the epiglottis the flap that sits at the base of the tongue, which keeps food from going into the trachea (windpipe). Due to its place in the airway, swelling of this structure can interfere with breathing and constitutes a medical emergency. The infection can cause the epiglottis to either obstruct or completely close off the windpipe.

- With the advent of the Hib vaccine, the incidence has been reduced, but the condition has not been eliminated.
- Epiglottitis involves bacterial infection of the epiglottis, most often caused by *Haemophilus influenzae* type B, although some cases are attributable to *Streptococcus pneumoniae*, *Streptococcus agalactiae*, *Staphylococcus aureus*, and *Streptococcus pyogenes*.

Epiglottitis typically affects children, and is associated with fever, difficulty in swallowing, drooling, hoarseness of voice, and stridor. However, it is important to note that since the introduction of the *H. infuenzae* vaccination in many Western countries (including the United Kingdom), the disease is becoming relatively more common in adults. The child often appears acutely ill, anxious, and has very quiet shallow breathing with the head held forward, insisting on sitting up in bed. The early symptoms are insidious but rapidly progressive, and swelling of the throat may lead to cyanosis and asphyxiation. Cases in adults are most typically seen among abusers of crack cocaine and have a more subacute presentation. George Washington is thought to have died of epiglottitis.

Seizures

- In children who have chronic seizures are rarely life threatening. However, seizures, including febrile, should be considered life threatening by the EMT.
- May be brief or prolonged.
- Assess for presence of injuries that may have occurred during seizures.
- Caused by fever, infections, poisoning, hypoglycemia, trauma, or decreased levels of oxygen, or could be idiopathic in children.
- History of seizures. Ask the following questions:
  - Has the child had prior seizure(s)?
  - If yes, is this the child's normal seizure pattern?
  - Has the child taken his antiseizure medications?

Emergency Management

- Ensure airway position and patency.
- Position patient on side, if no possibility of cervical spine trauma.
- Have suction ready.

- Provide oxygen and, if in respiratory arrest or severe respiratory distress, ensure airway position and patency and ventilate with bag-valve-mask.
- Transport. Although brief seizures are not harmful, there may be a more dangerous underlying condition.

Altered Mental Status

Can be caused by a variety of conditions:

- Hypoglycemia
- Poisoning
- Postseizure
- Infection
- Head trauma
- Decreased oxygen levels
- Hypoperfusion (shock)

Emergency Management

- Ensure patency of airway.
- Be prepared to artificially ventilate/suction.
- Transport to the appropriate hospital.

Poisonings

Identify suspected container through adequate history. Bring container to receiving facility if possible.

Emergency Management

RESPONSIVE POISONING PATIENT

- Contact medical control.
- Consider need to administer activated charcoal.
- Provide oxygen.
- Transport.
- Continue to monitor patient—May become unresponsive.

UNRESPONSIVE POISONING PATIENT

- Ensure patency of airway.
- Be prepared to artificially ventilate.
- Provide oxygen if indicated.
- Call medical control.
- Transport.
- Rule out trauma; trauma can cause altered mental status.

Fever

- Common reason for infant or child ambulance call.
- Many causes—rarely life threatening. A severe cause is meningitis.
- Fever with a rash is a potentially serious consideration.

Emergency Management

- Transport.
- Be alert for seizures.

Shock (Hypoperfusion)

It is rarely a primary cardiac event.

Common Causes

- Diarrhea and dehydration
- Trauma
- Vomiting
- Blood loss
- Infection
- Abdominal injuries

Less Common Causes

- Allergic reactions
- Congenital cardiac disease

Signs and Symptoms

- Rapid respiratory rate
- Pale, cool, clammy skin
- Weak or absent peripheral pulses
- Delayed capillary refill
- Decreased urine output, measured by asking parents about diaper wetting and looking at the diaper
- Mental status changes
- Absence of tears, even when crying

Emergency Management

- Ensure airway/oxygen.
- Be prepared to artificially ventilate.
- Manage bleeding if present.
- Elevate legs.
- Keep warm.
- Transport. Note—need for rapid transport of infant and child patients, with secondary examination completed en route, if time permits.

Near Drowning

- Artificial ventilation is a top priority.
- Consider possibility of trauma.
- Consider possibility of hypothermia.
- Consider possible ingestion, especially alcohol.
- Protect airway, suction if necessary.
- Secondary drowning syndrome—Deterioration after breathing normally from minutes to hours after event. All near-drowning victims should be transported to the hospital.

Sudden Infant Death Syndrome

Signs and Symptoms

- Sudden death of infants in the first year of life.
- Causes are many and not clearly understood.
- Baby most commonly discovered in the early morning.

Emergency Management
- Try to resuscitate unless rigor mortis.
- Parents will be in agony from emotional distress, remorse, and imagined guilt.
- Avoid any comments that might suggest blame to the parents.

Trauma

- Injuries are the number-one cause of death in infants and children.
- It is not uncommon for a child to be severely injured but display no early obvious signs.
- Blunt injury is most common.
- The pattern of injury will be different from adults.
  - Motor vehicle crashes
    - Unrestrained passengers have head and neck injuries.
    - Restrained passengers have abdominal and lower spine injuries.
  - Struck while riding bicycle—Head injury, spinal injury, abdominal injury
  - Pedestrian struck by vehicle—Abdominal injury with internal bleeding, possible painful, swollen, deformed thigh, head injury
  - Falls from height, diving into shallow water—Head and neck injuries
  - Burns
  - Sports injuries—Head and neck
  - Child abuse

REVIEW OF SPECIFIC BODY SYSTEMS
Head

- The single most important maneuver is to ensure an open airway by means of the modified jaw thrust.
- Children are likely to sustain head injury along with internal injuries. Signs and symptoms of shock (hypoperfusion) with a head injury should cause you to be suspicious of other possible injuries.
- Respiratory arrest is common, secondary to head injuries and may occur during transport.
- Common signs and symptoms are nausea and vomiting.
- Most common cause of hypoxia in the unconscious head injury patient is the tongue obstructing the airway. Jaw thrust is critically important.
- Do not use sandbags to stabilize the head because the weight on child's head may cause injury if the board needs to be turned for emesis.

Chest

- Children have very soft pliable ribs.
- There may be significant injuries without external signs.

Abdomen

- More common site of injury in children than adults.

- Often a source of hidden injury.
- Always consider abdominal injury in the multiple trauma patients who is deteriorating without external signs.
- Gastric distention can distend abdomen and interfere with artificial ventilation efforts.

Extremities

Extremity injuries are managed in the same manner as adults.

CHILD ABUSE AND NEGLECT

- Child abuse encompasses the most serious harm committed against children. An abused child is one whose parent or legal guardian inflicts serious physical injury, creates a risk for serious injury, or commits a sex act against the child.
- Maltreatment, including neglect, means the child's physical, mental, or emotional condition has been impaired, or placed in imminent danger by the parent or legal guardian.
- The EMT must be aware of condition to be able to recognize the problem.
- Signs and symptoms of abuse
  - Multiple bruises in various stages of healing.
  - Injury inconsistent with mechanism described.
  - Repeated calls to the same address.
  - Fresh burns.
  - Parents seem inappropriately unconcerned.
  - Conflicting stories.
  - Fear on the part of the child to discuss how the injury occurred.
  - Central nervous system (CNS) injuries are the most lethal—Shaken baby syndrome.
- Signs and symptoms of neglect
  - Lack of adult supervision.
  - Malnourished appearing child.
  - Unsafe living environment.
  - Untreated chronic illness.
- Do not accuse in the field.
  - Accusation and confrontation delay transportation.
  - Bring objective information to the receiving facility.
    - Objective—What you see and what you hear—*not* what you think.

SPECIAL NEEDS PEDIATRIC PATIENTS

This can include many different types of situations.

- Premature babies with lung disease
- Babies and children with heart disease
- Infants and children with neurological disease
- Children with chronic disease or altered function from birth

Often special needs children will be at home, technologically dependent.

Tracheotomy Tube

Common Complications

- Obstruction
- Bleeding
- Air leak
- Dislodged
- Infection

Emergency Management

- Maintain an open airway.
- Suction as needed.
- Maintain position of comfort.
- Transport.

Home Ventilators

Usually the parent or guardian is familiar with operation of a home ventilator.

Emergency Management

- Guarantee patent airway
- Artificially ventilate with high-concentration oxygen
- Transport

Central Lines

- Intravenous lines (IVs) that are placed near the heart for long-term use.
  - Complications include cracked line, infection, clotting off, or bleeding.

Emergency Management

- If bleeding is present, apply pressure.
- Transport.

Gastrostomy tubes and gastric feeding are placed directly into stomach for feeding. These patients usually cannot be fed by mouth.

- Be alert for breathing problems.
- Ensure adequate airway.
- Have suction available.
- If a diabetic patient, be alert for altered mental status. Infant will become hypoglycemic quickly if they cannot be fed.
- Provide oxygen.
- Transport.

Shunts are devices running from the brain to the abdomen to drain excess cerebral spinal fluid. It will find reservoir on side of the skull.

- Change in mental status
- Prone to respiratory arrest
  - Manage airway.
  - Ensure adequate artificial ventilation.
  - Transport.

FAMILY RESPONSE TO A CHILD'S ILLNESS OR INJURY

- A child cannot be cared for in isolation from the family; therefore, you have multiple patients.
- Striving for calm, supportive interaction with family will result in improved ability to deal with the child. Calm parents = calm child; agitated parents = agitated child.
- Anxiety arises from concern over child's pain; fear for child's well-being.
- Worsened by sense of helplessness.
- Parent may respond to EMT with anger or hysteria.
- Parents should remain part of the care unless child is not aware or medical conditions require separation.
- Parents should be instructed to calm the child; can maintain position of comfort and/or hold oxygen.
- Parents may not have medical training, but they are experts on what is normal or abnormal for their children and what will have a calming effect.

Provider Response

- Anxiety from lack of experience with treating children as well as fear of failure.
- Skills can be learned and applied to children.
- Stress from identifying patient with their own children.
- Provider should realize that much of what they learned about adults applies to children; they need to remember the differences.
- Infrequent encounters with sick children, advance preparation is important (practice with equipment and examining children).

? CHAPTER QUESTIONS

1. Emotional and physical characteristics of adolescents include:

   a. believing that, generally, nothing bad can happen to them
   b. concerns about death and disability first emerge in this age group
   c. believing the illness or injury that they have is some form of punishment
   d. having vivid imaginations and being able to dramatize events

2. When examining and caring for an infant:

   a. begin your assessment with the head and end with the feet
   b. complete your scene size-up and primary assessment from across the room
   c. explain each procedure that you are going to do to the infant
   d. separate the infant from the caregiver during assessment

3. An 8-year-old child:

   a. has no understanding of what EMS is about
   b. is preoccupied with his/her body and is extremely concerned about modesty
   c. is the most difficult to manage
   d. is able to rationalize, and may be curious about what you are doing

4. When treating a child which of the following you should keep in mind?

   a. The child's ribs are more rigid than an adult's.
   b. The tracheal diameter of a newborn is the same as that of an adult.
   c. The child's skin surface is small compared to body mass.
   d. Infants and children have a higher metabolic rate, so periods of poor oxygenation can be more dangerous.

5. Which of the following is correct regarding infants' and children's respiratory status?

   a. Compensatory mechanisms are the same as an adult's, and they will both gradually deteriorate.
   b. The leading cause of cardiac arrest in infants and children is failure of the respiratory system.
   c. It is not important to distinguish between an upper airway obstruction from a foreign body and an obstruction caused by a respiratory condition.
   d. Determining the origin of the child's respiratory dysfunction is essential in the pre-hospital setting to appropriately care for the patient.

6. A child is displaying nasal flaring and retractions, but is maintaining an adequate respiratory rate and depth. This child is in:

   a. decompensated respiratory failure
   b. compensated respiratory failure
   c. early decompensated failure
   d. late respiratory distress

7. Indications that a pediatric patient has a partial airway obstruction include:

   a. crowing or other noisy respirations
   b. ineffective or absent cough
   c. no crying or talking
   d. unresponsiveness

8. Important sounds to listen for include:

   a. stridor, which sounds like rolling a few strands of hair near the ear
   b. crackles, which are harsh, high-pitched sounds that occur during inspiration
   c. rales, which are loud, gurgling sounds occurring during exhalation
   d. wheezing, which is caused by air moving at a high rate through narrowed bronchioles

9. While assessing the circulation of a 2-year-old child, you should check all of the following *except*:

   a. warmth and color of hands and feet
   b. mental status
   c. blood pressure
   d. capillary refill

Chapter 31

Assessment of the Geriatric Patient

You and your partner are called to the scene of a home in a nearby neighborhood. Upon arrival you find an 85-year-old man unconscious, not breathing. His home health-care nurse states the patient "just stopped breathing." He is on home oxygen and has a garbage bag full of medications for chronic obstructive pulmonary disease (COPD). You begin your primary assessment, and attempt to ventilate. You find the patient difficult to ventilate. What would be your next action?

- The elderly population is at a greater risk for nearly all types of injuries and illnesses.
- They present with different signs and symptoms because of the changing physiology of the geriatric body system.
- In the United States, people over age 65 make the fastest growing segment of the population.
- Because of the aging process, there can be many subtle differences in how illness and injury present in geriatrics, when compared to their younger counterparts.
- Coexisting medical problems further hamper the emergency medical technician (EMT) assessment.
- The aging process is inevitable.
- Physiology starts to change as early as 30 years of age.
- Because of significant advances in medicine, there is an increase in longevity of people with chronic illnesses.
- It is important for the EMT to be able to differentiate chronic changes from aging, and acute changes due to illness or injury.

CARDIOVASCULAR SYSTEM

- Diminished pumping action of the heart due to loss of muscle strength.
- Progressive increases in heart rate, and slow degeneration of the conduction system.
- Loss of elasticity of the vascular system which causes diminished ability to constrict and dilate resulting in a weaker heart that must pump against higher resistance, with slowed electrical conduction within the heart.

RESPIRATORY SYSTEM

- Diminished size and strength of pulmonary musculature.
- Alveolar surfaces degenerate, impairing gas exchange.
- Lung elasticity is lost as ribs also become less pliable.
- The pulmonary system's ability to resist disease and infection decreases.
- Net effect is less gas exchange, increased infection, and a loss of muscle coordination.

MUSCULOSKELETAL SYSTEM

- Loss of minerals to the skeleton due to osteoporosis.
- Increased susceptibility to fractures from bones being brittle.
- Progressive loss of joint flexibility and muscle strength.
- Kyphosis will complicate spinal immobilization.
- In all, elderly patients fall more, fracture bones easier, take longer to heal, and may also be victim to additional medical problems.

NEUROLOGICAL SYSTEM

- Decrease in mass of brain (loss of neurons).
- Slowing of reflexes from nerve cell degeneration.
- Difficulty in being able to perceive body position.
- Decreased night vision and some loss of hearing.
- Deterioration of nervous system contributes to the high incidence of falls, and a general slowing in the body's adaptation to stressors.

GASTROINTESTINAL SYSTEM

- Loss in sense of appetite, smell, and thirst.
- Diminished function of the intestinal tract with less effective peristaltic waves and absorption of nutrients.
- Liver function diminishes, which also hampers digestion.
- Malnutrition and constipation are common results from the change in physiology due to aging.

RENAL SYSTEM

- Loss of nephrons decreases kidney size and function.
- Reduced renal blood flow from progressive stenosis of the renal vasculature.
- Electrolytes normally controlled by the kidneys may become disturbed.
- Overall changes may result in diminished filtration of waste products from the blood, which causes electrolyte disturbances and possible drug toxicity.

INTEGUMENTARY SYSTEM

- Thinning of skin from loss of subcutaneous layer.
- Replacement skin cells develop slower.
- Sense of touch dulled as are other sensory structures.
- Resultant changes include increased fragility of the skin and a loss in the protective barrier as the skin tears more easily.

LEADING CAUSES OF DEATH IN THE ELDERLY

- Cardiovascular diseases
- Cancer
- Fractures and falls
- Pulmonary diseases
- Diabetes
- Misuse of drugs

The manifestation of these emergencies may be altered due to more than one pathological process occurring at once in the body. Those especially at risk are geriatrics who:

- Live alone
- Are incontinent
- Are immobile
- Have recently been hospitalized
- Have recently been bereaved
- Have an altered mental status

ASSESSMENT: SCENE SIZE-UP

- Be attentive to body substance isolation (BSI) precautions—especially with concerns of TB in the geriatric population.
- Note the environmental conditions they live in.
- Watch for environmental influences when numerous geriatrics share living quarters.
- The ease in determining the mechanism of injury (MOI) versus nature of illness (NOI) is not as clear, as the precipitating event (ie, the fall or the heart attack) may have actually occurred days earlier.

THE PRIMARY ASSESSMENT

- Mental status
  - Important to differentiate acute from chronic alteration
- Airway
  - Diminished gag reflex increases risk of airway compromise.
- Breathing
  - Respiratory muscle failure occurs rapidly in light of pulmonary emergencies.
  - Carefully assess respiratory rate *and* tidal volume.
- Circulation
  - Assess central and peripheral pulses (noting rate and rhythm).
  - Indirect measures of circulatory adequacy may include mental status and skin characteristics.
- Skin condition and temperature
  - Dehydration is best assessed by evaluating mucous membranes of the eyes and mouth, rather than the skin.
  - Fever may not be present during infectious processes as this response is blunted in the geriatric patient.

SECONDARY ASSESSMENT

- Based on the assessment findings made during your primary assessment, first determine the patient criticality (priority or nonpriority).
- Secondly, perform a thorough secondary assessment.
- In any instance, however, certain characteristics may be present which make assessment difficult. These include failing eyesight and diminished hearing.
- Problems with diminished sight or blindness.
    - Increased anxiety occurs from an inability to see surroundings along with an inability to control the situation.
    - As an EMT, you should talk calmly and be positioned in front of the patient should they have any remaining eyesight.
    - Explain what you are doing fully.
- Problems with diminished hearing or deafness.
    - Hearing loss is not a direct result of aging.
    - Ask prior to assuming the geriatric patient is deaf.
    - Ensure hearing aid is turned on if used by the patient.
    - When speaking louder, increase volume rather than pitch of your voice.
    - Consider lip reading or note writing if the patient prefers.

Regarding Geriatric Trauma Patients

- Note mechanism of injury; remember that geriatrics are more prone to falls.
- Maintain a high index of suspicion at all times as the pain experienced by the geriatric patient may be masked.
- Consider a rapid trauma assessment on all trauma patients.
    - Inspect and palpate for DCAPBTLSC. (Deformities, Contusions, Abrasions, Punctures/Penetrations, Burns, Tenderness, Lacerations, Swelling, and Crepitation)
- Obtain a baseline set of vitals.
- Complete a SAMPLE (Signs/Symptoms, Allergies, Medications, Past medical problems, Last oral intake, Events) history from the geriatric patient.

Regarding Geriatric Medical Patients

- Remember to determine if presenting conditions are acute changes or chronic findings.
- Obtaining a history may be problematic with geriatrics, so be diligent with your task and patient with their responses.
- Always talk *to* the patient whenever possible instead of *about* the patient with other family members that may be present.
- During the SAMPLE history of a geriatric patient, remember the following points:
    - The patient may easily fatigue.
    - Clearly explain what you are doing.
    - Watch for the patient trying to minimize what is wrong.
    - Peripheral pulses may be difficult to assess.

- Watch for symptoms from numerous chronic illnesses.
- Differentiate findings from aging from findings due to an acute illness or injury.
- Questions that may help during your assessment of the geriatric patient:
  - Have you had any trouble breathing?
  - Have you had a cough lately?
  - Have you had any chest pain?
  - Have you been dizzy (vertigo)?
  - Have you fainted at all (syncopal episodes)?
  - Any history of headaches?
  - Any change with nutrition habits (eating and drinking)?
  - Any alterations in bowel or bladder habits?
  - Any recent history of falls?
- Completion of the physical examination considerations include:
  - Geriatric patients typically dress in layers (you must expose to assess!).
  - Perform a rapid medical assessment in cases of altered mental status.
  - Time and patient condition allowing, the detailed physical examination may provide additional clues as to what is underlying the patient's complaints.

EMERGENCY MANAGEMENT

- Maintain a patent airway.
- Watch for dentures.
- Suction any excess secretions or fluids.
- Consider a jaw thrust if neck is relatively inflexible.
- Insert a simple mechanical airway.
- Deterioration may occur rapidly.
- Insert an oral pharyngeal airway (OPA) when no gag reflex is present, or an nasopharyngeal airway (NPA) should airway maintenance be warranted in the patient with an intact gag reflex.
- Assess and be prepared to assist ventilations.
  - Respiratory muscles fatigue easily.
  - When providing positive-pressure ventilation (PPV), be cautious not to create excessive airway pressures which may promote gastric insufflation or cause pulmonary injury (barotrauma).
- Ensure adequate oxygenation.
  - Via non-rebreather (NRB) at 15 L/min with adequate ventilations
  - Via PPV with reservoir attached and liter flow at 15 L/min with inadequate breathing
- Monitor pulse oximetry constantly.
- Use a nasal cannula at 6 L/min only if the patient has adequate ventilations and cannot tolerate the NRB.

Optimal Patient Position

- Opt for position of comfort (Fowler probably) if patient's condition allows it.
- Use left lateral recumbent, should an altered mental status or airway aspiration concern exist.

- Full spinal precautions should be taken if there is a need based on MOI, or if the patient's circumstances are unknown.
- Use extra padding when immobilizing a geriatric with kyphosis of the spine.

Transport

- Perform ongoing assessment en route.
- Be attentive to changes in status as geriatrics can rapidly decompensate.
- Repeat and record assessment findings every 15 minutes if the patient is stable, or every 5 minutes with an unstable patient.

ASSESSMENT OF THE GERIATRIC CARDIOVASCULAR EMERGENCY

Myocardial Infarction/Acute Coronary Syndrome

- Typical chest pain from a myocardial infarction (MI) may not be present.
- Weakness, fatigue, and dyspnea are common initial findings seen with these "silent heart attacks."
- Common medication that may be prescribed is "nitro," and the EMT-B can assist in the administration if appropriate per medical direction.
- Refer to Chap. 11, Cardiovascular and Hematological Emergencies, for a thorough discussion.

Congestive Heart Failure

- Chronic weakening of the heart which causes blood to back up into the lungs.
- For these patients, ensure high concentrations of oxygen, place them in a Fowler position, and deliver PPV should their breathing become inadequate.

ASSESSMENT OF THE GERIATRIC RESPIRATORY EMERGENCY

- Dyspnea is an extremely common finding with the geriatric population.
- Since geriatric patients already have diminished pulmonary capacity, any additional disturbance could prove fatal.
- May be the primary symptom, or an associated complaint.

Pulmonary Edema

- Usually due to the heart's inability to pump blood, causing a backup of fluid.
- This results in excess fluid "leaking" into the lungs and severely hampering oxygen and carbon dioxide diffusion.
- May cause crackles, orthopnea, or blood-tinged sputum.
- Requires the administration of high-flow oxygen, Fowler positioning, and rapid transport.
- Severe cases may necessitate PPV.

Pulmonary Embolism

- Caused by a sudden blockage of a blood vessel carrying blood from the right side of the heart to the lungs (for oxygenation).
- The drop in perfusion to the lungs results in sudden onset of respiratory distress, sharp local chest pain, and possible fainting.
- Like other pulmonary disturbances, the major treatment includes high-flow oxygen, assistance with breathing if necessary, and rapid transport.

Chronic Obstructive Pulmonary Disease

- General name given to numerous disease etiologies that result in the deterioration of normal lung tissue.
- As the lung tissue is destroyed, the patient has a harder time maintaining normal oxygenation.
- They characteristically use oxygen at home as the disease advances.
- Pre-hospital management includes assuring adequate oxygenation and ventilation.

ASSESSMENT OF THE GERIATRIC ALTERED MENTAL STATUS PATIENT

- Not a result of aging, but the consequence of pathological condition(s) within the body.
- Be sure to determine if altered mental status is an acute change in the patient, or a chronic finding.
- Anything that can alter oxygenation, ventilation, perfusion, neuron activity, blood chemistry, and the like could cause an alteration in mental status.
- Although management is essentially the same despite cause, understanding common reasons for altered mental status may show the EMT what else to assess for.

Stroke

- Common medical emergency in the geriatric population.
- Results when a blood vessel in the brain is blocked or ruptures.
- Brain cells die from lack of oxygen and from rising pressure in the skull.
- The region of the brain affected determines the symptoms seen (please refer to Chapter 12).
- Key emergency care is identifying the emergency, providing oxygen therapy and airway maintenance, and rapidly transporting the patient.

Transient Ischemic Attack

- Also known as a "mini stroke."
- Is caused by a temporary diminishment of blood flow to a region of the brain.
- Region of the brain tissue affected malfunctions, causing the altered mentation and other signs.
- Resolves itself completely within 24 hours (but usually within the first few hours).
- Treatment is the same as recommended for a stroke.

Seizure

- Sudden alteration in the normal mental status of the patient caused by a massive electrical discharge in the brain.
- Results in abnormal muscular contraction which may cause inadequate breathing and airway compromise.
- Treatment goals include close attention to the airway status, suctioning as needed, provision of PPV if breathing is inadequate, and protection from injury if the seizure is still progressing.

Syncope

- "Fainting" episode which is relatively common to geriatrics.
- Usually reverses once patient is again horizontal.
- Any condition that causes a temporary decrease to blood flow in the brain can cause a syncopal episode.
- Treatment is mainly supportive to any lost function of the airway, breathing, or circulatory status.
- Ensure oxygenation, ventilation, and immobilization if warranted.

Drug Toxicity

- Defined as an adverse or toxic reaction to a drug.
- Common emergency also for geriatrics as they tend to be on multiple drugs simultaneously.
- Occasionally they overdose accidentally by forgetting that they previously took the medication.
- Abnormal reactions usually cause inadequate airway, breathing, circulation, or a combination thereof.
- Treatment is geared toward supporting any lost function of the airway, breathing, and circulation.

Dementia

- Irreversible malfunctioning of normal brain activity.
- Occurs in about 15% of the population over the age of 65.
- Results in impaired cognition, memory loss, and abstract thought.
- Could be caused by certain medications, brain tumors, heart disease, urinary retention, and many other underlying disease states.

Alzheimer Disease

- Thought to be the most common cause of dementia in the elderly population.
- Nerve cell disease where the brain tissue progressively deteriorates and dies.
- Results in changes in mental status, which may not be life threatening, but presents as a special challenge to pre-hospital care providers.
- Treatment supportive of airway, breathing, and circulation.

ASSESSMENT FINDING: TRAUMA OR SHOCK

- One of the leading causes of death to the elderly.
- Commonly from blunt trauma as a result of falls, motor vehicle collisions (MVCs), and pedestrians hit by a car.

- If fall related, ascertain if fall was preceded by a moment of dizziness.
- Other than specific treatment for isolated traumatic injuries, any indication of hypoperfusion should be considered as a serious sign of trauma.

ASSESSMENT OF THE GERIATRIC ENVIRONMENTAL EMERGENCY

- Geriatric patients have a harder time regulating normal core body temperature.
- Stay cognizant of environmental temperature when entering the scene of a geriatric patient.
- Remember that hypothermia or hyperthermia may occur in the presence of a normal ambient temperature.
- Refer to Chap. 28, Environmental Emergencies, for more details.

ASSESSMENT OF THE GERIATRIC ABUSE PATIENT

- Incidence of geriatric abuse has risen over the past several years.
- May be found in extended-care facilities or at the home of the individual.
- Abuse could be physical, mental, sexual, or financial.
- If you suspect geriatric abuse, carefully document your objective findings and be sure to notify the emergency department (ED).

? CHAPTER QUESTIONS

1. Changes in the geriatric body systems include:

   a. increased tendency for respiratory infection

   b. cough power intensifies

   c. frequent fevers with illness

   d. skin becomes tougher

2. Cardiovascular system changes in the geriatric patient include:

   a. widespread arteriosclerosis

   b. a decrease in resting heart rate

   c. an increase of electrical conducting cells

   d. increased elasticity of the arteries

3. You are caring for a 72-year-old female patient. Changes in her respiratory system may include:

   a. the body becoming more sensitive to hypoxia

   b. more air entering and exiting the lungs, and an increase in lung tissue elasticity

   c. calcium deposits where the ribs join the sternum, causing the rib cage to be less pliable

   d. a progressive increase in diffusion of oxygen and carbon dioxide across the alveolar membrane

4. The most significant musculoskeletal change resulting from aging is a loss of minerals in the bones, known as:

   a. osteoarthritis

   b. skeletal hypertrophy

   c. osteoporosis

   d. kyphosis

5. The neurological system becomes impaired by the normal effects of aging. Changes that occur include which of the following?

   a. The ability to discern lower frequency sounds is slowly lost.

   b. A decrease in the amount of cerebral spinal fluid in the skull.

   c. Nerve cells begin to degenerate and die as early as the mid-forties.

   d. The elderly have a harder time perceiving their body position.

6. The renal system is affected by the normal aging process. Which of the following are common changes in the elderly patient's renal system?

   a. The kidneys begin retaining more fluid, and increase in size and weight.

   b. There is a buildup of nephrons in the kidneys over time, decreasing their function.

   c. There is a greater amount of blood per minute passing through the kidneys for filtration.

   d. It is common for the elderly to suffer from drug toxicity due to kidney malfunction.

7. As a result of the normal aging process, the response to an illness is altered. Medical problems present with which of the following different signs and symptoms?

   a. A slowing respiratory rate, instead of increasing, may indicate respiratory failure rather than improved oxygenation.

   b. A lack of chest pain in a geriatric patient experiencing a heart attack is common.

   c. Because the geriatric patient is predisposed to peripheral vascular diseases, a diminished radial pulse may not be an abnormal sign.

   d. All of the above.

Chapter 32
Patients With Special Challenges

You are treating a 59-year-old morbidly obese woman, with a history of congestive heart failure, who presents with dyspnea that has gradually increased over the past week. She has a productive cough with brown sputum.

Vital signs are BP 110/66, HR 96, RR 20, and temperature is 100.6°F.

What would be the most likely assessment?

Emergency medical technicians (EMTs) frequently provide care to patients with special challenges. Patients who are physically challenged may require special considerations in patient assessment and management.

PHYSICAL CHALLENGES

Hearing Impairments

- Deafness is a complete or partial inability to hear. Total deafness is rare and usually congenital. Partial deafness may range from mild-to-severe, and most commonly is the result of disease, injury, or degeneration of the hearing mechanism that occurs with age.
- Conductive deafness refers to the faulty transportation of sound from the outer to the inner ear. This type of deafness is often curable and usually results from accumulation of earwax that blocks the outer ear canal, infection such as otitis media, or injury to the eardrum or middle ear.
- Sensorineural deafness is when sounds that reach the inner ear fail to be transmitted to the brain because of damage to the structures within the ear or to the acoustic nerve, which connects the inner ear to the brain. It is often incurable. Causes include:
  - Sensorineural deafness that is present in early life, may be congenital.
  - Birth injury or damage to the developing fetus.
  - Severe jaundice soon after birth.
- Sensorineural deafness that occurs in later life may be caused from:
  - Prolonged exposure to loud noise
  - Disease, such as Meniere disease
  - Tumors
  - Medications

- ○ Viral infections
- ○ Natural degeneration of the cochlea and/or labyrinth in old age
- Recognizing a patient with a hearing impairment may be possible by noting the following:
  - ○ Presence of hearing aids
  - ○ Poor diction
  - ○ Inability to respond to verbal communication in the absence of direct eye contact

Visual Impairments

- Normal vision depends on the uninterrupted passage of light from the front of the eye to the light-sensitive retina at the back.
- Any condition that obstructs the passage of light from the retina can cause vision loss. Visual impairments may be present at birth from a congenital disorder or result from:
  - ○ Cataracts
  - ○ Degeneration of the eyeball, optic nerve, or nerve pathways
  - ○ Eye or brain injury
  - ○ Infection (cytomegalovirus [CMV], herpes simplex virus [HSV], bacterial ulcers)
  - ○ Vitamin A deficiency in children living in poor countries
- Patients with visual impairment may be totally blind or have a partial loss of vision that affects central vision, peripheral vision, or both.
- Patient who has central loss of vision is usually aware of the condition.
- Those who have a loss of peripheral vision may be more difficult to identify since the loss often goes unnoticed by the person until it is well advanced.

Speech Impairments

- Speech impairments include disorders of language, articulation, voice production, or fluency (blockage of speech), all of which can lead to an inability to communicate effectively.
- Language disorders result from damage to the language centers of the brain (usually from stroke, head injury, or brain tumor). These patients often demonstrate aphasia with a slowness to understand speech, and problems with vocabulary and sentence structure.
- Aphasia can affect both children and adults and may affect their ability to speak, and/or comprehend written or spoken words.
- Delayed development of language in a child may result from hearing loss, lack of stimulation, or emotional disturbance.

Articulation Disorders (Dysarthria)—Inability to Produce Speech Sounds

- Result from damage to nerve pathways passing from the brain to the muscles of the larynx, mouth, or lips. Patient's speech will often be slurred, indistinct, slow, or nasal.
- Disorders of articulation may result from brain injury and from diseases such as multiple sclerosis and Parkinson disease.
- In children, they commonly are the result of delayed development from hearing problems.

Voice Production Disorders

- Characterized by hoarseness, harshness, inappropriate pitch, and abnormal nasal resonance, and often result from disorders that affect closure of the vocal cords.
- Some disorders are caused by hormonal or psychiatric disturbances, and by severe hearing loss.

Fluency Disorders

Marked by repetitions of single sounds or whole words, and by the blocking of speech. Stuttering is an example of a fluency disorder.

Obesity

- Abnormal increase in the proportion of fat and cells, mainly in the viscera and the subcutaneous tissues of the body. Although reasons for obesity in some people are unclear, known causes for the condition include the following:
  - Caloric intake that exceeds calories burned
  - Low basal metabolic rate
  - Genetic predisposition for obesity
- Obesity is associated with an increased risk for the following:
  - Hypertension.
  - Stroke.
  - Heart disease.
  - Diabetes.
  - Some cancers.
  - Osteoarthritis is also aggravated by increased body weight.
- Managed with weight-loss programs, exercise, counseling, medications, and sometimes surgery. The goal of long-term treatment is permanent weight loss.

Paraplegia/Quadriplegia

- Paraplegia is weakness or paralysis of both legs and sometimes part of the trunk.
- Quadriplegia is weakness or paralysis of all four extremities and the trunk.
- Conditions result from nerve damage in the brain and spinal cord, usually caused by the following:
  - Motor vehicle crash
  - Sports injury
  - Fall
  - Gunshot wound
  - Medical illness
- Both paraplegia and quadriplegia are accompanied by a loss of sensation and urinary control.
- Patients with extremity and trunk paralysis may require accommodations in patient care.
- Patient may have a halo traction device to stabilize the spine, which may complicate airway management and make patient transport difficult.
- Ostomies
  - Trachea

- ○ Bladder
- ○ Colon
- Priapism may be present in some male patients.
- Transport
  - ○ Additional manpower may be needed to move special equipment and prepare patient for transport.

MENTAL CHALLENGES

Mental illness refers to any form of psychiatric disorder.

- Psychoses—Comprises a group of mental disorders in which the individual loses contact with reality. Thought to be related to complex biochemical disease that disorders brain function. Examples include:
  - ○ Schizophrenia
  - ○ Bipolar disorder (manic-depressive illness)
  - ○ Organic brain disease
- Neuroses—Refers to diseases related to upbringing and personality in which the person remains "in touch" with reality. Neurotic symptoms generally do not limit work or social activity and tend to fluctuate in intensity with stress. Examples include:
  - ○ Depression
  - ○ Phobias
  - ○ Obsessive-compulsive behavior
- Recognizing a patient who is mentally challenged may be difficult, especially when caring for mildly neurotic patients whose behavior may be unaffected.
- Patients with more serious disorders may present with signs and symptoms consistent with mental illness.
- When obtaining the patient history, do not be hesitant to ask about:
  - ○ History of mental illness
  - ○ Prescribed medications
  - ○ Compliance with prescribed medications
  - ○ Concomitant use of alcohol or other drugs
- If the patient appears to be paranoid or shows anxious behavior, ask the patient's permission before beginning any assessment or performing any procedure. Once rapport and trust have been established, care should proceed in the same manner as for a patient who does not have mental illness. These patients experience illness and injury like all other patients.

Developmentally Disabled

- Person who is developmentally disabled has impaired or insufficient development of the brain that causes an inability to learn at the usual rate.
- Causes include the following:
  - ○ Unsatisfactory parental interaction (lack of stimulation)
  - ○ Severe vision or hearing impairment
  - ○ Mental retardation
  - ○ Brain damage before, during, or after birth; or in infancy
  - ○ Severe diseases of body organs and systems

Signs of Developmental Delay

- Delays may be of varying severity and may affect any or all of the major areas of human achievement, including development of the following abilities:
  - Walking upright
  - Fine hand-eye coordination
  - Listening, language, and speech
  - Social interaction

Down Syndrome

- Down syndrome results from a chromosomal abnormality that causes mild-to-severe mental retardation and a characteristic physical appearance.
- Features of the patient with Down syndrome typically include:
  - Eyes that slope upward at the outer corners
  - Folds of skin on either side of the nose that cover the inner corners of the eyes
  - Small face and small facial features
  - Large and protruding tongue
  - Flattening on back of the head
  - Hands that are short and broad
- Commonly, Down syndrome occurs from the failure of the two chromosomes numbered 21 in a parent cell to go into separate daughter cells during the first stage of sperm or egg cell formation.
- Results in a triplet of chromosome 21 (trisomy 21) rather than the usual pair.
- Extra number 21 chromosome is passed on to the child, leading to Down syndrome.
- Incidence of affected fetuses increases with increased maternal age (mothers over age 35), and those with a family history of Down syndrome.
- Persons with Down syndrome usually do not survive past their middle years.
- About 25% of children born with Down syndrome have a heart defect at birth.
- Many have congenital intestinal disorders, hearing defects, and other illnesses.
- Persons with Down syndrome are capable of limited learning, and are often affectionate and friendly.
- Extra time must be allowed for obtaining a history, and for performing assessment and patient care procedures.

Emotionally Impaired

- Persons with emotional impairments include those with the following:
  - Neurasthenia (nervous exhaustion)
  - Anxiety neurosis
  - Compulsion neurosis
  - Hysteria
- These disorders can result in a wide range of physical or mental symptoms attributed to mental stress in someone who is not psychotic.
- Signs and symptoms that may result from emotional impairment include somatic complaints such as chest discomfort, tachycardia, dyspnea, choking, and syncope.

- It is important to gather a complete history from the patient and perform a thorough examination to rule out serious illness.
- Pre-hospital care (in the absence of serious illness) is primarily supportive and includes calming measures and transport for physician evaluation.

Emotionally/Mentally Impaired

- Emotionally/mentally impaired (EMI) refers to persons who have impaired intellectual functioning (mental retardation) that results in an inability to cope with normal responsibilities of life.
- Mental retardation can be further classified with IQ assessment as:
  - Mild (IQ 50-70)
  - Moderate (IQ 35-59)
  - Profound (IQ <20)

Causes of Mental Retardation

- Genetic conditions
  - Phenylketonuria (PKU): a single-gene disorder caused by a defective enzyme
  - Chromosomal disorder (Down syndrome)
  - Fragile X syndrome: a single-gene disorder on the Y chromosome, the leading inherited cause of mental retardation
- Problems during pregnancy
  - Use of alcohol, tobacco, or other drugs by the mother
  - Illness and infection (toxoplasmosis, cytomegalovirus, rubella, syphilis, HIV)
- Problems at birth
  - Brain injury
  - Prematurity, low birth weight
- Problems after birth
  - Childhood diseases (whooping cough, chicken pox, measles, HIV disease)
  - Injury (head injury, near drowning)
  - Exposure to lead, mercury, and other environmental toxins
  - Poverty and cultural deprivation
  - Malnutrition
- Disease-producing conditions
  - Inadequate medical care
  - Environmental health hazards
  - Lack of stimulation
- Special considerations
  - Accommodations that may be necessary during patient care will vary by the patient's level of retardation.
  - Many with mild retardation will show no psychological symptoms apart from slowness in carrying out mental tasks.
- Those with moderate-to-severe retardation may have the following:
  - Limited-to-absent speech.
  - Neurological impairments are common.
  - These patients may require extra time and care in patient assessment, management, and transportation.

PATHOLOGICAL CHALLENGES

Physical injury and disease may result in pathological conditions that require special assessment and management skills.

Arthritis

- Arthritis refers to inflammation of a joint, characterized by pain, stiffness, swelling, and redness. Arthritis has many forms and varies widely in its effects.
- Osteoarthritis results from cartilage loss and wear and tear of the joints (common in elderly patients).
- Rheumatoid arthritis is an autoimmune disorder that damages joints and surrounding tissues.

Cancer

- A group of diseases that allow for an unrestrained growth of cells in one or more of the body organs or tissues.
- Malignant tumors most commonly develop in major organs, like the lungs, breasts, intestine, skin, stomach, and pancreas, but may also occur in cell-forming tissues of the bone marrow, and in the lymphatic system, muscle, or bone.
- Patients with cancer are often very ill. Signs and symptoms depend on the cancer's primary site of origin.
- Try to obtain a thorough history from the patient, including a list of all medications. Many cancer patients take anticancer drugs and pain medicine through surgically implanted ports, such as a Mediport. Transdermal skin patches that contain analgesic agents are also very common.

Cerebral Palsy

- Cerebral palsy (CP) is the general term for nonprogressive disorders of movement and posture resulting from damage to the fetal brain during later months of pregnancy, during birth, during the newborn period, or in early childhood.
- Most common cause is cerebral dysgenesis (abnormal cerebral development) or cerebral malformations.
- Less common causes include the following:
  - Fetal hypoxia
  - Birth trauma
  - Maternal infection
  - Kernicterus (excessive fetal bilirubin, associated with hemolytic disease)
  - Postpartum encephalitis, meningitis, or head injury

Spastic Paralysis

- Produces abnormal stiffness and contraction of groups of muscles.
- Child may be categorized as having one of the following conditions:
  - Diplegia—Affecting all four limbs; the legs more severely than the arms
  - Hemiplegia—Affecting limbs only on one side of the body; the arm usually more severely than the leg
  - Quadriplegia—Affecting all four limbs severely; not necessarily symmetrically

- ○ Athetosis—Producing involuntary writhing movements
- ○ Ataxia—Producing a loss of coordination and balance
- ○ Hearing defects, epilepsy, and other central nervous system (CNS) disorders are commonly present with the disease
- Weakness, paralysis, and developmental delay vary by the type and severity of disease.
- Some children with mild CP attend regular schools.
- Those with more severe forms of the disease never learn to walk or effectively communicate, and require lifelong skilled nursing care.
- Accommodations that may be required during an emergency call include allowing additional scene time for the physical examination and extra resources and manpower to facilitate transport.

Cystic Fibrosis (Mucoviscidosis)

- Cystic fibrosis (CF) is an inherited metabolic disease of the lungs and digestive system that manifests itself in childhood. It is caused by a defective recessive gene inherited from each parent. The defective gene causes the glands in the lining of the bronchi to produce excessive amounts of thick mucus and predisposes the individual to chronic lung infections. Additionally, the pancreas of a patient with CF fails to produce the enzymes required for the breakdown of fats and their absorption from the intestine.
- These alterations in metabolism cause classic symptoms of CF that include the following:
  - ○ Pale, greasy-looking, and foul-smelling stools (often noticeable soon after birth)
  - ○ Persistent cough and breathlessness
  - ○ Lung infections that often develop into pneumonia, bronchiectasis, and bronchitis
- Other features of the disease include stunted growth and sweat glands that produce abnormally salty sweat.
- In some cases, the child with CF may fail to thrive. Many patients survive into adulthood, although poor health is common.
- Older patients with CF are generally aware of their disease.
- Some may be oxygen-dependent and will require respiratory support and suctioning to clear the airway of mucus and secretions.
- Expect a lengthy history and physical examination due to the nature of the disease and associated medical problems.
- Some patients will have received heart and lung transplants, and may require transfer to specialized medical facilities for treatment.
- If parents are unaware of the possibility of CF in the presence of signs and symptoms described above, the EMT should advise the physician at the receiving hospital of his or her suspicions.

Multiple Sclerosis

- Multiple sclerosis (MS) is a progressive and incurable autoimmune disease of the CNS, in which scattered patches of myelin in the brain and spinal cord are destroyed.
- Scarring and destruction of the tissues cause symptoms that range from numbness and tingling to paralysis and incontinence.
- Cause of MS is unknown; however, it may have a heritable or viral component.

- Disease usually begins early in adult life, becomes active for a brief time, and then resumes years later.
- Symptoms vary with the affected areas of the CNS and may include:
  - Brain involvement
    - Fatigue
    - Vertigo
    - Clumsiness
    - Muscle weakness
    - Slurred speech
    - Ataxia
    - Blurred or double vision
    - Numbness, weakness, or pain in the face
  - Spinal cord involvement
    - Tingling, numbness, or feeling of constriction in any part of the body
    - Extremities that feel heavy and become weak
    - Spasticity
- Symptoms of MS may occur singly or in combination, and may last from several weeks to months.
- Attacks vary in intensity and may be precipitated by injury, infection, or physical or emotional stress.
- Some patients become disabled, bedridden, and incontinent early in middle life.
- Disabled patients also often suffer from painful muscle spasms, constipation, urinary tract infection, skin ulcerations, and mood swings.
- Disease is managed with medications, physical therapy, and counseling.
- Some patients with MS may be difficult to examine and may be unable to provide a complete medical history due to the nature of their illness.
- Allow extra time for patient assessment and to prepare the patient for transport. Patient should not be expected to ambulate.
- Respiratory support may be indicated in severe cases.

Muscular Dystrophy

- Inherited muscle disorder that results in a slow but progressive degeneration of muscle fibers.
- Classified according to the following:
  - Age that symptoms first appear
  - Rate at which the disease progresses
  - Way in which it is inherited
- Muscular dystrophy is incurable.
- Most common form of the disease is Duchenne muscular dystrophy.
  - Caused by a sex-linked, recessive gene that affects only males.
  - Rarely diagnosed before 3 years of age.
- Signs and symptoms include:
  - Child slow in learning to sit up and walk.
  - Unusual gait.
  - Curvature of the spine.
  - Muscles that become bulky as they are replaced by fat.

- ○ Eventually, most children will be unable to walk.
  - — Many do not live past their teenage years because of chronic lung infections and congestive heart failure.
- Accommodations that may be required during emergency care will depend on the person's age, weight, and severity of disease.
- Young children will be relatively easy to examine and prepare for transport.
- Older patients may require additional manpower and resources to assist with moving the patient to the ambulance.
- Respiratory support may be indicated in severe cases.

Poliomyelitis (Polio)

- Infectious disease caused by poliovirus hominis. Virus is spread through direct and indirect contact with infected feces and by airborne transmission.
- It attacks with variable severity, ranging from asymptomatic infection to a febrile illness without neurological sequelae to aseptic meningitis and finally to paralytic disease (including respiratory paralysis) and possible death.
- Incidence has declined since the Salk and Sabin vaccines were made available in the 1950s.
- May affect nonimmune adults and indigent children.
- Signs and symptoms of polio in both the nonparalytic and paralytic forms include the following:
  - ○ Fever
  - ○ Malaise
  - ○ Headache
  - ○ Intestinal upset
- Often, persons with the nonparalytic form of polio recover completely.
- In the paralytic form, extensive paralysis of muscles of the legs and lower trunk can occur.
- Caring for a patient with paralytic polio who has respiratory paralysis may require advanced airway support to ensure adequate ventilation.
- If the lower body is paralyzed, urinary catheterization may be indicated.
- Additional resources and manpower may be needed to prepare the patient for transport.

Previously Head-Injured Patients

- Traumatic brain injury can result from many mechanisms of trauma.
- These injuries can affect many cognitive, physical, and psychological skills.
- Cognitive deficits of language and communication, information processing, memory, and perceptual skills are common.
- Physical deficit can include ambulation, balance and coordination, fine motor skills, strength, and endurance.
- Psychological status also is often altered.
- Depending on the patient's area of brain injury, obtaining a history, and performing assessment and patient care procedures may be very difficult.
- Some patients may require restraint.
  - ○ Family members and other caregivers should:
  - ○ Be involved in managing the patient (when appropriate)

  ○ Be interviewed to determine if the patient's actions and responses are "normal" for the patient

  ○ Expect to spend additional time at the scene to provide care to these patients

Spina Bifida

- Congenital defect in which part of one or more vertebrae fails to develop, leaving part of the spinal cord exposed. Condition ranges in severity from minimal evidence of a defect to severe disability. In severe cases, the legs of some children may be deformed with partial or complete paralysis and loss of sensation in all areas below the level of the defect.
- Associated abnormalities may include:
  ○ Hydrocephalus with brain damage
  ○ Cerebral palsy
  ○ Epilepsy
  ○ Mental retardation
- Because of the varying degrees of spina bifida, pre-hospital care will need to be tailored to the patient's specific needs.
- Some patients will require no special accommodations.
- Others will need extended on-scene time for assessment and management, and perhaps additional resources and manpower to prepare the patient for transport.

Myasthenia Gravis

- Autoimmune disorder in which muscles become weak and tire easily.
- Damage occurs to muscle receptors that are responsible for transmitting nerve impulses, commonly affecting muscles of the eyes, face, throat, and extremities.
- Rare disease that can begin suddenly or gradually.
- Can occur at any age, but usually appears in women between age 20 and 30, and in men between 70 and 80 years of age.
- Classic signs and symptoms include:
  ○ Drooping eyelids, double vision
  ○ Difficulty in speaking
  ○ Difficulty in chewing and swallowing
  ○ Difficult extremity movement
  ○ Weakened respiratory muscles
- Affected muscles become worse with use, but may recover completely with rest.
- May be exacerbated by infection, stress, medications, and menstruation.
- Can often be controlled with drug therapy to enhance the transmission of nerve impulses in the muscles.
- In a small number of patients, the disease will progress to paralysis of the throat and respiratory muscles, and may lead to death.
- Accommodations required for care vary based on the patient's presentation.
- In most cases, supportive care and transport will be all that is required.
- In the presence of respiratory distress, measures should be taken to ensure adequate airway and ventilatory support.

CULTURALLY DIVERSE PATIENTS

- Individuals vary in many ways, and there is enormous diversity in populations of all cultures. Diversity (a term once used primarily to describe "racial awareness") now refers to differences of any kind: race, class, religion, gender, sexual preference, personal habitat, and physical ability.
- Experiences of health and illness vary widely because of different beliefs, behaviors, and past experiences may conflict with the EMT's learned medical practice.
- By revealing awareness of cultural issues, the EMT will convey interest, concern, and respect.
- When dealing with patients from different cultures, remember the following key points:
  - The individual is the "foreground"—the culture is the "background."
  - Different generations and individuals within the same family may have different sets of beliefs.
  - Not all people identify with their ethnic cultural background.
  - All people share common problems or situations.
  - Respect the integrity of cultural beliefs.
  - Realize that people may not share your explanations of the causes of their ill health, but may accept conventional treatments.
  - You do not have to agree with every aspect of another's culture, nor does the person have to accept everything about yours for effective and culturally sensitive health care to occur.
  - Recognize your personal cultural assumptions, prejudices, and belief systems and do not let them interfere with patient care.
- Regardless of the patient's cultural background, educational status, occupation, or ability to speak English, most patients will be anxious during an emergency event.
- Attempt to communicate in English first to determine whether the patient understands or speaks some English words or phrases.
- Bystanders, coworkers, or family members may be available to provide assistance.
- If the patient does not speak or understand English, attempt to communicate with signs or gestures.
- Notify the receiving hospital as soon as possible to arrange for an interpreter.
- If time permits, all assessment procedures should be performed slowly and with the patient's permission.
- Be aware that "private space" is culturally defined.
- Pointing to the area of the body to be examined before touching the patient is best.
- Respect the patient's need for modesty and privacy at the scene and during transport.

TERMINALLY ILL PATIENTS

EMTs will care for terminally ill patients (patients with advanced stages of disease with an unfavorable prognosis and no known cure). These will often be emotionally charged encounters that will require a great deal of empathy and compassion for the patient and his or her loved ones. If emotions at the scene are out of control, it will be important for the EMT to take control and to calm the people involved. If emergency medical services (EMS) have been summoned to assess late stages of a patient's terminal illness or a change in the patient's condition, gather a complete history and ask the patient or family about advance directives and the appropriateness of resuscitation procedures. Carefully review any documentation made available to the EMS crew (a do-not-resuscitate [DNR] order) and consult with medical direction so that appropriate patient care decisions can be made.

Special Considerations

- Care of a terminally ill patient will often be primarily supportive and limited to calming and comfort measures, and perhaps transport for physician evaluation.
- Pain assessment and management are important in caring for these patients.
- Attempt to gather a complete pain medication history.
- Examine the patient for the presence of transdermal drug patches or other pain-relief devices.
- Following an assessment of the patient's vital signs, level of consciousness, and medication history, medical direction may recommend the administration of analgesics or sedatives to ensure the patient's comfort.

PATIENTS WITH COMMUNICABLE DISEASES

- Exposure to some infectious diseases can pose a significant health risk to EMS providers. It is important to ensure personal protection on every emergency response. Required precautions will depend on the mode of transmission and the pathogen's ability to create pathological processes.
- In some cases, gloves will provide for necessary protection.
- In other cases, respiratory barriers will also be indicated.

Special Considerations

- Some infectious diseases (acquired immunodeficiency syndrome [AIDS]) will take a toll on the emotional well-being of affected patients, their families, and loved ones.
- Psychological aspects of providing care to these patients include an emphasis on the following:
  - Recognizing each patient as an individual with unique health-care needs
  - Respecting each person's personal dignity
  - Providing considerate, respectful care focused on the person's individual needs

FINANCIAL CHALLENGES

- It is estimated that 41 million Americans and one-third of persons living in poverty have no health insurance, and insurance coverage held by many others would not carry them through a catastrophic illness.
- Financial challenges for health care can quickly result from loss of a job and depletion of savings.
- Financial challenges combined with medical conditions that require uninterrupted treatment (tuberculosis [TB], HIV/AIDS, diabetes, hypertension, mental disorders) or that occur in the presence of unexpected illness or injury can deprive the patient of basic health-care services.

- In addition, poor health is closely associated with homelessness, where rates of chronic or acute health problems are extremely high.
- Persons with financial challenges are often apprehensive about seeking medical care.
- Fortunately, the patient's ability to pay for emergency health care generally is not a concern for EMS providers.
- When caring for a patient with financial challenges who is concerned about the cost of receiving needed health care, explain the following:
  - Patient's ability to pay should never be a factor in obtaining emergency health care.
  - Federal law mandates that quality emergency health care be provided, regardless of the patient's ability to pay.
  - Payment programs for health-care services are available in most hospitals.
  - Government services are available to assist patients in paying for health care.
  - Free (or near-free) health-care services are available through local, state, and federally funded organizations.
- In cases where no life-threatening condition exists, counsel the patient with financial challenges about alternative facilities for health care that do not require ambulance transport for emergency department evaluation.
- Consider providing an approved list of alternative health-care sites that can provide medical care at less cost than those charged by emergency departments.

? CHAPTER QUESTIONS

1. Cystic fibrosis is an inherited metabolic disease of the lungs and digestive system that manifests itself in childhood; it is caused by a defective recessive gene inherited from each parent.

   a. True
   b. False

2. Congenital defect, in which part of one or more vertebrae fails to develop, leaving part of the spinal cord exposed.

   a. Spina bifida
   b. Myasthenia gravis
   c. Polio
   d. None of the above

Suggested Reading

US Department of Transportation, National Highway Traffic Safety Administration. *EMT Paramedic: National Standard Curriculum.* Washington, DC: US Department of Transportation, National Highway Traffic Safety Administration; 1998.

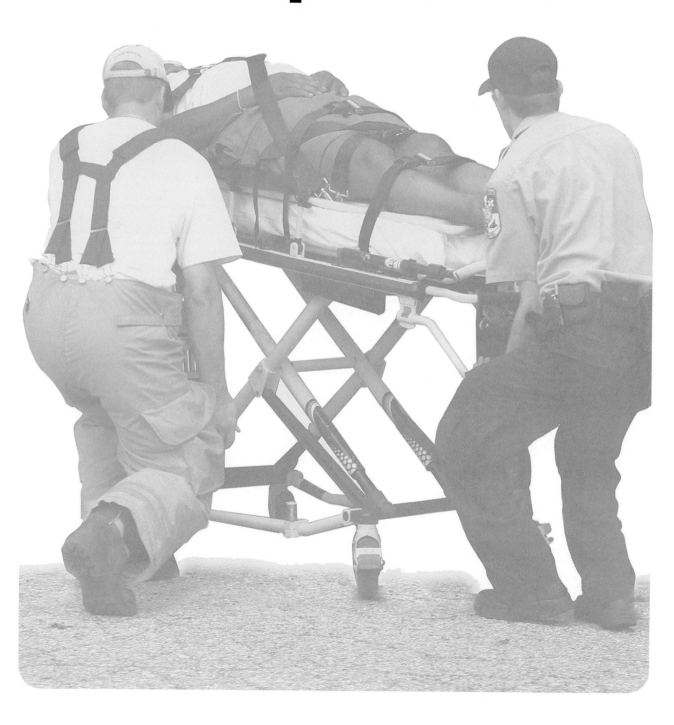

Section 8
EMS Operations

Chapter 33
Lifting and Moving Patients

Your ambulance is dispatched to an 18-story multiple dwelling. Dispatch data state you are responding for a person with abdominal pain in the hallway of the 17th floor. Upon arrival at the scene, you enter the lobby of the building and summon an elevator. The elevator arrives and you and your partner realize the stretcher will not fit in the elevator. Your partner runs out and gets the stair chair from the ambulance while you hold the elevator. When you arrive on the 17th floor, you find a patient in his 20s complaining of abdominal pain. You open the stair chair and have the patient sit down while you elicit a medical history. You begin to move the patient downstairs to the ambulance using a stair chair for patient transport.

BODY MECHANICS

- Proper body mechanics while lifting include:
  - Using your legs, not your back, to lift
  - Keeping weight as close to your body as possible
- Guidelines for lifting include:
  - Consider weight of patient and need for additional help.
  - Know physical ability and limitations.
  - Lift without twisting.
  - Have feet positioned properly.
  - Communicate clearly and frequently with partner.
- Safe lifting of cots and stretchers. When possible, use a stretcher having a mechanical lift (Fig. 33-1).
  - When possible, use a stair chair instead of a stretcher if medically appropriate.
  - Know or find out the weight to be lifted.
  - Use at least two people.
  - Ensure enough help is available. Use an even number of people to lift so that balance is maintained.
  - Know or find out the weight limitations of equipment being used. (Average new-style stretchers have a 700-lb maximum weight limit.)
  - Know what to do with patients who exceed weight limitations of equipment.
  - Using power-lift or squat-lift position (best defense against injury), keep back locked into normal curvature. The power-lift position is useful for individuals with weak knees or thighs. The feet are a comfortable distance apart. The back is tight and the abdominal muscles

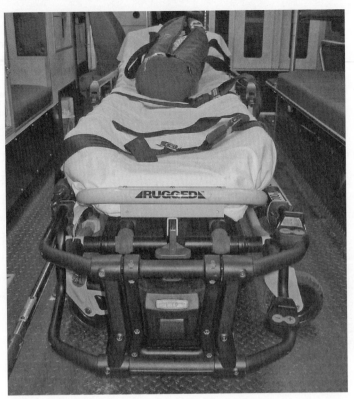

Figure 33-1   Mechanical lift stretcher (Stryker). *(Used with permission of Peter DiPrima)*

lock the back in a slight inward curve. Straddle the object. Keep feet flat. Distribute weight to balls of feet or just behind them. Stand by making sure the back is locked in and the upper body comes up before the hips.

- Use power grip to get maximum force from hands. The palm and fingers come into complete contact with the object and all fingers are bent at the same angles. The power grip should always be used in lifting. This allows for maximum force to be developed. Hands should be at least 10 in apart.
- Lift while keeping back in locked-in position.
- When lowering cot or stretcher, reverse steps.
- Avoid bending at the waist.

- Carrying precautions
  - Transport on devices that can be rolled.
  - Know or find out the weight to be lifted.
  - Know limitations of the crew's abilities.
  - Work in a coordinated manner and communicate with partners.
  - Keep the weight as close to the body as possible.
  - Keep back in a locked-in position and refrain from twisting.
  - Flex at the hips, not the waist; bend at the knees.
  - Do not hyperextend the back (do not lean back from the waist).

- One-handed carrying technique
  - Pick up and carry with the back in the locked-in position.
  - Avoid leaning to either side to compensate for the imbalance.

- Correct carrying procedure on stairs
  - When possible, use a stair chair instead of a stretcher.
  - Keep back in locked-in position.
  - Flex at the hips, not the waist; bend at the knees.
  - Keep weight and arms as close to the body as possible.
- Reaching
  - Keep back in locked-in position.
  - When reaching overhead, avoid hyperextended position.
  - Avoid twisting the back while reaching.
  - Avoid reaching in front of the body for long periods.
  - Avoid situations where prolonged (more than a minute) strenuous effort is needed in order to avoid injury.
- Log rolling a patient
  - Keep back straight while leaning over patient.
  - Lean from the hips.
  - Use shoulder muscles to help with roll.
- Pushing and pulling guidelines
  - Push, rather than pull, whenever possible.
  - Keep back locked-in position.
  - Keep line of pull through center of the body by bending knees.
  - Keep weight close to the body.
  - Push from the area between the waist and shoulder.
  - If weight is below waist level, use kneeling position.
  - Avoid pushing or pulling from an overhead position, if possible.
  - Keep elbows bent with arms close to the sides.

PRINCIPLES OF MOVING PATIENTS

- As a general rule, a patient should be moved immediately (emergency move) only when there is a/an:
  - Immediate danger to the patient if not moved.
  - Fire or danger of fire.
  - Explosives or other hazardous materials.
  - Inability to protect the patient from other hazards at the scene.
  - Inability to gain access to other patients in a vehicle who need life-saving care.
  - Life-saving care cannot be given because of the patient's location or position.
- A patient should be moved quickly (urgent move) when there is immediate threat to life.
  - Altered mental status
  - Inadequate breathing
  - Shock (hypoperfusion)
- If there is no threat to life, the patient should be moved when ready for transportation (nonurgent move).

Using Emergency Moves

- The greatest danger in moving a trauma patient quickly is the possibility of aggravating a spine injury.

- In an emergency, every effort should be made to pull the patient in the direction of the long axis of the body to provide as much protection to the spine as possible.
- It is impossible to remove a patient from a vehicle quickly and at the same time provide as much protection to the spine as can be accomplished with an interim immobilization device.
- If the patient is on the floor or ground, they can be moved by:
    - Pulling on the patient's clothing in the neck and shoulder area.
    - Putting the patient on a blanket and dragging the blanket.
    - Putting the emergency medical technician's (EMT's) hands under the patient's armpits (from the back), grasping the patient's forearms, and dragging the patient.
- Rapid extrication of a patient sitting in vehicle involves the following processes:
    - One EMT gets behind the patient and brings the cervical spine into a neutral in-line position and provides manual immobilization.
    - A second EMT applies a cervical immobilization device as the third EMT first places the long backboard near the door and then moves to the passenger seat.
    - The second EMT supports the thorax as the third EMT frees the patient's legs from the pedals.
    - At the direction of the second EMT, he (the first EMT) and the third EMT rotate the patient in several short, coordinated moves until the patient's back is in the open doorway and his feet are on the passenger seat.
    - Since the first EMT usually cannot support the patient's head any longer, another available EMT or a bystander supports the patient's head as the first EMT gets out of the vehicle and takes support of the head outside of the vehicle.
    - The end of the long backboard is placed on the seat next to the patient's buttocks. Assistants support the other end of the board as the first EMT and the second EMT lower the patient onto it.
    - The second EMT and the third EMT slide the patient into the proper position on the board in short, coordinated moves.
    - Several variations of the technique are possible, including assistance from bystanders. This must be accomplished without compromise to the spine.

Using Nonemergent Moves

Direct Ground Lift (No Suspected Spine Injury)

- Two or three rescuers line up on one side of the patient.
- Rescuers kneel on one knee (preferably the same for all rescuers).
- The patient's arms are placed on his chest, if possible.
- The rescuer at the head places one arm under the patient's neck and shoulder and cradles the patient's head. He places his other arm under the patient's lower back.
- The second rescuer places one arm under the patient's knees and one arm above the buttocks.
- If a third rescuer is available, he should place both arms under the waist and the other two rescuers slide their arms either up to the midback or down to the buttocks, as appropriate.

- On signal, the rescuers lift the patient to their knees and roll the patient in toward their chests.
- On signal, the rescuers stand and move the patient to the stretcher.
- To lower the patient, the steps are reversed.

Extremity Lift (No Suspected Extremity Injuries)

- One rescuer kneels at the patient's head and one kneels at the patient's side by his knees.
- The rescuer at the head places one hand under each of the patient's shoulders while the rescuer at the foot grasps the patient's wrists.
- The rescuer at the head slips his hands under the patient's arms and grasps the patient's wrists.
- The rescuer at the patient's foot slips his hands under the patient's knees.
- Both rescuers move up to a crouching position.
- The rescuers stand up simultaneously and move with the patient to a stretcher.

Transfer of Supine Patient From Bed to Stretcher Direct Carry

- Position cot perpendicular to bed with head end of cot at foot of bed.
- Unbuckle straps.
- Both rescuers stand between bed and stretcher, facing patient.
- First rescuer slides arm under patient's neck and cups patient's shoulder.
- Second rescuer slides hand under hip and lifts slightly.
- First rescuer slides other arm under patient's back.
- Second rescuer places arms underneath hips and calves.
- Rescuers slide patient to edge of bed.
- Patient is lifted/curled toward the rescuers' chests.
- Rescuers rotate and place patient gently onto cot.

Draw Sheet Method

- Loosen bottom sheet of bed.
- Position cot next to bed.
- Prepare cot-adjust height, lower rails, unbuckle straps.
- Reach across cot and grasp sheet firmly at patient's head, chest, hips, and knees.
- Slide patient gently onto cot.

Proper Patient Positioning During Transport

- An unresponsive patient without suspected spine injury should be moved into the recovery position by rolling the patient onto his side (preferably the left) without twisting the body.
- A patient with chest pain or discomfort or difficulty in breathing should sit in a position of comfort as long as hypotension is not present.
- A patient with suspected spine injury should be immobilized on a long backboard.
- A patient in shock (hypoperfusion) should have his legs elevated 8 to 12 in.

- For the pregnant patient with hypotension, an early intervention is to position the patient on her left side.
- A patient who is nauseated or vomiting should be transported in a position of comfort; however, the EMT should be positioned appropriately to manage the airway.

? CHAPTER QUESTIONS

1. When lifting a heavy object, avoid using the muscles of your:

   a. back
   b. arms
   c. shoulders
   d. legs

2. When performing a log roll, an EMT should:

   a. bend over the patient
   b. lean from the hips
   c. twist and pull simultaneously
   d. lean from the waist

3. The preferred device for carrying a conscious medical patient down a flight of stairs is the:

   a. stair chair
   b. reeves sleeve
   c. ambulance stretcher
   d. backboard

4. All of the following techniques will help prevent injuries when lifting or moving patients *except* the:

   a. power lift
   b. back lift
   c. power grip
   d. squat lift

Chapter 34
Ambulance Operations

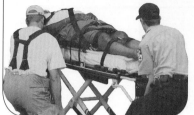

PHASES OF AN AMBULANCE CALL

Preassignment Operations and Check

- Preparation for the call
  - Necessary equipment needed for a medical assignment include:
    — Basic supplies
    — Patient transfer equipment
    — Airways
    — Suction equipment
    — Artificial ventilation devices
    — Oxygen inhalation equipment
    — Cardiac compression equipment
    — Basic wound care supplies
    — Splinting supplies
    — Childbirth supplies
    — Medications
    — Automated external defibrillator
  - Essential nonmedical equipment needed include:
    — Personal safety equipment per local, state, and federal standards
    — Preplanned routes or comprehensive street maps
- Personnel requirements
  - At least one emergency medical technician (EMT) in patient compartment is minimum staffing for an ambulance, two are preferred.
- Daily inspections of the vehicle systems include:
  - Fuel (Tank should be full.)
  - Oil (Level should be checked at the beginning of every tour/shift.) (Fig. 34-1)
  - Engine cooling system
  - Battery
  - Brakes (test)
  - Wheels and tires (Adequate tread should be on every tire for adequate traction.)

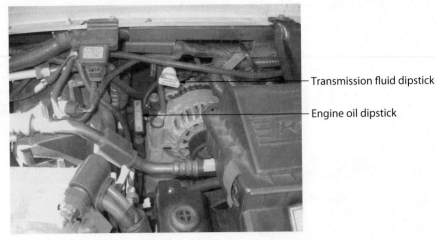

Figure 34-1 Under the hood of an ambulance.

- Headlights (working properly)
- Stoplights (working properly)
- Turn signals (working properly)
- Emergency warning lights (working properly)
- Wipers (working properly)
- Horn (working properly)
- Siren (working properly)
- Doors closing and latching (working properly)
- Communication system (working properly)
- Air conditioning/heating system/ventilation system (working properly)
- Equipment
  - Should be checked, maintained, restocked, and repaired as required.
  - Batteries for defibrillator, suction should be at full charge and ready for use.

Assignment Operations

Dispatch Center

- Central access
- Twenty-four-hour availability
- Trained dispatch personnel (emergency medical dispatch [EMD] certified)
- Dispatch information for responding units include:
  - Nature of call
  - Name, location, and callback number of caller
  - Location of patient
  - Number of patients and severity
  - Other special problems

En Route

- Seat belts should be worn.
- Notify dispatch (acknowledge assignment).

- Ascertain essential information.
  - Nature of the call
  - Location of the call
- Driving the ambulance with due regard for the public during emergency vehicle operations and nonemergency situations.
- Characteristics of good ambulance operators are:
  - Physically fit
  - Mentally fit
  - Able to perform under stress
  - Positive attitude about abilities
  - Tolerant of other drivers
- Safe driving is as important as providing emergency medical care to the ill or injured patient (Fig. 34-2).
  - The driver and all passengers should wear safety belts.
  - Become familiar with the characteristics of your vehicle.
  - Be alert to changes in weather and road conditions.
  - Exercise caution in use of red lights and siren.
  - Select appropriate route.
  - Maintain safe following distance.
  - Drive with due regard for safety of all others.
  - Know appropriateness of using lights and sirens.
  - Headlights are the most visible warning device on an emergency vehicle.
- Obtain additional information from dispatch.
- Assign personnel to specific duties.
- Assess specific equipment needs.
- Positioning the unit requires:
  - For safety.

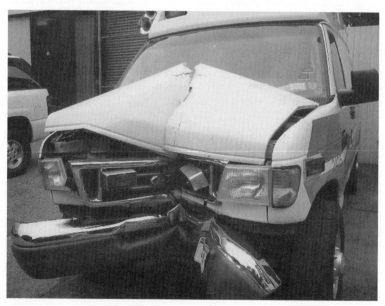

Figure 34-2 Ambulance accident. An ambulance on its way to a hospital swerved into an elevated train support attempting to avoid an oncoming vehicle. *(Used with permission of Peter DiPrima)*

- Uphill from leaking hazards.
- About 100 ft from wreckage.
- In front of the wreckage or beyond the wreckage.
- Set parking brake.
- Utilize warning lights.
- Shut off headlights unless there is a need to illuminate the scene.
- To exit the scene, avoid parking in a location that will hamper exit from the scene.
- Review state and local laws, regulations, or ordinances in the area relative to the operations of an emergency vehicle, including:
    - Vehicle parking or standing
    - Procedures at red lights, stop signs, and intersections
    - Regulations regarding speed limits
    - Direction of flow or specified turns
    - Emergency or disaster routes
    - Use of audible warning devices
    - Use of visual warning devices
    - Laws regarding a school bus

Escorts and Multiple Vehicle Response

- Extremely dangerous.
- Used only if unfamiliar with location of patient or receiving facility.
- No vehicle should use lights or siren.
- Provide a safe following distance.
- Recognize hazards of multiple vehicle response.

Intersection crashes (most common type of ambulance crash)

- Motorist arriving at intersection as light changes and does not stop.
- Multiple emergency vehicles following closely, and an awaiting motorist does not expect more than one, and vision is obstructed by vehicles.

Arrival at Scene

(Fig. 34-3)

- Notify dispatch.
- Size-up.
    - Body substance isolation
    - Scene safety—Assess the scene for hazards
    - Mechanism of injury/nature of illness includes:
        — Medical
            - Mass casualty incident.
            - Determine the number of patients.
            - Obtain additional help as needed.
            - Begin triage.
            - Provide C-spine stabilization as necessary.
        — Trauma
            - Mass casualty incident.
            - Number of patients.

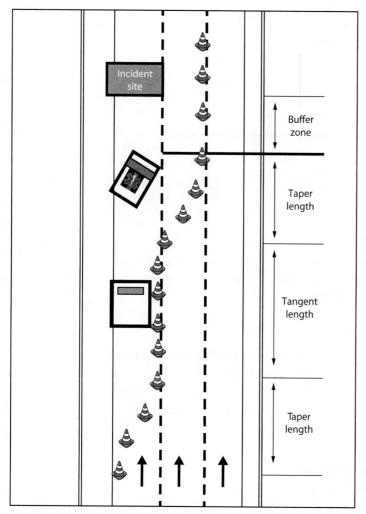

Figure 34-3 Proper rig placement at an accident scene. *(Used with permission of Peter DiPrima)*

- Obtain additional help.
- Begin triage.
- Spine stabilization if necessary.
- Total number of patients.
- Need for additional help or assistance.

Actions at the Scene

- Be organized.
- Perform rapid/efficient treatment.
- Goal of transport in mind.

Transferring the Patient to the Ambulance

- Prepare the patient for transport.
- Completion of critical interventions.
- Check dressings and splints.
- Patient is covered and secured to moving device.
- Lifting and moving is accomplished using the guidelines found in Chap. 33.

En Route to the Receiving Facility

- Notify dispatch.
- Ongoing assessment should be continued.
- Additional vital sign measurements should be obtained.
- Notify receiving facility.
- Reassure patient.
- Complete pre-hospital care reports.

At Receiving Facility

- Notify dispatch.
- Transfer the patient at the facility.

Reports

- A complete verbal report is given at bedside.
- A complete written report is completed, and left prior to returning to service.

En Route to Station

- At station or receiving facility, notify dispatch.
- Prepare for the next call. Restock supplies that were used.
- Clean and disinfect the ambulance as needed.
- Clean and disinfect ambulance equipment.

Post Run

- Refuel unit.
- File reports.
- Complete cleaning and disinfection procedures.
- Notify dispatch.

AIR MEDICAL CONSIDERATION—UTILIZATION, LANDING ZONES, AND SAFETY

- When requesting a Medevac, provide:
  - Your agency
  - Location of incident (cross streets)
  - Landing zone (LZ) information
  - LZ sector name
  - Patient information
  - Radio frequency you are operating on

LZ PREPARATION

- The LZ should be 100 × 100 ft, clear of overhead wires, free from debris, level flat, and clearly marked (Fig. 34-4).
- Turn off any lights that could blind the pilot during landing and takeoff.

During and After Landing

- Never approach the tail rotor.
- Protect the patient and yourself from rotor wash.

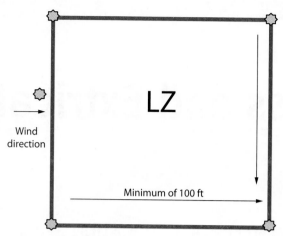

Figure 34-4 Landing zone.

? CHAPTER QUESTIONS

1. The phases of an ambulance call include all of the following *except*:

   a. daily vehicle and equipment inspection
   b. billing and collections
   c. en route to the receiving facility
   d. en route to the scene

2. Use of escort vehicles during an emergency response is often a:

   a. very quick way to respond
   b. more dangerous means of response and increases the chance for collision
   c. means of decreasing an ambulance collision
   d. way to make the driver's job easier

3. Emergency vehicle operators must drive with the safety of others in mind. This concept is known as driving:

   a. within the law
   b. with due regard
   c. in the emergency mode
   d. within intent

Chapter 35
Gaining Access and Extrication

FUNDAMENTALS OF EXTRICATION

- Role of the emergency medical technician (EMT) in nonrescue emergency medical services (EMS) includes:
  - Administer necessary care to the patient before extrication and assure that the patient is removed in a way to minimize further injury.
  - Patient care precedes extrication unless delayed movement would endanger life of the patient or rescuer.
  - Working with others includes:
    — The nonrescue EMS provider will need to work together with the providers of rescue.
    — The nonrescue EMT should cooperate with the activities of the rescuers, and not allow their activities to interfere with patient care.
- Role of the EMT in rescue EMS includes:
  - In some instances, the EMS providers are also the rescue providers.
  - A chain of command should be established to assure patient care priorities.
    — Administer necessary care to the patient before extrication and assure that the patient is removed in a way to minimize further injury.
    — Patient care precedes extrication unless delayed movement would endanger life of the patient or rescuer.

EQUIPMENT

- Basic equipment should be on the ambulance at all times (Fig. 35-1)

PERSONAL SAFETY

- The number-one priority for all EMS personnel.
- Protective clothing that is appropriate for the situation should be utilized.

PATIENT SAFETY

Following the safety of the EMS responders, the next priority is the safety of the patient.

- The patient should be informed of the unique aspects of extrication.
- The patient should be protected from broken glass, sharp metal, and other hazards, including the environment.

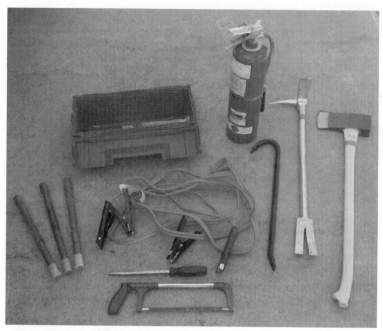

Figure 35-1 Basic equipment carried on an ambulance. *(Used with permission of Peter DiPrima)*

GETTING TO THE PATIENT

Simple access does not require equipment.

- Try opening each door.
- Roll down windows.
- Have patient unlock doors.

Complex access requires use of tools, special equipment. These are separate programs that should be taken (trench, high angle, and basic vehicle rescue).

REMOVING THE PATIENT

- Maintain cervical-spine stabilization. Immobilize spine securely.
- Complete initial assessment, provide critical interventions.

? CHAPTER QUESTIONS

1. When gaining access to a patient, the EMT should:

    a. try opening each door

    b. roll down windows

    c. have patient unlock doors, if capable

    d. all of the above are correct

2. The number-one priority at any EMS assignment is crew safety.

    a. True

    b. false

Chapter 36

Incident Management

We are in the middle of a very busy hurricane season. The National Weather Service (NWS) has issued a hurricane warning for your response area, with probable landfall in the late evening of the following day. The NWS estimates the hurricane to hit your location with sustained winds of over 140 mph (category 4 storm).

Category 4 is classified as:

Winds: 131 to 155 mph.

Damage: extreme, almost total destruction of doors, windows. Some wall and roof failure. Major damage to lower floors of oceanfront buildings. Evacuations up to 6 mi inland. Pressure 27.17 to 27.90 in accompanied by a storm surge of 13 to 18 ft.

Local government is calling for a mandatory evacuation of all coastal areas. You are assigned through dispatch to respond to one of the local nursing homes and report to the southwest evacuation officer in-charge of evacuating nonambulatory patients from this facility.

Upon arrival, you report to the command site of this facility and meet up with the southwest evacuation officer. She orders you and your partner to report to the third floor with your stretcher and necessary equipment to operate. Upon arrival on the third floor, you report what resources will be required for patient evacuation.

Who will you report your findings to, and who will be responsible for supplying the necessary equipment and staff to aid in the evacuation?

HOMELAND SECURITY PRESIDENTIAL DIRECTIVE 5

"To prevent, prepare for, respond to, and recover from terrorist attacks, major disasters, and other emergencies, the US Government shall establish a single, comprehensive approach to domestic incident management. The objective of the US Government is to ensure that all levels of government across the Nation have the capability to work efficiently and effectively together, using a national approach to domestic incident management."

WHAT IS THE NATIONAL INCIDENT MANAGEMENT SYSTEM?

National Incident Management System (NIMS) is a core set of:

- Doctrine
- Concepts
- Principles

- Terminology
- Organizational processes that is applicable to all hazards

NIMS has six components:

- Command and management
- Preparedness
- Resource management
- Communications and information management
- Supporting technologies
- Ongoing management and maintenance

Command and Management

NIMS standardizes incident management for all hazards across all levels of government. It is based on three key constructs:

- Incident command system
- Multiagency coordination systems
- Public information systems

Preparedness

It establishes measures and capabilities that all agencies should develop.

Resource Management

Standardization in describing and tracking inventory before, during, and after an incident

Communications and Information Management

Effective communications, information management, and intelligence sharing are paramount in operating at a domestic incident.

Supporting Technologies

Provide an architecture for science and technology support to incident management.

Ongoing Management

The Department of Homeland Security will establish a multijurisdictional, multidisciplinary NIMS integration center.

Disasters

It is important to remember that the term disaster has a specific legal meaning. States and localities declare "state of emergency." The President declares "major disasters."

Types of Disasters

Several events have the potential to cause mass casualty incidents (MCI):

- Natural disasters (floods, winter storms, hurricanes, tornados) (Figs. 36-1 and 36-2)

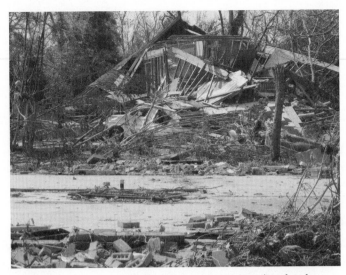

Figure 36-1   Destruction left by Hurricane Katrina. *(Used with permission of Peter DiPrima)*

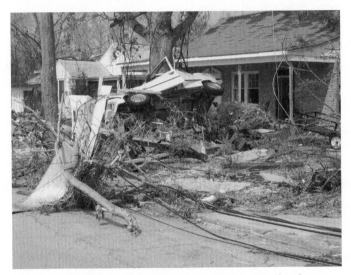

Figure 36-2   The aftermath of Hurricane Katrina. *(Used with permission of Peter DiPrima)*

- Technical hazards (hazardous materials [haz-mat] incidents, building collapse)
- Transportation accidents (road, rail, aircraft, ship, etc)
- Civil and political disorder (demonstrations, strikes, riots)
- Criminal or terrorist incidents (Fig. 36-3)

Mass Casualty Incidents

A mass casualty incident is any incident that injures or causes illness in enough people to overwhelm the resources usually available in a particular system or region.

Goals of MCI Management

- Do the greatest good for the greatest number.
- Manage scarce resources.

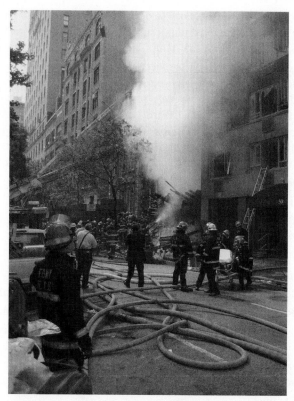

Figure 36-3 A building explosion/collapse was caused by an individual who filled the four-story building with natural gas. *(Used with permission of Peter DiPrima)*

- Do not relocate the disaster.
- MCIs place great demands on resources, including equipment, rescuers, and facilities. Our goal as responders is not to relocate the disaster!
- Patient prioritization at the scene is important for effective patient distribution.
- Don't send all of the red tag patients to one hospital.

STAGES OF AN INCIDENT

- Initial notification
- Implementation
- Operations
- Escalation
- Stabilization
- De-escalation
- Termination

EMS INITIAL RESPONSE ROLES AND RESPONSIBILITIES

Initial response roles—Emergency medical services (EMS) is a specific component of the overall incident management system. The first arriving unit should start the following actions:

- *First arriving unit*—The first emergency response unit to arrive at a mass casualty incident is by default "in charge" (the incident commander) until relieved. As a result, the individuals on the first emergency response unit must take immediate actions to begin to manage the entire incident. These actions may be the most important steps taken in the entire incident. The initial unit must resist the "temptation" to begin one-on-one patient care.

- *Assess scene for safety*—The object is to ensure no one else gets hurt. Assess the scene for safety much as you would for a normal response to any EMS incident, except that the scene is much bigger and requires a wider look. The following may pose a hazard: (1) fire, (2) electrical hazards, (3) spilled or contained flammable liquids, (4) hazardous materials, (5) nuclear, chemical, or biological agents, (6) other life threats, (7) debris that poses a threat to rescuers or their vehicles, and (8) secondary explosions.
- *Scene size-up*—How big is the incident and how bad is it?
  - Type of incident
  - Approximate number of patients
  - Severity of injuries
  - Area involved, including problems with scene access
- *Confirmation of incident*
  - Report situation—Contact dispatch with your size-up information.
  - Request assistance—Resources and mutual aid if needed.
  - Notify the Medical Command Center to ensure rapid hospital notification.
- *Set up*—Set up the scene for the best management of mass casualties by on-scene and responding resources, including:
  - Staging.
  - Secure access and egress.
  - Secure adequate space for work areas.
    - Triage, treatment, transportation

SIMPLE TRIAGE AND RAPID TREATMENT

Triage

Triage is a French word meaning "to sort."

Purpose of Triage

- Assigns treatment priorities.
- Separates MCI victims into easily identifiable groups.
- Determines required resources for treatment, transportation, and definitive care.
- Prioritizes patient distribution and transportation.

Benefits of Triage

- Identifies patients who require rapid medical care to save life and limb.
- Provides rational distribution of casualties.
- Separating the minor injuries reduces the urgent burden on each hospital— An average of 10% to 15% of MCI patients are serious enough to require extended hospitalization.

What Is START?

Simple triage and rapid treatment (START) was developed by Hoag Hospital and the Newport Beach Fire Department to be used in the event of an MCI.

- START enables EMS providers to triage patients at an MCI in less than 60 seconds and is based on three observations:
  - Respirations
  - Circulation
  - Mental status

This triage method assures rapid initial assessment of all patients as the basis for assignment to treatment and as the first medical assessment of the incident.

So how does it work?

- Begin where you are.
- Relocate green (minor) tag patients.
- Move in an orderly pattern, tagging patients as you go.
- Maintain count (how many red, yellow, black, and green tags).
- Provide minimal treatment.

START permits rescuers to quickly and accurately categorize patients into four treatment groups:

- *Red*—Immediate (highest priority). Typical problems are:
  1. R = Respirations/airway
  2. P = Perfusion/pulse
  3. M = Mental status
- *Yellow*—Delayed (second priority). Typical problems are:
  1. Burn patients without airway problems
  2. Major or multiple bone or joint injuries
  3. Back and spine injuries
- *Green*—Minor (third priority). Typical problems are:
  1. "Walking wounded" (The ability to "walk" does not necessarily mean that this is a "minor" patient. Minor cuts and bruises are acceptable criteria for this type of patient.)
  2. Minor painful swollen deformities
  3. Minor soft tissue injuries
- *Black*—Dead/nonsalvageable (lowest priority) (These are nonbreathing patients whose resuscitation would normally be attempted but who are not salvageable given the resources available early in an MCI response.)

The START Process

1. Begin where you stand.
2. Identify those injured who can walk. Make a clear announcement that those who can walk should get up and do so to an easily recognized point.

Relocate Green Patients

1. Relocate to a designated area (away from immediate danger and outside the initial triage area).
2. Tag each of these as a green patient.

Triage Patients in an Orderly Pattern

1. Move through the patients in an orderly pattern.
2. Assess each casualty and mark the category using triage ribbons or triage tags.

Maintain a Patient Count

1. Maintain a count of the casualties.
2. Mark on 2 to 3 in tape on thigh.
3. Save a small piece of triage ribbon and place in your pocket.

Steps in START Assessment

(Fig. 36-4)

- *Step 1—Move green tag patients.*
- *Step 2—Respiration.* Check for respiratory compromise.
    - If airway is closed, open the airway.
    - *None—black* tag (dead).
    - More than 30 breaths/min—*red* tag (immediate).
    - Less than 30 breaths/min—*further evaluation required*—go to Step 3 (perfusion).
- *Step 3—Perfusion.* Radial pulse check.
    - Not palpable—*red* tag (immediate).
    - Control severe bleeding—bystanders use direct pressure, raise legs.
    - Palpable—*further evaluation required*—go to Step 4 (mental status).
- *Step 4—Mental status.* Check for compromise of mental status.
    - Altered mental status—*red* tag (immediate).
    - Mental status appropriate—*yellow* tag (delayed) or green (minor) according to other findings (obvious injuries or illnesses).

Secondary Triage

Secondary triage and tagging can be done:

- On a stretcher on the way to a treatment area

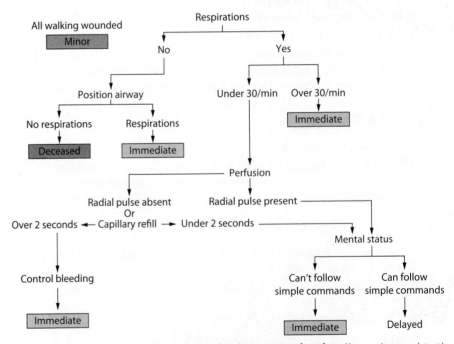

Figure 36-4 START flowchart. *(Reproduced with permission from http://www.citmt.org/start/flowchart.htm. Reprinted with permission from the Critical Illness and Trauma Foundation)*

- In the treatment area
- In the ambulance on the way to the hospital
  - Secondary triage is an in-depth reassessment based on clinical experience and judgment.
  - Triage is an on-going process and should be done continuously.

? CHAPTER QUESTIONS

1. The first phase of an incident is called:

   a. stabilization
   b. initial notification
   c. operations
   d. de-escalation

2. You are completing the START triage evaluation on a 27-year-old man who is complaining of difficulty breathing secondary to being involved in a building explosion. There are 53 patients that need to be triaged; all green tag patients have already been removed. The patient presents with the following during triage:

- Respiratory rate of 28.
- Radial pulses are present and capillary refill is less than 2 seconds.
- Follows simple commands.

   What color triage tag should this patient receive?

   a. Red
   b. Yellow
   c. Green
   d. Black

3. START stands for:

   a. slow triage and ridiculous treatment
   b. simple teaching and rapid transport
   c. simple triage and rapid treatment
   d. simple triage and rapid transport

Chapter 37

Response to Hazardous Materials and Terrorism

It is a midsummer day; the temperature has peaked at 98°F, and the humidity is 58%. Dispatch summons your ambulance to an overturn on Interstate 1 involving a tanker tractor trailer. As information is gathered by the dispatcher, she relays the information to your unit. Reports are coming in to central dispatch of rollover motor vehicle collision with people trapped. Upon arrival, you find an overturned 18-wheel tanker truck. Your partner notices during your scene survey that a green haze is emanating from the tanker portion of the truck. You notify dispatch that you are relocating to a safe location, and set up a staging area about half-mile away. You let incoming units know of the staging area and request the response of the county hazardous materials unit. Bystanders are reporting the driver is trapped and is seriously injured. You use the binoculars to survey the scene from a distance and confirm the driver is pinned in the vehicle. You also notice a UN placard number on the side of the vehicle. The UN number is 3355.

Is this the appropriate response for this incident so far?

HAZARDOUS MATERIALS

Any substance or material that is capable of posing a risk to health, safety, and property. Traditionally, the fire service was called to manage these events. In 1986, emergency medical services (EMS) involvement was mandated by Congress when they passed the Superfund Amendments and Reauthorizations Act (SARA), Title III.

- In 1989, the Occupational Safety and Health Administration (OSHA) required specific training for all EMS personnel who might respond to hazardous materials (haz-mat) incidents.
- The Department of Transportation (DOT) regulates all aspects of transporting haz-mat in the United States. This also includes design and type of container that must be used for transport.

EMT Response to Hazardous Materials

- Incident size-up (First priority is scene safety.)
- Recognition and/or confirmation that incident involves hazardous materials

Maintain a high index of suspicion when responding to incidents involving:

- Transportation
- Highway crashes
- Storage facilities
- Manufacturing plants
- Acts of terrorism

Use one of the following resources to identify the substance:

- DOT North American Emergency Response Guide (NAERG)
- UN numbers
- National Fire Protection Agency (NFPA) 704 placard system
- DOT placards
- Shipping papers (found in the driver's compartment of tractor trailers, also known as the shipping manifest)
- Material safety data sheets (MSDS)

The above resources will assist the first responder in determining:

- Immediate need for evacuation
- Immediate action with ambulatory patients
- Zones, such as:
  - Hot zone—Dangerous area
  - Warm zone—Entry/decontamination point
  - Cold zone—Safe area
- Assessment of toxicological risk
- Type of chemical
- Specific actions of a chemical and its reactivity to water
- Potential for secondary contamination
- Specific out-of-hospital medical treatment
- Appropriate techniques in decontamination of patients

Priority is to treat decontaminated patients and to transport patients that pose no risk of contaminating you or your equipment.

NFPA outlines levels of response, including what level of training is required by all personnel who may arrive first. All first responders must be trained to an awareness level.

- Emergency medical technicians (EMTs) who may transport "semidecontaminated patients" must be trained to the NFPA 473 Level-1.
- EMTs who may have to rapidly "decon" and assist in the decontamination corridor must be trained to the 473 Level-2.

Hazardous materials scene size-up includes a high degree of awareness. Responding to any one of the following could be a potential hazardous materials incident and should be approached with caution:

- Vehicle crashes
- Commercial vehicles
- Pest control vehicles
- Tankers
- Cars with alternative fuels
- Tractor-trailers

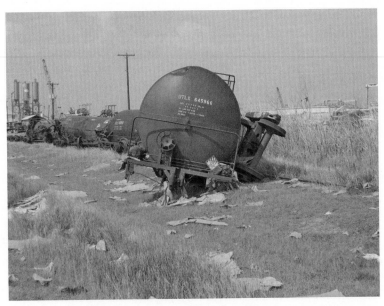

Figure 37-1   Derailed train car carrying hazardous materials. The aftermath of Hurricane Katrina included one of many derailed train cars carrying hazardous materials (UN 3257).

- Mass transportation
  - Railroads (Fig. 37-1)
  - Pipelines
- Mass storage facilities
  - Tanks/storage vessels
  - Warehouses
  - Hardware/agricultural stores
  - Agriculture
  - Manufacturing operations
  - Chemical plants
- Terrorism
  - Shopping centers
  - Other public environments
  - Health-care facilities
  - Laboratories

Recognizing Hazards

- Placarding of vehicles (required by law, some vehicles not placarded).
- Use of the NAERG could assist the paramedic in determining the specific chemical.

Common UN/DOT placard classifications are listed below:

- Explosives
- Gases
- Flammable liquids
- Flammable solids
- Oxidizers and organic peroxides
- Poisonous and etiologic agents

- Radioactive materials
- Corrosives
- Miscellaneous hazardous materials

NFPA 704 system for fixed facilities (Fig. 37-2A and B)

- Blue = health hazard
- Red = fire hazard
- Yellow = reactivity hazard

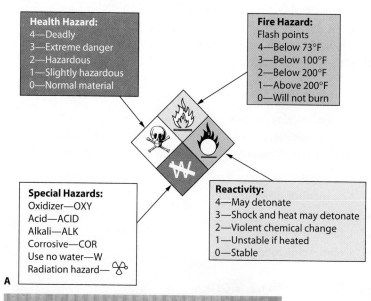

Health Hazard:
4—Deadly
3—Extreme danger
2—Hazardous
1—Slightly hazardous
0—Normal material

Fire Hazard:
Flash points
4—Below 73°F
3—Below 100°F
2—Below 200°F
1—Above 200°F
0—Will not burn

Special Hazards:
Oxidizer—OXY
Acid—ACID
Alkali—ALK
Corrosive—COR
Use no water—W
Radiation hazard—

Reactivity:
4—May detonate
3—Shock and heat may detonate
2—Violent chemical change
1—Unstable if heated
0—Stable

A

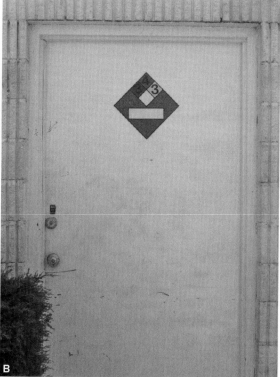

B

Figure 37-2 A. NFPA 704 placard. B. Example of the NFPA 704 on the entry-way to a factory.

Identification of Substances

The origin of dealing with a hazardous material is often difficult—especially with unknown substances. Using resources such as the MSDS may reveal detailed substance information. Shipping papers may also assist in revealing substance identification. Other resources used in responding to hazardous materials include:

- Poison control centers
- CAMEO (computer-aided management of emergency operations) computer database information
- Computer modeling for plumes
- CHEMTREC (Chemical Transportation Emergency Center) (1-800-424-9300; 24-hour toll-free hotline)
- Other reference sources include:
  - Textbooks
  - Handbooks
  - Technical specialists

Hazardous material response teams utilize specialized recognition equipment to monitor and recognize unknown chemicals. This equipment includes:

- Air monitoring equipment
- Gas monitoring equipment
- Ph testing
- Chemical testing
- Colorimetric tube testing

Hazardous Material Zones

(Fig. 37-3)

Hot Zone

- Contamination actually present
- Site of incident/release
- Entry with high-level personal protective equipment (PPE)
- Entry limited to trained hazardous materials team members

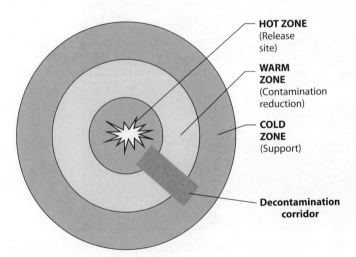

Figure 37-3   Hazardous materials zones.

Warm Zone

- Buffer zone outside of hot zone
- Where decontamination corridor is located
- Corridor has "hot" and "cold" ends
- Authorized trained hazardous materials team members

Cold Zone

- Safe area
- Staging for personnel and equipment
- Where medical monitoring occurs
- One end of corridor
- Safe operation area for EMS personnel

Specific Terminology for Medical Hazardous Materials Operations

- Boiling point (BP)—The temperature at which the vapor pressure of the material being heated equals atmospheric pressure.
- Flammable/explosive limits—The highest and lowest concentrations of a substance that can explode or burn.
- Flash point (FP)—The lowest temperature at which the vapor given off by a substance forms an ignitable mixture with air.
- Ignition temperature—Minimum temperature to which a substance must be heated before it will spontaneously burn independently of the source of heat.
- Specific gravity—The ratio of the density of a solid or liquid to the density of water.
- Vapor density (VD)—The relative density of a vapor compared to air.
- Vapor pressure—A measure of how readily a solid or liquid mixes with air at its surface. Vapor pressure approaching 760 mm Hg indicates a volatile substance and suggests that there will be high concentration in the air.
- Water solubility—The degree to which a material or its vapors dissolve in water.
- Alpha radiation—Massive and travel only 3 to 4 in from their radioactive source.
- Beta radiation—More energetic and less massive than alpha particles. Beta particles can travel up to 100 ft from their source.
- Gamma radiation is not particles but forms of pure energy and can travel great distances from its source.

Specific Toxicological Terms

- Threshold limit value (TLV)—A TLV reflects the level of exposure that the typical worker can experience without an unreasonable risk of disease or injury. TLVs are not quantitative estimates of risk at different exposure levels or by different routes of exposure.
- Lethal concentration and doses (LD_{50})—An LD_{50} value is the amount of a solid or liquid material that it takes to kill 50% of test animals (eg, mice or rats) in one dose.
- Parts per million (PPM)—PPM is defined as the mass of the component in solution divided by the total mass of the solution multiplied by 10^6 (one million).

- Immediately dangerous to life and health (IDLH)—This concentration is considered to be the limit beyond which an individual will not be capable of escaping death or permanent injury without help in less than 30 minutes.
- Permissible exposure limit (PEL)—A PEL is the maximum amount or concentration of a chemical that a worker may be exposed to under OSHA regulations.
- Short-term exposure limit (TLV-STEL)—A short-term exposure limit (STEL) is defined as the concentration to which workers can be exposed continuously for a short period of time without suffering from:
  - Irritation
  - Chronic or irreversible tissue damage
  - Narcosis of sufficient degree to increase the likelihood of accidental injury, impair self-rescue, or materially reduce work efficiency
- Ceiling level (TLV-C)—At no time should this exposure limit be exceeded.

TYPES OF CONTAMINATION

- Primary contamination
  - Exposure to substance
  - Only harmful to individual
  - Little chance of exposure to others
- Secondary contamination
  - Exposure to substance.
  - Substance easily transferred.
  - Touching patient results in contamination.
  - Key concept in hazardous materials medical operations.
  - Gas exposure rarely results in secondary contamination.
  - Liquid and particulate matter more likely to result in secondary contamination.

HOW POISONS ARE ABSORBED

- Topical absorption
  - Skin and mucous membranes.
  - Not all skin absorbs at the same rate and not all poisons are easily absorbed.
- Respiratory inhalation
  - Absorption through bronchial tree
  - Oxygen-deficient atmospheres
- Gastrointestinal ingestion
  - Ingestion of substances
  - Factors affecting absorption
- Parenteral injection
  - Injection
  - Wound entry
  - Invasive medical procedures

CYCLE OF POISON ACTIONS

- Absorption
  - Time to delivery into blood stream
- Distribution
  - Distribution to target organs
  - Poison or drug binds to tissues/molecules
  - Actions
  - Deposits
- Biotransformation
  - Liver
- Elimination through
  - Gastrointestinal (GI)
  - Kidneys
  - Respiratory system
- Actions of poisons are determined by several factors including:
  - Acute toxicity
    — Immediate effect from substance
  - Delayed toxicity
    — No immediate effect
    — Later appearance of symptoms
    — Delayed pathology or disease
  - Local effects
    — Effect immediate at the contaminated site
    — Burn model
    — Progression of effects like burn
    — Topical or respiratory
    — Skin irritation—Acute bronchospasm
  - Systemic effects
    — Cardiovascular
    — Neurological
    — Hepatic
    — Renal
  - Dose response
    — Physiological response to dosage
    — How much to get an effect
    — Essential concept for decontamination
  - Synergistic effects
    — Combinations may react synergistically.
    — Standard pharmacological approach.
    — Standard treatment can result in synergy.
    — Medical control/poison control reference.

COMMONLY ENCOUNTERED HAZARDOUS MATERIALS

- Corrosives (acids/alkalis)
- Pulmonary irritants (ammonia/chlorine)

- Pesticides (carbamates/organophosphates)
- Chemical asphyxiants (cyanide/CO)
- Hydrocarbon solvents (xylene/methylene chloride)

CONSIDERATIONS FOR PERFORMING INVASIVE PROCEDURES

Risk versus benefit (Will treating the patient contaminate you or further contaminate the patient?)

- The primary purpose of decontamination is to reduce the patient's dosage of material, decrease the threat of secondary contamination, and reduce the risk of rescuer injury and contamination.
- Environmental considerations are a consideration if there are no life threats. Trained hazardous materials response team members will prevent runoff of material. If there are life threats, patient comes first. Remember, only trained and fully protected haz-mat response team members should rescue victims of a hazardous materials incident.

Modes of Decontamination

- Dilution
  - Lavage with copious amounts of water.
  - Water is universal decontamination solution.
  - Dilution decreases dose and action.
  - Reduction of topical absorption.
- Absorption
  - Use of pads to "blot" up the material
  - Towels to dry the patient after lavage
  - Usually a secondary method to lavage
  - Common for environmental cleanup
- Neutralization
  - Almost never used in patient decontamination.
  - Hazard of exothermic reactions.
  - Time to determine neutralizing substance.
  - Lavage usually dilutes and removes faster.
- Disposal/isolation
  - Removal of clothing
  - Removal of substances

Decontamination Decision Making

- Field considerations include flight of walking contaminated victims to rescuers—"fast break" event—action required now.
- Conscious, contaminated people will "self-rescue" by walking out of hot zone.
- Immediate decontamination often not avoidable.
- Speed of hazardous materials team response may hinder walking contaminated.

EMS Gross Decontamination and Treatment

- All EMS need gross decontamination capability.
- EMS should be prepared for quick decontamination.
- Need for rapid EMS PPE.
- Need quick transport isolation methods.

"Fast Break" Incident Decision Making

- Critical patient—Unknown/life-threatening material (remember patients who are contaminated are a risk to the EMS crew as well as equipment and the emergency department).
- Decontamination and treatment should be simultaneous.
- Remove clothing (80% of contamination is removed by having the patient remove their clothing).
- Treat life-threatening problems.
- Lavage—Water is universal decontamination solution.
- Contain/isolate patient.
- Transport.
- Noncritical—Unknown/life-threatening material.
  - More contemplative approach
  - Decontamination and treatment simultaneous
  - Remove clothing
  - Treat life-threatening problems
  - Lavage—Water is universal decontamination solution
  - Contain/isolate patient
  - Transport
- Noncritical—Substance known.
  - Slower approach
  - Environmental/privacy considerations
  - More thorough decontamination
  - Clothing removal
  - Thorough lavage/wash
  - Drying/reclothing PRN
  - Medical monitoring
  - Patient isolation PRN
  - Transport

Longer-Duration Event Decision Making

- Patients in hot zone—Nonambulatory
  - No rescue attempted.
  - Wait for hazardous materials team.
  - Team will set up decontamination corridor.
- Haz-mat team will not make entry until:
  - Medical monitoring of entry team
  - Decontamination corridor established
  - Longer duration event

○ Often 60 minutes for team deployment
○ Set up time
○ Better opportunity for thorough decontamination
○ Better PPE
○ Less chance of secondary contamination
○ Better environmental protection

Decontamination Methods Used by Trained Personnel

- Decontamination and PPE is driven by the substance encountered.
- Decontamination solutions.
  ○ Do not attempt to neutralize.
  ○ Lavage with copious amounts of water.
  ○ Water is the universal solution.
  ○ Tincture of green soap used to improve wash.
  ○ Isopropyl alcohol is used for some isocyanates.
  ○ Vegetable oil is used for some water-reactive substances.
- Remove the clothing.
  ○ Also remove rings and jewelry.
  ○ Remove shoes and socks.
  ○ Cut off clothing PRN.
- Thorough wash and rinse.
  ○ Allow fluid to drain away.
  ○ Do not allow them to stay in the runoff.
- Rewash and rinse.
  ○ Pay careful attention to difficult areas to decontaminate:
    — Scalp/hair
    — Ears/ear canals/nostrils
    — Axilla
    — Fingernails
    — Navel
    — Groin/buttocks/genitalia
    — Behind knees
    — Between toes, toenails

LEVELS OF TRAINED HAZARDOUS MATERIALS PERSONAL PROTECTION EQUIPMENT

There are four levels of protection (Fig. 37-4).

- Level "A" protection
  ○ Highest level of personal protection
  ○ Highest degree of protection from chemical breakthrough
  ○ Fully encapsulated suit
  ○ Covers everything including self-contained breathing apparatus (SCBA)
  ○ Impermeable/sealed
  ○ Typically used by hazardous materials team for entry into hot zone

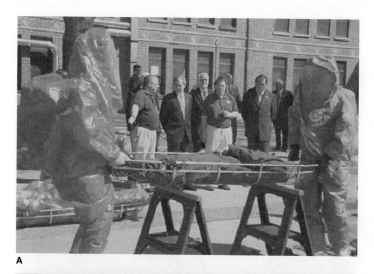

A

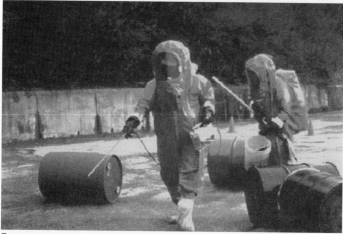

B

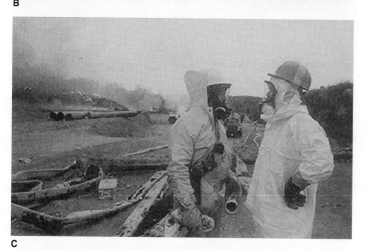

C

Figure 37-4   Levels of protection. A. Level A protective haz-mat suit. *(Used with permission of the Georgia Institute of Technology)* B. Level B protective haz-mat suit. *(Reproduced with permission from http:// www.epa.gov/superfund/programs/er/ resource/d1_04.htm)* C. Level C protective haz-mat suit. *(Used with permission of the National Library of Medicine)* D. Level C suit with personnel using powered air purifying respirators (PAPR) and chemical, biological, radiological, nuclear, explosive (CBRNE) gas masks. *(Used with permission of Peter DiPrima)*

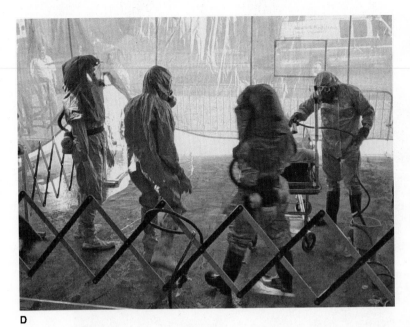

D

Figure 37-4 *(Continued)*

- Level "B" protection
  - Level of protection typically worn by decontamination team
  - Decontamination wears one level below entry
  - Usually nonencapsulating protection
  - SCBA worn outside suit
  - Easier entry and SCBA bottle changes
  - Easier to work in
  - High degree of repellency
- Level "C" protection
  - Nonpermeable clothing.
  - Eye, hand, and foot protection.
  - Used during transport of patients with potential of secondary contamination.
- Level "D" protection
  - Firefighter turnout clothing

Determining Appropriate PPE

- Depends on whether the chemical is known.
- A permeability chart is consulted to determine "breakthrough" time.
- Double or triple gloves or chemical-resistant gloves are used.
- Nitrile gloves have a high resistance to chemicals.
- If situation is emergent, take maximal barrier precautions—Full turnouts or Tyvek suit/gowns.
- Use high-efficiency particulate air (HEPA) filters and eye protection.
- Remove leather shoes, use rubber boots.
- Ideally, at least level "B" protection should be used.
- Ideally, use disposable protection.

PROCEDURES IN TRANSPORTING A SEMIDECONTAMINATED PATIENT (AS A LAST RESORT)

- Use as much disposable equipment as possible.
  - Reduces decontamination later
- Practicality of lining an ambulance interior with plastic:
  - Impractical
  - Time consuming

If airborne contaminants can permeate cabinets, it is unsafe for the driver to operate the ambulance. Patients who are "off-gassing" should not be placed in the patient compartment of the ambulance because of the risk of injuring the crew.

Medical Monitoring and Rehabilitation

Entry team/decontamination team readiness prior to entry:

- Assessment of vital signs and documentation.
- Team members should have normal values on file.
- Documentation flow sheet must be started.
  - Blood pressure
  - Pulse
  - Respiratory rate
  - Temperature
  - Body weight
  - Mental/neurological status
- Rescuer PPE can cause considerable heat stress.
- Prehydration prior to entry.
  - About 8 to 16 oz of water or sport drink

After Exit, Personnel Should Return to the Medical Sector for "Rehab"

- Reassessment of vital signs and documentation.
- Documentation flow sheet must be started.
  - Blood pressure
  - Pulse
  - Respiratory rate
  - Temperature
  - Body weight
  - Mental/neurological status
- Rehydration at exit.
  - About 8 to 16 oz of water or sport drinks (such as Gatorade)
- Use weight to estimate fluid losses.
  - Medical control/protocol determination
    — PO fluids
- No reentry until:
  - Vitals are back to normal.
    — Nontachycardic

— Alert

— Normotensive

— Body weight within percentage of normal

Heat stress factors include prehydration of the member, degree of physical fitness, ambient air temperature, degree of activity, and duration in the PPE.

Response to Weapons of Mass Destruction Incidents

It is a particularly busy day for the local emergency medical services (EMS) units, humidity is at 75% and it feels like it is 100°F, and you are working on your 10th assignment for the shift. A known terrorist group has successfully detonated an explosive device in a tanker truck that was transporting liquefied chlorine across a well-known bridge in your response area. Multiple calls are coming into the 911 system regarding this assignment.

Moments later, your unit is dispatched to the staging area of this scene. Due to the close proximity of this assignment, you and your partner will be the first arriving EMS unit.

What type of scene size-up should you perform, and should you enter the scene?

TERRORISM

"The unlawful use of or threatened use of force or violence against individuals or property to coerce or intimidate governments or societies, often to achieve political, religious, or ideological objectives."—US Department of Defense

Throughout history, terrorism has been a global threat from which no community is free. Terrorism surpasses all geographic and demographic boundaries; suburban, urban, and rural neighborhoods are at risk.

Terrorists have demonstrated the ability to strike anywhere in the world.

- International terrorists continue to pose a threat to the interests of the United States (Fig. 37-5). Many terrorist groups and loosely affiliated extremists view the United States as an enemy.
- Increasingly, emergency responders must deal with incidents arising from domestic sources. According to the Federal Bureau of Investigation (FBI), domestic groups or individuals are more likely to be the source of an incident involving weapons of mass destruction (WMD) than are international organizations.

THE THREAT OF TERRORISM

Terrorists have the knowledge, capability, and patience to strike anywhere, and at any time. In the past, we have seen that when properly motivated they will perform any task to achieve their goals. All communities, especially those of free societies, are vulnerable to terrorism. Any community in the United States has some form of high-profile target.

Examples of critical infrastructures that become targets for criminal terrorist activity include:

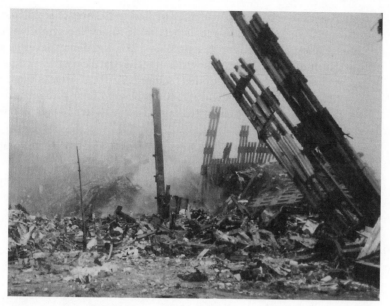

Figure 37-5 World Trade Center, September 11, 2001. *(Used with permission of Peter DiPrima)*

- Places of public assembly
- Public buildings (ie, schools)
- Mass transit systems
- Places of high economic impact
- Telecommunications centers
- Information and communications
- Banking and finance
- Water supplies
- Electrical power, oil, and gas production and storage
- Places of historical or symbolic significance
- Apartment buildings
- Medical clinics (abortion clinics)
- Research facilities
- Transportation hubs
- Emergency services

WHY WMD: TERRORISM?

- Chemical and biological agents are relatively easy to manufacture. Most agents can be produced by knowledge gained in college. Weapons of mass destruction (WMD) are readily available and are cheap to produce. Libraries contain the "recipes" required. Chemicals are readily available in school laboratories. Biological pathogens can be obtained from nature, hospital laboratories, and university research facilities. Radiological materials are found in industry and in research laboratories.
- WMD terrorism is spread relatively easy by air. A clever person can easily devise methods to disseminate a chemical, biological, or radiological weapon that results in little, if any, signature. For example, the first indication of a chemical attack may be when people begin to

collapse, as in the Tokyo incident. The first indication of a biological attack may be an influx of people beginning to develop symptoms of disease hours to days after infection. And last, there may never be any obvious indication of a radiological attack. Regardless of what type of agent is used, decontamination is required. Terrorist attacks cause a psychological impact that will extend far beyond their actual effects. Psychological effects of terrorism cause people to live in fear. A few examples of this were:

- During the Gulf War, when Israeli citizens boarded up their homes fearful of Iraqi chemical attacks.
- Post September 11, 2001, when after strong media coverage, many people feared planes flying overhead, traveling on mass transit, and being in large crowded areas.

Limitations of WMD

- Chemical weapons need large quantities in open areas.
- Delayed effects can detract from impact.
- Potentially hazardous to the terrorists.
- Development and use require skill.

INDICATORS OF WMD ATTACK

Primary Indicators

- Similar symptoms of victims
- Mass casualties
- Casualty patterns
- Finding a dissemination device, and observing its functioning
- Detectors
- Warning given or credit taken

Secondary Indicators

- Dead animals or birds
- Statements of victims
- Unexplained liquids or strange smells
- Confirmed test results

POTENTIAL OUTCOMES OF TERRORIST WMD EVENT

- Mass casualties
- The overwhelming of emergency response systems
- Disruption of normal routine
- Shutdown and decontamination of contaminated facilities
- Panic and confusion
- Loss of faith in government
- Loss of faith in emergency services

WEAPONS OF MASS DESTRUCTION: CHEMICAL AGENTS

Classes of Chemical Agents

- Choking agents

- ○ *Choking agents (lung-damaging agents)* include phosgene (CG), diphosgene (DP), chlorine, and chloropicrin (PS). These agents produce injury to the lungs and irritation of the eyes and respiratory tract. They may cause intractable pulmonary edema and predispose to secondary pneumonia.
- Blister agents
  - ○ *Blister agents (vesicants)* include sulfur mustard (H/HD), nitrogen mustard (HN), arsenicals (Lewisite [L]), and phosgene oxime (CX). Blister agents produce pain and injury to the eyes, reddening and blistering of the skin, and when inhaled, damage to the mucous membranes and respiratory tract. Mustard may produce major destruction of the epidermal layer of the skin.
- Blood agents
  - ○ *Blood agents (cyanogens)* include hydrogen cyanide (AC) and cyanogen chloride (CK). These agents are transported by the blood to all body tissues, where the agent blocks the oxidative processes, preventing tissue cells from utilizing oxygen. The central nervous system (CNS) is especially affected and leads to cessation of respiration followed by cardiovascular collapse.
- Nerve agents
  - ○ *Nerve agents (anticholinesterase)* include tabun (GA), sarin (GB), soman (GD), GF, and V-agent (VX). They inhibit cholinesterase enzymes. The cholinesterase enzymes are responsible for the hydrolysis of acetylcholine (ACh), a chemical neurotransmitter. The inhibition creates accumulation of ACh at the cholinergic synapses that disrupts the normal transmission of nerve impulses. Cholinergic synapses are located in the CNS, neuromuscular end plates of the peripheral voluntary nervous system, parasympathetic endings, and sympathetic presynaptic ganglia of the autonomic nervous system (Table 37-1).

WEAPONS OF MASS DESTRUCTION: BIOLOGICAL AGENTS

Biological Warfare Agents

Biological warfare involves the use of several broad categories of agents. Two of these are infectious microbial pathogens—bacteria and viruses, both

TABLE 37-1: Signs and Symptoms of Nerve Agent Exposure

	Signs/Symptoms	Vapor Exposure	Liquid Exposure
Mild	P Pin point pupils (miosis)	X	
	S Salivation	X	
	L Lacrimation	X	
Severe	U Urination	X	X
	D Defecation	X	X
	G Gastrointestinal distress pain/gas	X	X
	E Emesis	X	X
	M Muscle twitching	X	X
	C Convulsions	X	X

of which cause disease in humans, animals, and plants. The third is known as biological toxins, which are poisons extracted from biological sources previous to their use as weapons.

Characteristics of Biological Agents

- Do not penetrate unbroken skin.
- Nonvolatile.
- More toxic than chemicals by weight.
- Undetectable by senses.
- Some detection devices are available depending on the agent involved.
- Disseminate as aerosols.

Types of Biological Agents

- *Bacteria* are single-cell, free-living organisms that reproduce by division. Bacteria cause disease in humans by invading tissues and/or producing toxins; this causes the body's immune system to be overcome.
- *Viruses* cannot replicate by themselves. Viruses require a host cell in order to reproduce, and are technically described as obligate intracellular parasites. Viruses cause epidemics.
- *Toxins* are poisonous substances produced as a by-product of pathogens or plants and even some animals. (Snake venom is an example of a toxin.)

Potential Biological Agents

- Anthrax (bacteria)
- Plague (bacteria)
- Q fever (rickettsia)
- Small pox (virus)
- Ebola (virus)
- Venezuelan equine encephalitis (VEE) (virus)
- Staphylococcal enterotoxin B
- Botulinum (neurotoxin)
- Ricin (cytotoxin)

WEAPONS OF MASS DESTRUCTION: RADIOLOGICAL/ NUCLEAR WEAPONS

Characteristics of Nuclear Agents

- Of the three categories, chemical, biological, or nuclear, nuclear agents in the past were considered to be the least likely of the threats. However, the potential risk is increasing with current intelligence. Threats of using a "dirty bomb" with radioactive material are on a steady increase.
- In its simplest definition, radiation can be defined as either electromagnetic or particulate emission of energy.
- This energy, when impacting on or passing through material, including us, can cause some form of reaction. This radiation is referred to as *ionizing radiation.*
- When absorbed by our bodies, it can cause changes in our cells. Small amounts can be tolerated; larger amounts can be harmful.

For EMS purposes, radiation can be classified as:

- Alpha particles—Slow moving

- Beta particles—Higher in energy
- Gamma particles—Highly energized

Ionizing radiation cannot be seen, felt, or heard. Therefore, a detection device is required to measure the radiation being emitted by the radioactive source. The most commonly used device is the Geiger counter. The rate of radiation is measured in roentgens per hour (R/h) or milliroentgens per hour (mR/h).

- The unit of local tissue energy deposition is called radiation absorbed dose (RAD) (See Table 37-2). Roentgen equivalent in man measure (REM) provides a gauge of the likely injury to the irradiated part of the organism. Simply stated, ionizing radiation causes alterations in the body's cell, primarily the DNA. Depending on dosage received, the changes can be in cell division, cell structure, and cellular biochemical activities.

Ways to Limit Exposure

- *Time*—Cutting down your time reduces your exposure
- *Distance*—The farther you are from the source the better
- *Shielding*—Through various materials

DISSEMINATION DEVICES

There are five types of dissemination devices:

- Direct deposit
- Breaking devices
- Bursting/exploding devices
- Spraying devices
- Vectors

Direct Deposit

- Mechanical
- Point source
- No collateral damage
- Easily controlled
- Fitted into cans, umbrellas, pens, and the like

TABLE 37-2: Dose-Effect Total Body Exposure

Radiation Absorbed Dose (RAD)	Effect
5-25	Asymptomatic, normal blood studies
50-75	Asymptomatic, minor depression in WBC
75-125	Anorexia, nausea, vomiting, fatigue within 2 days
125-200	Nausea, vomiting, diarrhea, anxiety, tachycardia
200-600	Nausea, vomiting, diarrhea within several hours, 50% fatal within 6 weeks, untreated
600-1000	Severe nausea, vomiting, diarrhea within several hours, fatal 100% within 2 weeks, untreated
1000+	Burning sensation within minutes, nausea and vomiting, confusion, ataxia, and prostration within 1 hour

Fatal 100% within short time without prompt treatment!

Breaking Devices

- Mechanical.
- Point source.
- Breaking devices are those mechanical weapons which encapsulate the agent and release it when broken (small drilled hole in the base, agent inserted, and hole sealed).

Bursting/Exploding Devices

Bursting or exploding devices are those which employ an explosive to break the agent container and disseminate the agent.

Spraying Devices

Mechanical spraying devices also contain an agent reservoir, but rather than an explosive charge, they employ pressure to disseminate the agent.

Vectors

Usually disseminate living biological agents. A vector is a carrier of the bacteria, and may be an insect or a contaminated item such as clothing, food, or water.

PERSONAL PROTECTION

- As stated earlier, personal safety takes precedence. If we become incapacitated, injured, or even die responding to an incident, we will be unable to provide the services needed to control the scene. Becoming a victim at an incident endangers your partners and other rescuers involved.
- We must understand that nuclear, biological, and chemical agents were deliberately developed to cause injury or death to individuals. They are all very toxic to humans and animals; however, they are not the end of the world. The majority of agents can be detected, protected against, and can be treated and decontaminated.

Regulations Involving Personal Protective Equipment

OSHA standards mandate specific training. OSHA's final rule (March 6, 1989, 29 CFR [1910.120]) as it applies to emergency medical personnel: Training shall be based on the duties and functions to be performed by each responder of an emergency response organization. No single combination of protective equipment and clothing is capable of protecting against all hazards. PPE should be used in conjunction with other protective measures. So training is essential before any individual attempts to use PPE.

Protecting Yourself against Chemical Agents

- Self-contained breathing apparatus
- Protective clothing

Protecting Yourself Against Biological Agents

- Mask (HEPA filters or SCBA)[*]
- Clothing

> ► Note:
>
> Clothing contaminated with nerve agents can "OFF-GAS," creating a problem for individuals around undecontaminated clothing and who are unprotected.

---

[*] Depends on biological agent involved.

- Sanitation measures
- Decontamination
- Medical treatment
- Bloodborne pathogen universal precautions

If you know you are responding to a potential biological agent incident:

- *SCBA or protective mask combined with your clothing and unbroken skin are your first line of defense.*
- *Use good sanitation measures, which include not eating or drinking in the immediate area. Wash your hands with soap and water if you touch something.*
- *Decontaminate with 0.5% hypochlorite solution.*
- *Do not ignore early flu-like symptoms, seek medical attention immediately.*

Levels of Protection

The Environmental Protection Agency (EPA) designated four levels of respiratory protection and protective clothing. (See Fig. 37-4)

- Level A protection should be worn when the highest level of respiratory, skin, eye, and mucous membrane protection is needed. It consists of a fully encapsulated, vapor-tight, chemical-resistant suit, chemical-resistant boots, chemical-resistant inner/outer gloves, coveralls, hard hat, and SCBA.
- Level B protection should be worn when the highest level of respiratory protection is needed and a lesser degree of skin and eye protection. It differs from a Level A suit in which it provides splash protection through the use of chemical-resistant clothing (two-piece chemical splash suit, or fully encapsulated non-vapor tight suit and SCBA).
- Level C protection should be selected when the type of airborne substances is *known*, concentration measured, and all criteria for air purifying systems are met, and skin and eye exposures are unlikely.
- Level D is a primary work uniform.

Protecting Yourself Against Nuclear Agents

- Time
  - Cutting down your time reduces your exposure.
- Distance
  - *Distance*—Referring back to forms of radiation, alpha particles only travel a little over an inch in air. Beta particles will not travel for more than a few yards in air. However, gamma particles will travel extensive distances and this is the radiation we are the most concerned with. The farther you are from the source, the better.
- Shielding
  - Radiation can also be blocked or partially blocked by various materials. A sheet of paper stops alpha particles; beta particles are stopped by aluminum foil or clothing; and gamma rays are only reduced by dense materials such as lead or earth.

▶Note:

Because of the ease of protecting from alpha and beta radiation, our main concern from these substances is inhalation and ingestion of actual radioactive material in the form of dust or contaminated food or water. Gamma is more difficult to protect against, so time, distance, and shielding are vital.

? CHAPTER QUESTIONS

For questions 1 to 4, match the following definitions with the correct terms.

  a. Level "A" protection
  b. Level "B" protection
  c. Level "C" protection
  d. Level "D" protection

1. Nonpermeable clothing

2. Highest level of personal protection

3. Level of protection typically worn by decontamination team

4. Firefighters' gear

5. Through which of the following routes are poisons absorbed?

  a. Topical
  b. Respiratory
  c. Gastrointestinal
  d. Injection
  e. All of the above

6. Decontamination occurs in the cold zone.

  a. True
  b. False

7. The unlawful use of force to intimidate or coerce a segment of a population for political or social reasons is:

  a. terrorism
  b. conflict
  c. warfare
  d. negotiation

8. Biological weapons target all but:

  a. utilities
  b. animals
  c. people
  d. agriculture

9. Explosives are the terrorist's weapon of choice.

  a. True
  b. False

10. Which weapon's material is easiest to obtain?

  a. Biological
  b. Chemical
  c. Nuclear
  d. Incendiary

End of Book Crosswords

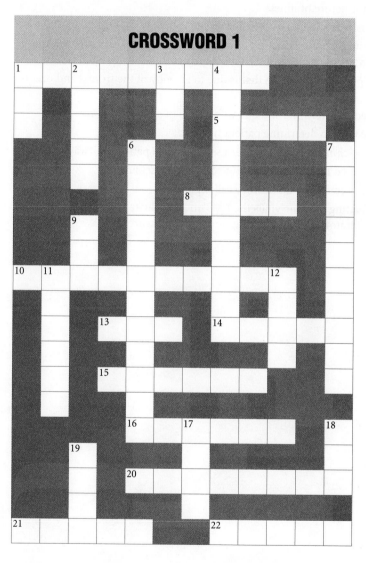

CROSSWORD 1

Across

1. _____ of injury is the manner in which an injury occurred.

5. Physical _____ is when an emergency medical technician (EMT) performs systematic hands-on approach to evaluating a patient.

8. The mnemonic for performing cervical spinal immobilization.

10. Patient _____.

13. During the general impression it is important to determine the patient's _____.

14. A baseline vital sign _____.

15. The medical term used for the hip.
16. _____ assessment is used for patients with a mechanism of injury (MOI).
20. A _____ forwards a radio transmission and increases its strength.
21. _____ is the medical term for the absence of breathing.
22. In the mnemonic DCAPBTLS, the "B" stands for?

Down

1. Acronym for 1 across.
2. ____ complaint is why the patient called the ambulance.
3. Acronym for nature of illness.
4. The process of evaluating a scene for safety.
6. Medical term that describes two or more rib fractures on each affected rib resulting in paradoxical chest wall movement.
7. A form of presenile dementia that is due to atrophy of the frontal and occipital lobes.
9. A scale used to determine and quantify a level of a patient's coma.
11. Mnemonic used to determine patient history.
12. Head-_____-chin-lift is a maneuver used to open a patient's airway manually.
17. Mnemonic used to evaluate a patient's level of consciousness.
18. Mnemonic used for the ambulance call report.
19. When evaluating baseline vitals the EMT must evaluate _____, pulse rate and quality, respiratory rate and quality, and blood pressure.

CROSSWORD 2

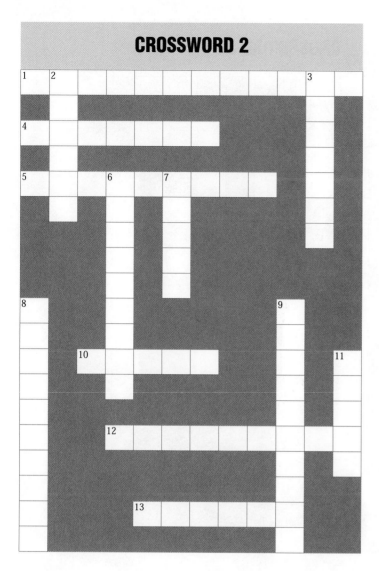

Across

1. The device of choice for assisting ventilations during rescue breathing.
4. The trachea bifurcates into the right and left mainstem _____.
5. The maneuver used to open a patient's airway with a suspected spinal injury.
10. Adequate _____ volume for the adult patient is approximately 500 cc.
12. The major muscle that separates the chest cavity from the abdominal cavity.
13. A medication given to all patients.

Down

2. An _____ adjunct is placed in the oropharynx.
3. When testing a suction unit, the minimum required _____ is 300 mm Hg.
6. Another name for the Yankauer suction catheter.
7. The medical term used to describe fluid in the lungs.
8. When lungs' sounds are difficult to hear on one or both sides they are said to be?
9. Portion of the pharynx that extends from the mouth to the oral cavity at the base of the tongue.
11. An artificially created opening that is found in the neck.

CROSSWORD 3

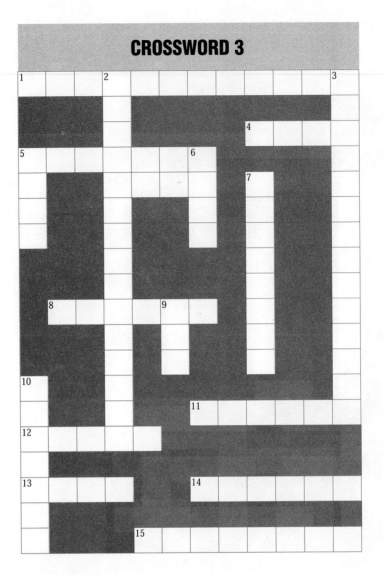

Across

1. The medical term used for listening to lung sounds.
4. _____ medical history.
5. To check for a pulse on an unconscious adult patient, the EMT should palpate the _____ pulse.
8. During evaluation of a patient who is exhibiting signs of a stroke, the EMT should use the Cincinnati Pre-hospital Stroke Scale. Using this scale includes evaluating _____ droop, arm lift, and speech.
11. Another name for a cerebral vascular accident.
12. The medical term "renal calculus" is known as a kidney _____.
13. The "L" in SAMPLE stands for _____ meal or oral intake.
14. The medication used most frequently in an EMS system.
15. The heart has four _____ that prevent blood from flowing back into a specific chamber.

Down

2. Situations in which a drug should not be used because it may harm the patient.

3. A medication that is given to patients who are experiencing signs/symptoms of a myocardial infarction.

5. The mnemonic used to describe various respiratory distress syndromes.

6. How much of a drug should be administered.

7. An abnormal curvature of the spine.

9. The mnemonic used for the defibrillator.

10. The medication diabetic patients administer to themselves to lower blood sugar.

CROSSWORD 4

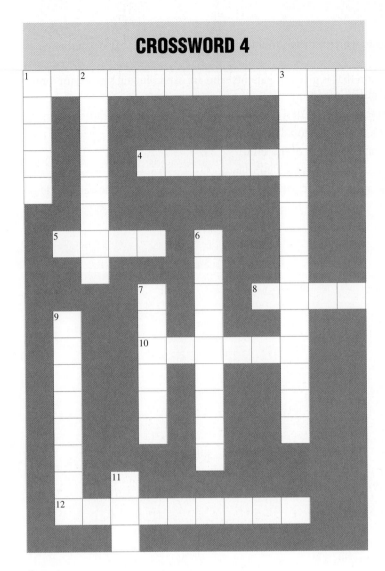

Across

1. Listening with a stethoscope.
— 4. Away from the attached limb or origin.
5. The pneumonic for stress debriefing.
8. _____ substance isolation.
10. The middle layer of the skin.
12. An agency that coordinates emergency care as part of the continuum of care.

Down

1. The patient may project feelings of _____ at family of emergency medical services (EMS).
2. The top number of the blood pressure.
3. Permission obtained from a parent or legal guardian for emergency treatment of a patient, who is not of legal age or is unconscious.
6. When lifting use the _____ _____ to maintain control of the device.
7. Toward the middle.
9. EMS should be a patient _____.
11. An abnormal sign found when evaluating the skin (diaphoresis).

CROSSWORD 5

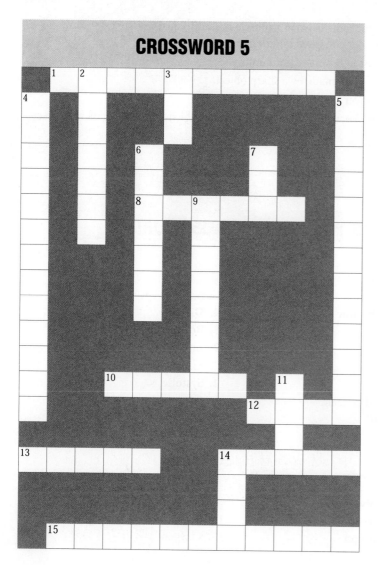

Across

1. Movement of segments of the body without regard to the forces that caused the movement to occur.
8. A form of shock that presents with tachycardia, hypoperfusion, fever, tachypnea, and altered mental status.
10. The rule of _____ is used to estimate the total body surface area burned.
12. Superficial, partial, and full thickness _____.
13. _____ pressure.
14. _____ segment is two or more ribs broken in two or more places.
15. _____ shock is a form of shock that is defined by hypoperfusion from fluid or blood loss.

Down

2. _____ object is a foreign body that penetrates the skin and remains imbedded in body tissue.
3. The acronym for mechanism of injury.
4. The amount of blood discharged from the right and left ventricles per minute, or stroke volume multiplied by heart rate.
5. Another term used for shock.

6. _____ syndrome is when a muscle has prolonged pressure, for example, a leg stuck under collapsed building material.

7. Acronym for a traumatic brain injury.

9. A hole or wound made by a sharp object.

11. Innermost layer that surrounds the brain.

14. _____ thickness burns are burns that have blisters and redness with severe pain.

ANSWERS TO CHAPTER CROSSWORDS

Crossword 1
Across

1. Auscultation	4. Distal
5. CISD	8. Body
10. Dermis	12. Emergency

Down

1. Anger	2. Systolic
3. Implied consent	6. Power grip
7. Medial	9. Advocate
11. Wet	

Crossword 2
Across

1. Bag-valve-mask	4. Bronchi
5. Jaw thrust	10. Tidal
12. Diaphragm	13. Oxygen

Down

2. Airway	3. Suction
6. Tonsil tip	7. Rales
8. Diminished	9. Oropharynx
11. Stoma	

Crossword 3
Across

1. Mechanism	5. Examination
8. CSIC	10. Assessment
13. Age	14. Pulse
15. Pelvis	16. Trauma
20. Repeater	21. Apnea
22. Burns	

Down

1. MOI	2. Chief
3. NOI	4. Scene size-up
6. Flail segment	7. Alzheimer
9. GCS	11. SAMPLE
12. Tilt	17. AVPU
18. PCR	19. Skin

Crossword 4

Across

1. Auscultation
5. Carotid
11. Stroke
13. Last
15. Chambers

4. Past
8. Facial
12. Stone
14. Oxygen

Down

2. Contraindication
5. COPD
7. Kyphosis
10. Insulin

3. Nitroglycerin
6. Dose
9. AED

Crossword 5

Across

1. Kinematics
10. Nines
13. Blood
15. Hypovolemic

8. Sepsis
12. Burn
14. Flail

Down

2. Impaled
4. Cardiac output
6. Cushing
9. Puncture
14. Full

3. MOI
5. Hypoperfusion
7. TBI
11. Dura

End of Chapter Answers

Chapter 1

1. **The correct answer is d.** A patient advocate is one who speaks on behalf of the patient, protects the patient, and assures that the rights of the patient are not violated.
2. **The correct answer is a.** The emergency medical technician (EMT) is a physician extender of the system's medical director.
3. **The correct answer is b.**

Chapter 2

1. **The correct answer is b.** The five stages of death and dying are *Denial* ("Not me.") Defense mechanism creating a buffer between shock of dying and dealing with the illness/injury. *Anger* ("Why me.") EMTs may be the target of the anger. Do not take anger or insults personally, be tolerant, and do not become defensive. Employ good listening and communication skills. Be empathetic. *Bargaining* ("OK, but first let me…") Agreement that, in the patient's mind, will postpone the death for a short time. *Depression* ("OK, but I haven't…") Characterized by sadness and despair. The patient is usually silent and retreats into his own world. *Acceptance* ("OK, I am not afraid.") Does not mean the patient will be happy about dying. The family will usually require more support during this stage than the patient.
2. **The correct answer is a.** *Depression* ("OK, but I haven't…"), characterized by sadness and despair. The patient is usually silent and retreats into his own world.

Chapter 3

1. **The correct answer is d.**
2. **The correct answer is d.**
3. **The correct answer is a.**
4. **The correct answer is c.**
5. **The correct answer is b.**
6. **The correct answer is a.**
7. **The correct answer is c.**
8. **The correct answer is d.**
9. **The correct answer is d.**
10. **The correct answer is b.**
11. **The correct answer is b.**

Chapter 4

1. **The correct answer is a.**
2. **The correct answer is d.** To prove negligence, the following three elements need to be established: (1) The EMT's action or lack of action incurs injury to the patient. (2) The EMT has violated the standard of care. (3) There was a duty to act.

3. **The correct answer is d.** The EMT can act under implied consent. This means the EMT can assume the patient would want emergency treatment while unconscious or unable to express verbal consent.

4. **The correct answer is c.** Abandonment refers to leaving a patient without transition of care within a hospital or medical facility, or handing over care to a lesser level of care (handing care over to a first responder).

5. **The correct answer is a.** Release of confidential information should never be made to anyone in the press. Information can be released if the EMT is subpoenaed to testify; another health-care provider needs information for the continuity of care, or for billing purposes.

Chapter 5

1. **The correct answer is a.** Physiology refers to the study of the functioning of living organisms.

2. **The correct answer is a.** *Lateral* means away from the midline, *posterior* means located in the rear, and *anterior* means located on the front.

3. **The correct answer is d.** The trachea carries oxygenated air to the lungs and expired air containing carbon dioxide back outside the body.

4. **The correct answer is d.** The left ventricle is responsible for pumping oxygenated blood to all the tissues of the body via the aorta.

5. **The correct answer is d.** The dorsalis pedis is located on the anterior portion of the foot.

Chapter 6

1. **The correct answer is a.**

2. **The correct answer is a.**

Chapter 7

1. **The correct answer is c.** Penicillin can only be prescribed by a physician. There are no pre-hospital emergency uses for penicillin.

2. **The correct answer is c.** The medication that EMTs can assist in administration that can be given this route is nitroglycerin.

3. **The correct answer is c.**

4. **The correct answer is d.** The universal medication administered by all emergency medical services (EMS) personnel is oxygen.

5. **The correct answer is b.**

6. **The correct answer is d.**

7. **The correct answer is b.**

Chapter 8

1. **The correct answer is b.** The top number of the blood pressure refers to the systolic blood pressure.

2. **The correct answer is d.** SAMPLE refers to signs/symptoms, allergies, medications, past/present medical history, last oral intake, events leading to what happened.

3. **The correct answer is c.**

4. **The correct answer is b.** The blue/gray appearance occurs from inadequate tissue perfusion.

5. **The correct answer is b.** Mechanism of injury refers to what caused the injury or how the patient was injured.

6. **The correct answer is e.**

7. **The correct answer is d.**

8. **The correct answer is a.**

9. **The correct answer is e.**

10. **The correct answer is a.**

11. **The correct answer is c.**

12. **The correct answer is c.**

13. **The correct answer is d.**

14. **The correct answer is c.**

15. **The correct answer is b.**

16. **The correct answer is c.**

17. **The correct answer is b.**

18. **The correct answer is c.**

19. **The correct answer is d.**

20. **The correct answer is d.** Scene size-up should be performed on every call.

21. **The correct answer is b.**

22. **The correct answer is c.**

23. **The correct answer is b.**

24. **The correct answer is c.** Every EMS response has the possibility of being dangerous to operate at.

Chapter 9

1. **The correct answer is d.**

2. **The correct answer is a.** The number-one cause of airway compromise in an unconscious patient is airway obstruction from the tongue.

3. **The correct answer is d.**

4. **The correct answer is b.**

5. **The correct answer is b.**

6. **The correct answer is c.**

7. **The correct answer is c.**

8. **The correct answer is d.**

9. **The correct answer is c.**

10. **The correct answer is d.**

Chapter 10

1. **The correct answer is d.**

2. **The correct answer is a.**

3. **The correct answer is c.**

4. **The correct answer is b.**

Chapter 11

1. **The correct answer is b.** High-concentration oxygen should always be administered to any patient experiencing cardiac compromise.

2. **The correct answer is d.**

3. **The correct answer is a.**

4. **The correct answer is d.**

5. **The correct answer is a.**

6. **The correct answer is a.**

7. **The correct answer is c.**

8. **The correct answer is a.**

9. **The correct answer is c.** Always check medicine for the expiration date. If it is expired, do not use it.

10. **The correct answer is c.** Nitroglycerin is a vasodilator and may cause hypotension.

11. **The correct answer is a.**
12. **The correct answer is c.**
13. **The correct answer is c.**
14. **The correct answer is c.**
15. **The correct answer is d.**

Chapter 12

1. **The correct answer is c.**
2. **The correct answer is d.**
3. **The correct answer is b.** Seizures lasting greater than 10 minutes or seizures occurring without a lucid interval are considered a "true emergency."
4. **The correct answer is a.**
5. **The correct answer is c.**
6. **The correct answer is d.** This is a commonly prescribed antiseizure medicine.
7. **The correct answer is b.** Seizures lasting for long periods do not allow the patient to breathe properly. This causes hypoxia, in turn causing further complications.
8. **The correct answer is c.**

Chapter 13

1. **The correct answer is b.** Massive vasodilation causes hypotension, tachycardia, and altered mental status.
2. **The correct answer is d.**
3. **The correct answer is c.** Edematous tissue is a common finding from allergic reactions. Edema is caused by fluid leaking from the tissues.
4. **The correct answer is d.** After any medication administration, the EMT-Basic should reassess the patient.
5. **The correct answer is b.** Epinephrine is an adrenergic medicine that causes bronchodilation and peripheral venous constriction.
6. **The correct answer is c.**

Chapter 14

1. **The correct answer is a.**
2. **The correct answer is c.**
3. **The correct answer is a.** As with any patient with inadequate ventilation, positive-pressure ventilation is the priority treatment.

Chapter 15

1. **The correct answer is b.**
2. **The correct answer is c.**

Chapter 16

1. **The correct answer is d.**
2. **The correct answer is a.**

Chapter 17

1. **The correct answer is d.** Any insult to the central nervous system may cause a change in mental status.
2. **The correct answer is b.** A common finding when evaluating a seizure patient is lacerations on the tongue from the patient biting down during seizure activity.
3. **The correct answer is a.** The inability of insulin to take glucose into the cells causes an increase in blood sugar.
4. **The correct answer is d.** It is imperative that the patient has an intact gag reflex. A patient with a compromised gag reflex increases the risk of aspiration.

Chapter 18
1. The correct answer is d.

Chapter 19
1. The correct answer is a.
2. The correct answer is a.

Chapter 20
1. The correct answer is d.
2. The correct answer is a.

Chapter 21
1. **The correct answer is a.** Hypovolemic shock is the loss of bodily fluid (blood or plasma from injury).
2. **The correct answer is b.**
3. **The correct answer is b.** Myocardial infarction causes death of cardiac muscle tissue; this results in the inability of the heart's "pump" to pump blood effectively.

Chapter 22
1. The correct answer is a.
2. The correct answer is a.

Chapter 23
1. **The correct answer is d.**
2. **The correct answer is b.** Body substance isolation should be used on every EMS assignment.
3. **The correct answer is c.**
4. **The correct answer is b.**
5. **The correct answer is c.**
6. **The correct answer is b.** Puncture and penetrating wounds tend to have little or no external bleeding.
7. **The correct answer is d.** controlling bleeding and ensuring air does not enter the wound is vital.

Chapter 24
1. **The correct answer is d.** You should always have a high index of suspicion when treating a patient with a traumatic injury to the face.
2. **The correct answer is b.**
3. **The correct answer is d.** The cervical spine has 7 vertebrae, thoracic 12, lumbar 5, sacral 5, and the coccyx 4.
4. **The correct answer is a.**
5. **The correct answer is a.**
6. **The correct answer is a.**
7. **The correct answer is a.** This discoloration is indicative of a significant injury (basal skull fracture).
8. **The correct answer is a.**
9. **The correct answer is b.**

Chapter 25
1. **The correct answer is d.**

Chapter 26
1. **The correct answer is c.**

Chapter 27

1. The correct answer is a.
2. The correct answer is a. A strain is damage or tearing to the tendons. A sprain is overextending or stretching of the ligaments.
3. The correct answer is d.
4. The correct answer is a.
5. The correct answer is a.
6. The correct answer is b.

Chapter 28

1. The correct answer is a.
2. The correct answer is d.
3. The correct answer is d.

Chapter 29

1. The correct answer is a. Swelling is an indication of toxemia.
2. The correct answer is a. Never insert anything into the vaginal opening.
3. The correct answer is d.
4. The correct answer is c.
5. The correct answer is c.
6. The correct answer is c.
7. The correct answer is b.
8. The correct answer is a. This usually means the infant is in distress. It is an ominous sign; advanced life support (ALS) should be requested.
9. The correct answer is c.
10. The correct answer is b.
11. The correct answer is c.
12. The correct answer is c.
13. The correct answer is a. Ectopic pregnancy can cause severe hemorrhage and death.
14. The correct answer is d.
15. The correct answer is a.
16. The correct answer is c.
17. The correct answer is d.
18. The correct answer is b.
19. The correct answer is c.
20. The correct answer is d.

Chapter 30

1. The correct answer is a. Adolescents usually think they are invincible.
2. The correct answer is b.
3. The correct answer is b.
4. The correct answer is d.
5. The correct answer is b.
6. The correct answer is d.
7. The correct answer is a. A partial airway obstruction in a pediatric patient will cause upper airway sounds such as crowing and/or stridor.
8. The correct answer is d.

9. **The correct answer is c.** Obtaining the blood pressure of a 2-year-old child would be difficult. The best indication of adequate circulation is to evaluate mental status, skin color, moisture, and temperature.

Chapter 31

1. The correct answer is a.
2. The correct answer is a.
3. The correct answer is c.
4. The correct answer is c.
5. The correct answer is d.
6. The correct answer is d.
7. The correct answer is d.

Chapter 32

1. The correct answer is a.
2. The correct answer is a.

Chapter 33

1. **The correct answer is a.** Avoiding using your back in lifting will reduce back injuries.
2. The correct answer is d.
3. The correct answer is a.
4. The correct answer is b.

Chapter 34

1. The correct answer is b.
2. The correct answer is b.
3. The correct answer is b.

Chapter 35

1. The correct answer is d.
2. The correct answer is a.

Chapter 36

1. The correct answer is b.
2. The correct answer is b.
3. The correct answer is c.

Chapter 37

1. The correct answer is c.
2. The correct answer is a.
3. The correct answer is b.
4. The correct answer is d.
5. The correct answer is e.
6. The correct answer is b.
7. The correct answer is a.
8. The correct answer is a.
9. The correct answer is a.
10. The correct answer is d.

Index

Page numbers followed by *f* or *t* indicate figures or tables, respectively.

A

Abandonment, 29
Abdomen
    anatomy, 170*f*, 259
    dialysis patient, assessment
        of, 173–174
    examination/inspection, 204, 205
    gastrointestinal system emergencies,
        169–172
    pediatric considerations, 303–304
Abdominal injuries, 235
    assessment, 259–260
    evisceration, 260
    hemorrhage, 170–171
    perforation, 170
Abnormal uterine bleeding, 208
Abortion, 282. *See also* Spontaneous
    abortion
Abrasion, 234
Abruptio placenta, 284
    emergency management, 285
    signs/symptoms, 285
Absence seizure, 146
Absorbed poisoning, 159–160, 364
Absorption, as decontamination
    mode, 366
Abuse. *See* Alcohol abuse; Child
    abuse; Geriatric patients,
    abuse, assessment of
Acceptance, grieving process stage, 12
"Accidental Death and Disability: The
    Neglected Disease of Modern
    Society" (report), 5
Activated charcoal, 61, 62*f*,
    160–161, 160*f*
Acute bacterial prostatitis, 199
Acute coronary syndrome, in geriatric
    patients, 313
Acute renal failure (ARF), 197
Adenomyosis, 209
Adolescents, 294
    endocrine changes, 53–54
    growth rate, 53

psychosocial development, 54
Adrenal cortex, 182
Adrenal gland, 182, 182*f*
Adrenal medulla, 183
Adult respiratory distress syndrome
    (ARDS), 119–120
Adults
    older. *See* Older adults
    psychosocial development,
        54–55
Advance directives, 27–28
AED. *See* Automated external defibril-
    lator (AED)
Aerobic metabolism, 218
Affective disorders, 190
Afterload, 216
Agoraphobias, 191
Air ambulance service, 346, 347*f*
Airlift. *See* Medivac
Airway, 38
    assessment of, 117
    compromise, 118–119
    and head injuries, 238
    head-tilt-chin lift, 99, 99*f*, 105–106
    lower, 95–96
    management
        allergic reactions and, 155
        poisoning and, 160
    modified jaw-thrust, 99, 100*f*, 106
    nasopharyngeal, 109, 109*f*
    obstructions
        in pediatric patients, 297–298
    opening, 99, 99–100*f*
    oropharyngeal, 108–109, 108*f*, 109*f*
    pediatric patients, 294–295
    status, assessment of, 78
    upper, 95
Alarm stage, of stress, 193
Albuterol sulfate, 64–65
Alcohol abuse
    and behavioral emergencies, 190
    delirium tremens, 166–167
    emergency management, 167

and poisoning, 166
    and somatization, 192
Allergens, pathways for, 153
Allergic reactions
    and airway management, 155
    anaphylaxis, 153–154
    and cardiac arrest, 153
    causes of, 154
    emergency management,
        154–155
    insects and, 154
    medications, 155–156
    and patient assessment, 154
Alpha radiation, 363
Altered mental status. *See also*
        Behavioral emergencies
    in geriatric patients, 314–315
    in pediatric patients, 301
Alveolar/capillary exchange, 38, 116
Alzheimer disease, in geriatric
        patients, 315
Ambulance, first vehicle as, 3
Ambulance call reports, 20–21
Ambulance operations
    assignment operations, 342–344
    daily inspection of vehicle systems,
        341–342, 342*f*
    dispatch center, 342
    en route to receiving facility, 346
    en route to scene, 342–344
    escorts and multiple vehicle
        response, 344
    post run, 346
    preassignment operations and
        check, 341–342
    scene arrival, 344–345, 345*f*
Ambulance services. *See* Emergency
        medical services (EMS)
Ambulance volante, 3
American Civil War, and emergency
        services, 4
Amnesic psychogenic dissociative
        disorder, 191

Amniotic sac, 281
Amphetamines, 163
Amputations, 235, 236
Anaerobic metabolism, 219
Anaphylactic shock, 223
Anaphylaxis, 153–154
Anatomical position, 35, 36f
Anatomical terms, 35–36
Anger, grieving process stage, 11
Animal bites. See Bites
Anterior, anatomical term, 36
Antigens. See Allergic reactions
Aorta, 42, 129
Aortic aneurysm, 171
APGAR scoring, 287–288, 288t
Aphasia, 319
Appendicitis, 170
ARDS. See Adult respiratory distress
        syndrome (ARDS)
ARF. See Acute renal failure (ARF)
Arteries
    aorta, 42, 129
    arteriole, 43, 130
    brachial, 43, 130
    carotid, 43, 130
    coronary, 42, 129
    dorsalis pedis, 43
    femoral, 43, 130
    posterior tibial, 43, 130
    pulmonary, 42, 129
    radial, 43, 130
Arteriole, 43, 130
Arthritis, 324
Articulation disorders, 319
Artificial ventilation, 296
    adequate, 98
    bag to stoma/tracheotomy tube, 108
    bag-valve-mask (BVM) for. See
        Bag-valve-mask (BVM)
    flow-restricted, oxygen-powered
        devices, 106–107
    inadequate, 98–99
Aspirin, 61, 63f, 69
Assault/battery, 28
Asthma, 121–122
Asymptomatic inflammatory prosta-
        titis, 199
Ataxia, 325
Athetosis, 325
Atrioventricular (AV) node, 42, 129
Atrium, 40
Atropine, 67–68
Auscultation, 205
Automated external defibrillator (AED)
    advantages of, 134

age and weight guideline, 135
and cardiac rhythms analysis,
        133–134
    examples of, 133f
    importance to EMT, 132–133
    maintenance, 136–137
    medical direction for usage, 136
    operational procedures, 134–135
    and recurrent ventricular fibrilla-
        tion, 135, 135f
    types of, 133
Automaticity, 41
Automatisms, 146
Automobile accident. See Motor vehi-
        cle crash (MVC)
Autonomic nervous system, 242
Avulsion, 235

B
Bacteria, 376
Bag-valve-mask (BVM), 103–105f,
        103–106
    adult, 104f
    with head-tilt-chin-lift, 103f,
        105–106
    infant, 105f
    with modified jaw-thrust, 103f, 106
    pediatric, 105f
    pros/cons of, 103
    to stoma, 108
Bargaining, grieving process stage, 11
Baroreceptors, 217
Baseline vital signs
    assessment of, 85–88, 85t
    blood pressure, 88
    breathing, 86
    pulse, 86–87
    pupils, 87–88
    skin, 87
Base station, communication system
        component, 15
Basilar Artery, blockage, and stroke, 144
Bees sting, 274, 276
Behavior, patient, causes of
        alteration, 189
Behavioral emergencies
    causes, 189
    defined, 189
    management of, 196
    medical/legal considerations, 194
    patients
        assessment of, 194–195
        methods to calm, 195–196
    psychiatric disorders, 190–192. See
        also specific disorders

somatoform disorders, 192–193
    suicide, 190, 193–194
    violence assessment in, 195
Bell clapper deformity, 198
Beta radiation, 363
Bilateral, anatomical term, 36
Bio-hazards, and body substance iso-
        lation, 175–177
Biological agents
    characteristics, 376
    protection against, 378–379
    types of, 376
    as weapons of mass destruction,
        375–376
Birth canal, 281
Bites
    bees, 274, 276
    cats, 274, 275
    dog, 273–274, 275
    emergency management, 277
    humans, 274, 275–276
    jellyfish, 275, 276–277
    snakes, 274–275, 276
    spider, 274, 276
    stingrays, 275, 277
    wasps, 274, 276
Blast injury, 231
Bleeding
    characteristics of, 220
    external, 221
    internal, 220
    and shock, 220–221
Bleeding diverticulosis, 170
Blister agents, 375
Blood, 217
    composition, 43, 130
    flow, 40, 217
Blood agents, 375
Blood pressure, 44
    assessment of, 88, 118
    defined, 216
    diastolic, 131
    systolic, 131
Blood vessels. See also Arteries;
        Capillaries; Veins
    older adults, 55
    and perfusion, 217–218
    severed, in neck, 252
    types of, 42–43, 129–130
"Bloody show," 281
Blunt trauma, 227–230. See also
        Motor vehicle crash (MVC)
Bodily fluids, infectious, 179–180
Body mechanics, for lifting and
        moving patients, 335–337

Body substance isolation (BSI), 76, 175–177
Boiling point (BP), 363
Bone injuries, 263–265
    emergency management, 263–265
    signs/symptoms, 263
Bowel obstruction, 170
BP. *See* Boiling point (BP)
Brachial arteries, 43, 130
Brain, 141, 142*f*
    injuries. *See* Traumatic brain injuries (TBIs)
Brain attack. *See* Stroke
Brand name, medications. *See* Trade/brand name, medications
Breaking dissemination devices, 378
Breastbone, 37
Breathing, 38
    abnormal sounds, 117–118
    adequate, 97–98
    assessment of, 78, 86, 117
    head injuries and, 238
    inadequate, 98
    normal rate/ranges, 38
    normal sounds, 117
    pediatric patients, 295
Breech birth, 289
Bronchi, 38, 95
Bronchitis, chronic, 120–121
Bruise. *See* Contusion
BSI. *See* Body substance isolation (BSI)
Bundle branches, 42, 129
Bundle of His, 42, 129
Bursting/exploding dissemination devices, 378
BVM. *See* Bag-valve-mask (BVM)

C
Cancer, 324
    cervical, 211–212
    fallopian tubes, 212
Capillaries, 43, 130
Capillary/cellular exchange, 38, 116
Car accident. *See* Motor vehicle crash (MVC)
Carbatrol, 148
Carbon monoxide (CO), poisoning, 161, 162*f*
Carboxyhemoglobin (COHb), 161
Carcinoma, colon, 170
Cardiac compromise, 131
Cardiac conduction system, 41–44, 126, 128*f*, 129
    electrical impulses, 41–42

Cardiac emergency. *See also* Automated external defibrillator (AED)
    allergic reaction and, 153
    in geriatric patient, 313
    management, 131–132
    syncope, 150
    witnessed, 135–136
Cardiac muscles, 44
Cardiac One (ambulance), 4–5
Cardiac output, 216
Cardiac rhythms, analysis of, 133–134
Cardiogenic shock, 221–222
Cardiopulmonary resuscitation (CPR), 105, 131–132
    interruption of, 134
Cardiovascular system
    anatomy, 126–130, 127–128*f*
    geriatric patients, 308
    heart, 39–40, 41*f*
    infants, 47
    older adults, 55–56
    physiology, 43, 131
    pump of, 216
    toddlers, 50
Carotid arteries, 43, 130
    blockage, and stroke, 143–144
Cat bites, 274, 275
Catheters, suction, 102
Ceiling level (TLV-C), 364
Central circulation, 44
Central lines, and special needs pediatric patients, 305
Central nervous system, 45
Central pulses, 131
Cerebral hemorrhage, 144
Cerebral herniation, 240–241
Cerebral palsy (CP), 324
Cerebral vascular accident (CVA). *See* Stroke
Cervical cancer
    signs/symptoms, 211
    staging, 212
    types, 211
Cervical spine immobilization devices (CSIDs), 245–246
CF. *See* Cystic fibrosis (CF)
Chain of survival, 132–133
Chambers, of heart, 40
Cheek, impaled object to, 251
Chemical agents
    protection against, 378
    as weapons of mass destruction, 374–375. *See also* specific agents
Chemical burn injury, eyes, 250

Chest
    anatomy of, 254, 255*f*
    injuries, 235
        assessment, 256–257
        emergency management, 257–258
        flail segment, 256, 258
        hemothorax, 256
        open, 254, 258
        pneumothorax, 255
        "sucking chest wound," 254
        tension pneumothorax, 255–256
    pediatric considerations, 303
Child abuse
    and neglect, 304
    report of suspected, 32*f*
Childbirth emergency
    abnormal delivery, 288–289
    normal delivery, 286–287, 286*f*
Children. *See also* Pediatric patients
    developmental considerations, 293–294
    divorce impact on, 52
    organophosphate poisonings in, treatment of, 68–69
    and respiratory considerations, 39, 98
    seizures in, 300–301
    spastic paralysis in, 324–325
    as trauma patients, 81–82
Choking agents, 374–375
Cholecystitis, 171
Cholinergic poisonings, 68
Chronic bacterial prostatitis, 199
Chronic obstructive pulmonary disease, in geriatric patients, 314
Cincinnati Pre-hospital Stroke Scale (CPSS), 145*t*
Circulation
    head injuries and, 238–239
    inadequate, 131
    pediatric patients, 295
Circulatory system. *See* Cardiovascular system
CISD/CISM. *See* Critical incident stress debriefing/management (CISD/CISM)
Civilian ambulance services, 3–4
Closed soft tissue injuries, 233–234. *See also* specific injuries
Cocaine, 163
Cogentin, 191
Cognitive development, toddlers, 51
Cold, exposure to. *See* Environmental emergencies, local cold injuries; Hypothermia

Cold zone, hazardous materials, 359, 362f, 363
Colon, carcinoma, 170
Coma
    causes of, 187
    defined, 186
    Glasgow Coma Scale, 187, 187t
Common cold, 124
Communicable diseases
    patients with, 330
    protection from, 179–180
Communications, 15–18
    interpersonal, 18
    issues with elderly patients, 18
    with medical direction, 16
    and patient reporting, 16–17
    radio, 15–16
    with receiving facilities, 16
    system components, 15
    verbal, 18
Compazine, 191
Compensated shock, 219
Complex partial seizures (CPS), 146
Conductive deafness, 318
Conductivity, 41
Confidentiality, patient, 30
Congestive heart failure, in geriatric patients, 313
Consent, forms of, 28
Contamination, types of, 364
Contractile force, 216
Contusion, 233–234
Conversion disorder, 191
Coricidin HBP (CCC), 165
Coronary arteries, 42, 129
CP. See Cerebral palsy (CP)
CPR. See Cardiopulmonary resuscitation (CPR)
CPS. See Complex partial seizures (CPS)
CPSS. See Cincinnati Pre-hospital Stroke Scale (CPSS)
Cricoid cartilage, 38
Crime scene
    evidence preservation, 33
    violent, 179
Critical incident stress debriefing/ management (CISD/CISM), 13
Croup, 124, 299–300, 299t
Crowning, 281
Crush injuries, 234, 235
Crying, infants, 50
CSIDs. See Cervical spine immobilization devices (CSIDs)
Cyanide poisoning, 162

Cystic fibrosis (CF), 325
Cystolithiasis, 198

D
Deafness, 318. See also specific types
Decompensated shock, 219
Decontamination
    decision making, 366
    gross, 367
    methods used by trained personnel, 368
    modes, 366
Defibrillation, 133. See also Automated external defibrillator (AED)
Delirium tremens, 166–167
Delivery procedures, normal childbirth, 286–287, 286f
Dementia, in geriatric patients, 315
Denial, grieving process stage, 11
Dental appliances, and oxygen administration, 111
Dental system
    infants, 49
    toddlers, 51
Depakene, 148–149
Depakote, 148–149
Depersonalization, 191
Depression
    grieving process stage, 11
    and suicide, 190
Dermis, 45, 45f, 233, 234f
Developmental delay, 321–322
Diabetes
    defined, 184
    effects of, 184–185
    pathophysiology, 184
    signs/symptoms, 185
Dialysis
    complications of, 173–174
    hemodialysis, 173
    patient management, 174
    peritoneal, 173
Diaphragm physiology, 115
Diastolic blood pressure, 44, 131
DIC. See Disseminating intravascular coagulopathy (DIC)
Diethylstilbestrol (DES), 211
Dilution, as decontamination mode, 366
Diplegia, 324
Direct deposit dissemination devices, 377
Direct ground lift, 338–339
Direct pressure, to control bleeding, 221

Disasters. See also Mass casualty incident (MCI); Terrorism; Weapons of mass destruction (WMD)
    hurricane, 354
    natural, 355, 356f
    technical hazards, 356, 357f
Dispatch center, 342
Dispatcher, and scene assessment, 75
Disposal/isolation, as decontamination mode, 366
Disseminating intravascular coagulopathy (DIC), 220
Distal, anatomical term, 36
Diverticulitis, 169
Diverticulosis, bleeding, 170
Divorce, impact on children, 52
DNR order. See Do not resuscitate (DNR) order
Documentation, 18–22
    ambulance call reports, 20–21
    crime scene, 33
    at multiple casualty incidents, 22
    of patient refusal, 21–22
    pre-hospital care report, 19f, 20–21
    special situations/reports/incident reporting, 22, 23f
    Unusual Occurrence Report, 23f
Dog bites, 273–274, 275
Donor/organ harvesting, 31
Do not resuscitate (DNR) order, 27, 27f
Dorsal, anatomical term, 36
Dorsalis pedis artery, 43
Down syndrome, 322
Draw sheet method, 339
Drowning/near drowning, 302
Drug abuse. See also Alcohol abuse
    and behavioral emergencies, 191
    defined, 163
    emergency management, 167
    street drugs and, 163–165. See also specific drugs
    and withdrawal of drugs, 165
Drugs. See Medications
Drug toxicity, in geriatric patients, 315
Duchenne muscular dystrophy, 326
Duty to act, 30
Dysarthria, 319
Dysmenorrhea, 208
Dystonia, 191

E
Ear, injuries to, 252
Eclampsia, 284

Ectopic pregnancy, 173
emergency management, 283
signs/symptoms, 283
Electrical impulses, cardiac, 41–42
Elevation, to control bleeding, 221
Elimination patterns, toddlers, 51
Emergency medical services (EMS)
civilian, 3–4
communication. *See*
Communications
components of, 7–8
defined, 7
documentation. *See* Documentation
early history of, 3–4
evolution and growth, 6–7
public discovery of, 5–7
quality improvement system and, 9
roles/responsibilities, mass casualty
incident and, 357–358
Technical Assistance Program
Standards (NHTSA), 7
Emergency medical technicians
(EMTs)
Code of Ethics, 26
and emotional aspects of emergency
care, 11–12
immunizations, 180
legal duties of, 26–27
and medications. *See* Medications
and needs of dying patient, 12
paramedics *vs.*, 6
personal protection, 175–180,
368–370, 369–370f. *See also*
Personal protective
equipment (PPE)
professional attributes, 8–9
protection against false
accusations, 194
and quality improvement, 9
response to pediatric patients, 306
roles/responsibilities, 8
in extrication, 348
at rescue hazardous material incidents, 178–179
safety of, 76
and stress management, 12–13
systems medical director and, 9
and terminally ill patients, 329–330
training
formal origins, 4
specialty, 176
Emergency moves, 337–338
Emergency Response Guidebook,
177, 178f
Emergency! (television show), 5–6

EMI. *See* Emotionally/mentally
impaired (EMI)
Emotional impairments, 322–323
Emotionally/mentally impaired
(EMI), 323
Emphysema, 120
EMS. *See* Emergency medical
services (EMS)
EMTs. *See* Emergency medical technicians (EMTs)
Endocrine system
adrenal cortex, 182
adrenal gland, 182, 182f
adrenal medulla, 183
anatomy, 181–184, 182f
changes in, adolescence and, 53–54
function of, 46
homeostasis, 46
older adults, 56
ovaries, 182f, 183
pancreas, 182f, 184
parathyroid gland, 182, 182f
physiology, 181–184
pituitary gland, 181, 182f, 183f
testes, 182f, 183–184
thyroid gland, 182, 182f
Endometriosis, 209
Endometritis, 210
Environmental emergencies
bites and stings. *See* Bites
and geriatric patients, 316
hyperthermia, 267, 271–273
hypothermia, 267, 268–270
local cold injuries, 270–271
Epidermis, 45, 45f, 233, 234f
Epididymitis, 173, 199
Epiglottis, 38, 95
Epiglottitis, 124, 300
Epilepsy
and Lennox-Gastaut syndrome, 147
and seizures, 145, 146. *See also*
Seizures
and West syndrome, 147
Epinephrine, 65
Epipen auto-injector, 61, 62f, 155–156
Esophageal varices, 169
Estrogen, 183, 206
decreased, consequences of, 207
Ethical development, adolescents
and, 54
Ethics. *See* Medical ethics
Evisceration, 260
Excitability, 41
Exhalation, 38, 96
Exhaustion stage, of stress, 193

External bleeding, and shock, 221
Extremities
pediatric considerations, 304
and respiratory system
assessment, 118
Extremity lift, 339
Extrication
access to patient during, 349
fundamentals, 348
and patient safety, 348
removing patient, 349
rescue equipment, 348, 349f
Extruded eyeball, 250
Eyes
anatomy of, 247f
foreign object in, 250
impaled object in, 251
injuries
assessment of, 248, 249–250
removing contact lenses, 251
types, 250–251
protection, 175, 176f
surrounding structures of, 247f

F
Face, anatomy, 248
Facial bones, 36
Facial injuries
assessment of, 248–249
emergency management, 251
and oxygen administration, 110–111
Fainting. *See* Syncope
Fallopian tubes, cancer of, 212
Falls, as cause of trauma, 231
Families
and psychosocial development
in adolescents, 54
in school-age children, 53
response to child's illness/injury, 306
"Fast break" incident decision
making, 367
Felbatol, 148
Female
endocrine changes in, 53
genitalia
anatomy, 261f
assessment, 262
injuries, 262
treatment, 262
genitourinary system diseases, 203
reproductive system
anatomy and physiology,
281–282, 282f
emergencies. *See* Gynecological
emergencies

Femoral arteries, 43, 130
Fetus, 281
Fever, in pediatric patients, 301
Fibroids, 209
Fick principle, 218
Financial challenges, for health care, 330–331
Flail segment, 256, 258
Flammable/explosive limits, 363
Flash point (FP), 363
Fluency disorders, 320
Fontanelles, infants, 48
Foreign object, in eye, 250
Fowler, anatomical term, 36
FP. *See* Flash point (FP)
Frank-Starling mechanism, 216
Fugue disorder, 191
Fully automated defibrillator, 133

G

Gabitril, 148
Gamma hydroxybutyrate (GHB), 163
Gamma radiation, 363
Gastritis, 169
Gastrointestinal (GI) system
    diseases, 202–203
    family history, 203
    geriatric patients, 309
    older adults, 56
    personal and social history, 204
Gastrointestinal hemorrhage
    lower, 171
    upper, 170–171
GCS. *See* Glasgow Coma Scale (GCS)
Generalized hypoxia, 39
Generalized seizures, 146. *See also* specific types
Generic name, medications, 61
Genitalia. *See* Female, genitalia; Male, genitalia
Genitourinary and renal emergencies
    acute renal failure, 197
    cardinal signs/symptoms, 200–202
    epididymitis, 199
    history of present illness, 200
    patient assessment in, 200–205
    priapism, 199–200
    prostatitis, 199
    testicular torsion, 198
    urinary calculi, 198
    urinary tract infections, 197–198
Genitourinary (GU) system
    diseases, 203
    emergencies. *See* Genitourinary and renal emergencies

family history, 203
personal and social history, 204
Geriatric patients
    abuse, assessment of, 316
    altered mental status, 314–315
    assessment, 310–312
    cardiac emergency, 313
    cardiovascular system, 308
        emergency, 313
    causes of death in, 310
    emergency management, 312–313
    environmental emergency and, 316
    gastrointestinal system, 309
    integumentary system, 309
    musculoskeletal system, 309
    neurological system, 309
    positioning, 312–313
    renal system, 309
    respiratory system, 309
        emergency, 313–314
    shock and, 315–316
    transporting, 313
    trauma and, 315–316
GHB. *See* Gamma hydroxybutyrate (GHB)
GI system. *See* Gastrointestinal (GI) system
Glands. *See* Endocrine system
Glasgow Coma Scale (GCS), 187, 187t
Globe injury, 250
Gloves, protective, 175, 176f, 177
Glucagon, 184
Glucose
    oral, 64
    and osmotic diuresis, 184
Gonadotropin, 53, 54
Gowns, protective, 175, 176f
Grand mal seizure, 146
Grieving process, stages of, 11–12
GU system. *See* Genitourinary (GU) system
Gynecological emergencies, 172–173, 206–212. *See also* Childbirth emergency; Pregnancy
    abnormal uterine bleeding, 208
    cervical cancer, 211–212
    endometriosis, 209
    endometritis, 210
    fallopian tubes cancer, 212
    incontinence, 210–211
    ovarian tumors, 212

pelvic inflammatory disease, 210
postmenopausal bleeding, 209
premenstrual syndrome, 207–208
sexually transmitted diseases, 209–210
toxic shock syndrome, 210

H

Haldol, 191
Hallucinogens, 164
Hand washing, 76
Hazardous materials
    common, 365–366
    contamination, 364
    decontamination
        decision making, 366
        gross, 367
        methods used by trained personnel, 368
        modes, 366
    EMT response, 358–360
    and "fast break" incident decision making, 367
    identification, 362
    incidents
        protective clothing for, 178
        rescue, responsibility at, 178–179
    medical operations terminology, 363
    personal protection, 177, 368–370, 369–370f
    recognizing, 360–361, 361f
    scene size-up, 359
    tagging with placards, 177, 177f
    toxicological terms, 363–364
    zones, 359, 362–363, 362f
Hazardous Waste Operations and Emergency Response (HAZWOPER) training, 176
Head
    injuries. *See also* Traumatic brain injuries (TBIs)
        brain and skull, 238
        emergency management, 241
        nontraumatic brain injuries, 239
        open, 240
        types, 239–240
    pediatric considerations, 303
Head-tilt-chin-lift, 99, 99f
    bag-valve-mask with, 103f, 105–106
Health-care system, components of, 8–9
Health Insurance Portability and Accountability Act (HIPAA), 30–31

Hearing, toddlers, 51
Hearing impairments, 318–319
Heart, 39–40
    anatomy of, 41f, 127–128f
    atrium, 40
    blood flow through, 40
    chambers, 40
    muscle, 40
    older adults, 55–56
    and perfusion, 215–217
    ventricle, 40
Heart attack. See Cardiac emergency
Heart rate, and respiratory system
        assessment, 118
Heat index (National Weather
        Service), 271f
Hematoma, 234
Hemiplegia, 324
Hemodialysis, 173
Hemorrhagic stroke, 143, 143t
    signs/symptoms, 144–145
Hemothorax, 256
Hepatitis, 171
Heroin, 164
HIPAA. See Health Insurance
        Portability and Accountability
        Act (HIPAA)
Homeland Security Presidential
        Directive 5, 354
Homeostasis, 46
Home ventilators, and special needs
        pediatric patients, 305
Hormone, defined, 181
Hospital, communication
        with, 16–18
Hot zone, hazardous materials, 359,
        362, 362f, 367–368
Huffing, 164
Human bites, 274, 275–276
Hurricane, 354
Hyperglycemia, 186
Hyperthermia
    defined, 267
    emergency management, 272–273
    risk factors, 272
    signs/symptoms, 272
Hyperventilation syndrome, 123
Hypochondriasis, 191
Hypoglycemia, 185–186
Hypoperfusion. See Shock
Hypothermia
    defined, 267
    emergency management, 270
    environmental conditions and, 269
    injuries, 270–271

risk factors, 268
signs/symptoms, 269
Hypovolemic shock, 220–221
Hypoxia, 39
Hypoxic drive, 115

I
ICH. See Intracerebral
        hemorrhage (ICH)
Identity development, adolescents
        and, 54
IDLH. See Immediately dangerous to
        life and health (IDLH)
Ignition temperature, 363
Imidazolines, 164–165
Immediately dangerous to life and
        health (IDLH), 364
Immune system
    infants, 48
    toddlers, 51
Immunizations, EMTs, 180
Incontinence, 210
    infertility, 211
    polycystic ovarian syndrome, 211
    stress, 211
Infantile spasm. See West syndrome
Infants
    cardiovascular system, 47
    dental system, 49
    developmental considerations, 293
    growth and development, 49–50
    immune system, 48
    musculoskeletal system, 49
    nervous system, 48–49
    psychosocial development, 50
    pulmonary system, 47
    renal system, 48
    weight of, 47
Inferior, anatomical term, 36
Infertility, 211
Ingested poisoning
    emergency management, 159
    signs/symptoms, 158
Inhalants, huffing, 164
Inhalation, 38, 96
Inhaled poisoning, 159
Injury assessment
    eyes, 248, 249–250
    facial, 249–250
    neck, 248–249
    soft tissue, 233–236
    spinal, 244
    trauma, 79–83, 80t
Insects, and allergic reactions, 154
Instaglucose gel, 63, 63f

Insulin, 184
Integumentary system, 45. See also Skin
    geriatric patients, 309
Internal bleeding, and shock, 220
Interpersonal communication, 18
Intracerebral hemorrhage (ICH), 143
Involuntary (smooth) muscles, 44
Irreversible shock, 219–220
Ischemic phase, menstrual cycle, 207
Islets of Langerhans, 184

J
Jellyfish bites, 275, 276–277
Joints, 37
    injuries, 263–265
        emergency management, 263–265
        signs/symptoms, 263
        splinting, 264
Journal of Emergency Medical Services
        (JEMS), 6

K
KE. See Kinetic energy (KE)
Keppra, 148
Ketoacids, renal secretion of, 185
Ketone bodies, 185
Ketone body formation, 185
Kidney stones, 171–172
Kinetic energy (KE), 227
Klonopin, 149

L
Labor, 281
Laceration, 235
Lamictal, 148
Landing zone (LZ), 346, 347f
Late adulthood. See Older adults
Lateral, anatomical term, 35
Legal issues
    abandonment, 29
    advance directives, 27–28
    with behavioral emergencies, 194
    crime scene/evidence
        preservation, 33
    donor/organ harvesting, 31
    duty to act, 30
    EMT's duties, 26–27
    forms of consent, 28
    Health Insurance Portability and
        Accountability Act, 30–31
    medical alert tag, 31, 31f
    negligence, 29
    patient confidentiality, 30
    refusals of treatment and/or trans-
        port, 28–29

Lennox-Gastaut syndrome, 147
Lethal concentration and doses (LD$_{50}$), 363
Letterman, Jonathan, 4
Lid injury, 250
Life span, development of, 47–57, 48t
　　adolescence, 53–54. See also Adolescents
　　early adulthood, 54–55. See also Adults
　　infancy, 47–50. See also Infants
　　middle adulthood, 55
　　older adults, 55–57. See also Older adults
　　school-age children, 52–53
　　toddlers, 50–52. See also Toddlers
Lifestyle changes, and stress management, 13
Lifting and moving patients, 335–340
Limb presentation, 289
Lower airway, 95–96
Lower extremities, 37
Lower GI hemorrhage, 170–171
Low-flow priapism, 199
Lyrica, 148
LZ. See Landing zone (LZ)

M
Male
　　endocrine changes in, 54
　　genitalia
　　　anatomy, 261f
　　　assessment, 262
　　　injuries, 261
　　　treatment, 262
　　genitourinary system diseases, 203
　　reproductive system, emergencies, 173
Manual suction device, 102f
Mark-I auto-injector, 61, 62f, 65–66
Masks
　　non-rebreather, 110
　　protective, 175, 177f
Mass casualty incident (MCI)
　　causes of, 355–356
　　defined, 356
　　documentation at, 22
　　EMS roles and responsibilities, 357–358
　　management, goals of, 356–357
　　stages of, 357
　　triage, 358–361
Mechanical lift stretcher, 335–336, 336f

Mechanism of injury (MOI)
　　abdominal injuries, 259–260
　　bone and joint injuries, 263
　　determination of, 77
　　history and secondary assessment, 80t
　　injuries associated with specific, 226
　　spinal injuries, 243–245
Meconium, 289
Medial, anatomical term, 35
Medical alert tag, 31, 31f
Medical direction
　　for AED use, 136
　　during behavioral emergencies, 194
　　communication with, 16
Medical ethics
　　defined, 26
　　duty to act, 30
　　and ethical responsibilities, 27
　　Health Insurance Portability and Accountability Act, 30–31
　　and legal duties, 26–27
　　patient confidentiality, 30
　　and patient refusals, 28–29
Medical Orders for Life-Sustaining Treatment (MOLST) form, 28
Medical patient. See also Nature of illness (NOI)
　　geriatric, 311
　　history and secondary assessment, 83–84
　　physical examination, 84–85, 85t
　　unresponsive, 84
Medications, 61–63. See also specific drugs
　　allergic reactions, 155–156
　　on EMS unit, 61, 62–63f
　　forms of, 63–64
　　names, 61
　　overdose. See Drug abuse; Poisoning
　　in patient history, 89
　　pre-hospital. See Pre-hospital medications
　　seizures, 148–149
Medivac, 346
Menopausal phase, menstrual cycle, 207
Menorrhagia, 208
Menstrual cycle
　　ischemic phase, 207
　　menopausal phase, 207
　　proliferation phase, 206–207
　　secretory phase, 207
Mental illness, defined, 321
Mental retardation. See Emotionally/mentally impaired (EMI)

Mental status, patient's
　　altered. See Altered mental status
　　assessment of, 78
Methamphetamines, 163
Metrorrhagia, 208
Microcirculation, 217
Midclavicular, anatomical term, 36
Military conflict, and development of ambulance services, 3–4
Mini stroke. See Transient ischemic attack
Miscarriage. See Spontaneous abortion
Mittelschmerz, 173
Mobile two-way radios, communication system component, 15
Modeling, toddlers and, 52
MOI. See Mechanism of injury (MOI)
Moral development, school-age children and, 53
Motor vehicle crash (MVC)
　　ambulance, 343f
　　and hazardous materials, 358–360, 360f
　　kinematics, 227
　　and spinal injuries, 241
　　types of, 228, 228–230f
Movements, infants, 48
MS. See Multiple sclerosis (MS)
Mucoviscidosis. See Cystic fibrosis (CF)
Multiple births, 289
Multiple sclerosis (MS), 325–326
Muscle, heart, 40
Muscular dystrophy, 326–327
Musculoskeletal system
　　functions of, 44
　　geriatric patients, 309
　　infants, 49
　　toddlers, 51
MVC. See Motor vehicle crash (MVC)
Myasthenia gravis, 328
Myocardial infarction (MI). See Cardiac emergency
Myoclonic seizures, 147

N
NAEMT. See National Association of Emergency Medical Technicians (NAEMT)
Nasal cannula, 110
Nasopharyngeal (nasal) airways, 109, 109f
Nasopharynx, 95
National Association of Emergency Medical Technicians (NAEMT), 6

National Fire Protection Agency 704
    placard system, 361*f*
National Incident Management
    System (NIMS), 354–355
National Registry of Emergency
    Medical Technicians
    (NREMT), 6
National Weather Service
    heat index, 271*f*
    Wind Chill chart, 268*f*
Natural disasters, 355, 356*f*
Nature of illness (NOI)
    determination of, 76–77
    history and secondary assessment, 80*t*
Neck
    anatomy, 248
    injuries
        assessment of, 248–249
        care to, 252
        open, 236
        severed blood vessel, 252
Negligence, 29
Nephrolithiasis, 198
Nerve agents, 375, 375*t*
Nervous system, 242
    autonomic, 242
    central, 45
    functions of, 45
    infants, 48–49
    older adults, 57
    parasympathetic, 242
    peripheral, 45, 242
    sympathetic, 242
    toddlers, 51
Neurogenic shock, 222
Neurological system, geriatric
    patients, 309
Neurontin, 148
Neuroses, 321
Neutralization, as decontamination
    mode, 366
Newborns
    developmental considerations, 293
    initial care, 288*f*
NIMS. *See* National Incident
    Management System (NIMS)
Nitroglycerin, 61, 63, 63*f*, 69–70
NOI. *See* Nature of illness (NOI)
Nonemergent moves, 338–340
Non-rebreather mask, 110
Nontraumatic brain injuries, 239
Nose, injuries to, 251
NREMT. *See* National Registry
    of Emergency Medical
    Technicians (NREMT)

Nuclear agents
    characteristics, 376–377
    limiting exposure, 377
    protection against, 379

O
Obesity, 320
Obstetrical emergencies
    abruptio placenta, 284–285
    eclampsia, 284
    ectopic pregnancy, 283
    placenta previa, 285
    preeclampsia, 283–284
    spontaneous abortion, 283
    uterine rupture, 285
Obstructive lung disease
    chronic bronchitis, 120–121
    emphysema, 120
Older adults, 55–57
    cardiovascular system, 55–56
    endocrine system, 56
    gastrointestinal system, 56
    nervous system, 57
    psychosocial development, 57
    renal system, 56
    respiratory system, 56
    sensory changes in, 56–57
    as trauma patients, 81
Oligomenorrhea, 208
Onboard suction unit, 101*f*
Open injuries
    chest, 254, 258
    head, 240
    neck, 236
    soft tissue injuries, 234–236
Open soft tissue injuries, 234–236. *See
    also* specific injuries
Oral glucose, 64
Orbit injury, 250
Organic disorders, 192
Organophosphate poisonings, treat-
    ment of, 68–69
Oropharyngeal (oral) airways,
    108–109, 108*f*, 109*f*
Oropharynx, 95
Orthopedic trauma, bone and joint
    injuries, 263–265
Osmotic diuresis, 184
Osteoarthritis, 324
Outcome-based research, 6–7
Ovarian cyst, 172
Ovarian tumors, 212
Ovaries, 182*f*, 183
Overdose. *See* Drug abuse;
    Poisoning

Ovulation. *See* Secretory phase, men-
    strual cycle
Oxygen, 64
    administering. *See also* Artificial
        ventilation
        dental appliances and, 111
        cylinders, 109–110
        equipment for delivery, 110–111
Oxygen flow formula, 110
Oxygen therapy, pediatric patients, 296
Oxygen transport, 217–218

P
Page, James O., 5–6
Palmar, anatomical term, 36
Pancreas, 182*f*, 184
Pancreatitis, 171
Panic attacks, 191
Paralysis, spastic, 324–325
Paramedics, 5–7
    vs emergency medical technician, 6
Paranoid disorder, 192
Paraplegia, 320–321
Parasympathetic nervous system, 242
Parathyroid gland, 182, 182*f*
Parenchymal hemorrhage. *See*
    Cerebral hemorrhage
Parenting styles, and toddlers, 52
Partial seizures, 146. *See also* specific
    types
Parts per million (PPM), 363
Patient assessment, 77–89, 77*t*
    acute abdomen dialysis, 173–174
    allergic reactions and, 154
    baseline vital signs, 85–88, 85*t*
    in behavioral emergencies, 194–195
    cardiac emergency, 131–132
    in genitourinary and renal emer-
        gencies, 200–205
    geriatric, 310–312, 316
    inadequate breathing, 98
    injuries. *See* Injury assessment
    pediatric patients, 295*t*, 296–297
    during pregnancy, 282
    primary, 77–79
    respiratory system, 116–118
    shock patient, 223–224
    spinal injuries, 244
    for suicide risk, 190
    trauma, 231–232
Patient history
    allergies, 88
    events, 89
    last oral intake, 89
    medications in, 89

Patient history (*Cont.*):
  pertinent past history, 89
  SAMPLE, 88–89
  signs/symptoms, 88
Patients. *See also* Medical patient;
      Trauma patients
  access, during extrication, 349
  assessment of. *See* Patient assessment
  with communicable diseases, 330
  confidentiality/confidential infor-
      mation, 30
  culturally diverse, 329
  dying, needs of, emergency medical
      technicians and, 12
  elderly, communications issues
      with, 18
  geriatric. *See* Geriatric patients
  lifting and moving, 335–340
  pediatric. *See* Pediatric patients
  positioning during transport,
      339–340
  principles of moving, 337–340
  priority, identification of, 79
  refusal to treatment, 21–22, 28–29
  reporting concepts, 16–17
  respiratory system assessment,
      38–39
  restraining, 195–196
  safety during extrication, 348
  semidecontaminated, procedures in
      transporting, 371–372
  transferring to ambulance, 345
Patients with special challenges
  arthritis, 324
  cancer, 324
  cerebral palsy, 324
  communicable diseases, 330
  culturally diverse patients, 329
  cystic fibrosis, 325
  developmental delay, 321–322
  Down syndrome, 322
  emotional impairments, 322–323
  emotionally/mentally impaired, 323
  hearing impairments, 318–319
  multiple sclerosis, 325–326
  muscular dystrophy, 326–327
  myasthenia gravis, 328
  obesity, 320
  paraplegia/quadriplegia, 320–321
  poliomyelitis, 327
  spastic paralysis, 324–325
  speech impairments, 319–320
  spina bifida, 328
  traumatic brain injury, 327–328
  visual impairments, 319

PCR. *See* Pre-hospital care
      report (PCR)
Pediatric patients. *See also* Children
  airway concerns, 294–295
  assessment, 296–297
  body systems, review of, 303–304
  child abuse and neglect, 304
  developmental considerations,
      293–294
  newborn care, 288*f*
  and oxygen administration, 111
  oxygen therapy, 296
  problems
    airway obstructions, 297–298
    altered mental status, 301
    croup, 299–300, 299*t*
    epiglottitis, 300
    fever, 301
    near drowning, 302
    poisonings, 301
    respiratory emergencies,
      298–299
    seizures, 300–301
    shock, 302
    sudden infant death syndrome,
      302–303
    trauma, 303
  with special needs, 304–305
Peer group, toddlers and, 52
PEL. *See* Permissible exposure
      limit (PEL)
Pelvic inflammatory disease (PID),
      172, 210
Pelvis, 37
Penetrating trauma, 231
Penetration/puncture, 235
Peptic ulcer disease, 169
Perfusion
  assessment of, 79
  defined, 44
  physiology of, 215–216
  tissue, 218
Perineum, 281
Peripheral circulation, 44
Peripheral nervous system, 45, 242
Peripheral pulse, 131
Peritoneal dialysis, 173
Permissible exposure limit (PEL), 364
Personal protective equipment (PPE)
  eye protection, 175, 176*f*
  gloves, 175, 176*f*
  gowns, 175, 176*f*
  hazardous materials, 368–370,
      369–370*f*
  masks, 175, 177*f*

protective clothing, 178, 368–370,
      369–370*f*
  training, 378–379
Petit mal seizure, 146
Pharynx, 95
Phenytoin, 148
Phobias
  classifications, 191
  symptoms, 192
Physical examination. *See also*
      Injury assessment; Patient
      assessment
  in genitourinary and renal emer-
      gencies, 204–205
  geriatric patients, 312
  medical patient, 84–85, 85*t*
PID. *See* Pelvic inflammatory
      disease (PID)
Pituitary gland, 181, 182*f*, 183*f*
Placenta, 281
Placenta previa, 285
Plantar, anatomical term, 36
Plasma, 43, 130
Platelets, 43, 130
Play, toddlers, 52
Pleural effusion, 123
Pneumonia, 124
Pneumothorax, 122–123, 255
Poisoning
  absorbed, 159–160, 364
  action cycle, 365
  acute cyanide, 162–163
  and airway management, 160
  alcohol, 166
  carbon monoxide, 161, 162*f*
  cholinergic, 68
  emergency management, 158–161
  ingested, 158–159
  inhaled, 159
  medications for treatment, 160–161
  organophosphate, treatment
      of, 68–69
  in pediatric patients, 301
  toxic injection, 159
Poliomyelitis, 327
Polycystic ovarian syndrome, 211
Polydipsia, 185
Polymenorrhea, 208
Polyphagia, 185
Polyuria, 185
Portable radios, communication sys-
      tem component, 15
Portable suction unit, 101*f*
Posterior, anatomical term, 36
Posterior tibial artery, 43, 130

Posttraumatic stress disorder (PTSD), 192
PPE. *See* Personal protective equipment (PPE)
PPM. *See* Parts per million (PPM)
Pralidoxime, 66–67
Preeclampsia
    emergency management, 284
    signs/symptoms, 283–284
Pregnancy
    ectopic, 173, 283
    emergency childbirth
        abnormal delivery, 288–289
        normal delivery, 286–287, 286f
    patient assessment, 282
Pre-hospital care report (PCR), 19f, 20–21
Pre-hospital medications, 4–5, 64–70
    albuterol sulfate, 64–65
    aspirin, 69
    cholinergic poisonings, 68
    epinephrine, 65
    Mark-I auto-injector, 65–66
    nitroglycerin, 69–70
    oral glucose, 64
    organophosphate poisonings, treatment of, 68–69
    oxygen, 64
    pralidoxime, 66–67
Preload, 216
Premature birth, 289
Premenstrual syndrome
    causes, 207
    signs/symptoms, 207–208
Prerenal acute renal failure, 197
Pressure points, controlling bleeding through, 221
Priapism
    low-flow, 199
    risk factors, 200
Primary contamination, 364
Progesterone, 183
Prolapsed cord, 288–289
Proliferation phase, menstrual cycle, 206–207
Prone, anatomical term, 36
Prostatitis, 173, 199
Protective barriers. *See* Personal protective equipment (PPE); Universal precautions
Protective clothing, 178, 368–370, 369–370f
Proventil, 64–65
Proximal, anatomical term, 36

Psychiatric disorders, 190–192. *See also* specific disorders
Psychological crises. *See* Behavioral emergencies; Psychiatric disorders
Psychoses, 321
Psychosocial development
    adolescents, 54
    adults, 54–55
    infants, 50
    older adults, 57
    school-age children, 53
    toddlers, 51–52
PTSD. *See* Posttraumatic stress disorder (PTSD)
Pulmonary arteries, 42, 129
Pulmonary edema, in geriatric patient, 313
Pulmonary embolism, 123
    in geriatric patient, 314
Pulmonary system
    infants, 47
    toddlers, 51
Pulmonary vein, 43, 130
Pulse
    administering CPR in absence of, 131
    assessment of, 86–87
    central, 131
    generation of, 43
    peripheral, 131
Pulse oximetry, and respiratory system assessment, 118
Pupils, assessment of, 87–88
Purkinje fibers, 42, 129
Pyelonephritis, 172, 198

Q

QI. *See* Quality improvement (QI)
Quadriplegia, 320–321, 324
Quality improvement (QI), 9
    continuous, 22

R

Radial arteries, 43, 130
Radiation absorbed dose (RAD), 377t
Radio communication system, 15–16
Red blood cells, 43, 130
Reflexes, infants, 48
Refusal of medical assistance, 28–29, 29f
Renal failure, 172
Renal system
    emergencies. *See* Genitourinary and renal emergencies
    geriatric patients, 309

infants, 48
    older adults, 56
    toddlers, 51
Repeater/base station, communication system component, 15
Reports. *See* Documentation
Reproductive system emergencies. *See also* Gynecological emergencies
    female, 172–173
    male, 173
Rescue, hazardous material incidents, 178–179
Research, outcome-based, practice driven by, 6–7
Resistance stage, of stress, 193
Respiratory disorders
    adult respiratory distress syndrome, 119–120
    asthma, 121–122
    chronic bronchitis, 120–121
    common cold, 124
    croup, 124
    emergencies
        in geriatric patient, 313–314
        in pediatric patients, 298–299
    emphysema, 120
    epiglottitis, 124
    hyperventilation syndrome, 123
    management of, 118–119
    pediatric, 299–300
    pleural effusion, 123
    pneumonia, 124
    pneumothorax, 122–123
    pulmonary embolism, 123
Respiratory rate, assessment of, 118
Respiratory system
    anatomy, 95–96, 96f, 115, 116f
    assessment of, 38–39, 116–118, 154
    disorders. *See* Respiratory disorders
    exhalation, 38
    function of, 37
    geriatric patients, 309
    inhalation, 38
    older adults, 56
    pediatric considerations, 39, 98
    physiology, 38, 96, 97f, 116
Rheumatoid arthritis, 324
Ribs, 36
Ritalin, 165
Robitussin DM, 165

S

Safety, scene, 175–177
SAH. *See* Subarachnoid
    hemorrhage (SAH)
SAMPLE history, 88–89, 117
    geriatric patient, 311–312
SARA. *See* Superfund Amendments
    and Reauthorizations
    Act (SARA)
Scene size-up
    body substance isolation, 76
    dispatcher and, 75
    and EMT safety, 76
    and geriatric patient, 310
    hazardous materials, 359
Schizophrenia, 192
School-age children, 52–53
    bodily functions, 52
    growth rate of, 52
    psychosocial development, 53
Secondary contamination, 364
Secretory phase, menstrual cycle, 207
Seizures
    causes of, 147
    in children, 300–301
    emergency management, 149,
        300–301
    generalized, 146
    in geriatric patients, 315
    medications, 148–149
    myoclonic, 147
    partial, 146
    statistics, 145–146
    status epilepticus, 147–148
    types of, 146–147
Self-concept development, school-age
    children and, 53
Sellick maneuver, 38
Semiautomated defibrillator, 133
Semidecontaminated patients, proce-
    dures in transporting, 371–372
Sensorineural deafness, 318–319
Sensory changes, in older adults,
    56–57
Septic shock, 222
Serotonin syndrome, 165
Sexually transmitted disease (STD),
    209–210
Shock, 131
    anaphylactic, 223
    cardiogenic, 221–222
    at cellular level, 218–219
    defined, 44, 215
    and geriatric patients, 315–316
    hypovolemic, 220–221

inappropriate delivery, causes of, 134
management, 224
neurogenic, 222
pathophysiology, 215
patient assessment, 223–224
pediatric patients, 302
physiological response, 218
septic, 222
stages of, 219–220. *See also* specific
    stages
Shock position, anatomical term, 36
Short-term exposure limit
    (TLV-STEL), 364
Sibling relationships, toddlers and, 52
Sickle cell anemia, 137
    signs/symptoms, 137–138
    treatment, 138
Simple partial seizures, 146
Simple phobias, 191
Simple triage and rapid treatment
    (START), 358–359
    and patients categorization, 359
    process of, 359–360
    steps in assessment, 360, 360*f*
Sinoatrial (SA) node, 41, 42, 129
Skeletal system. *See also*
    Musculoskeletal system
    components of, 36–37, 36*f*. *See also*
        specific components
    function in relation to spine, 242
Skin
    assessment of, 79, 87, 154
    function of, 233
    functions of, 45
    layers of, 45, 45*f*, 233, 234*f*. *See also*
        specific layers
Skull, 36, 239*f*
    injuries. *See* Head, injuries
    skeletal system of, 243
Sleep, infants, 49
SLUDGEM syndrome, 61
Snakes bites, 274–275, 276
Social phobias, 191
Soft tissue injuries
    closed, 233–234
    emergency management, 234, 235
    open, 234–236
Somatization, 192–193
Somatoform disorders, 192–193
Spastic paralysis, 324–325
Special needs patients, pediatric,
    304–305
Specific gravity, 363
Speech impairments, 319–320
Spider bites, 274, 276

Spina bifida, 328
Spinal column, 36
Spinal cord, 242
    injuries. *See* Spinal injuries
    skeletal system and, 242, 243*f*
    skeletal system of, 243
Spinal injuries, 241
    complications of, 245
    emergency management, 245
    mechanism of injury, 243–245
    moving patient and, 337–338
    patient assessment, 244
    signs/symptoms, 244
Splinting, 263
    complications, 264
    joint injury, 264
    rules, 264
    traction, 264–265
Spontaneous abortion, 283
Spraying dissemination devices, 378
START. *See* Simple triage and rapid
    treatment (START)
Status epilepticus, 147–148
STD. *See* Sexually transmitted
    disease (STD)
Sternum, 37
Stingrays, 275, 277
Stress
    incontinence, 211
    management, EMTs and, 12–13
    physical changes during, 193
    warning signs of, 12
Stretcher
    mechanical lift, 335–336, 336*f*
    transferring supine patient from
        bed to, 339
Stroke
    basilar artery blockage and, 144
    carotid artery blockage and,
        143–144
    Cincinnati Pre-hospital Stroke
        Scale, 145*t*
    classifications, 142–145, 143*t*
    in geriatric patients, 314
    hemorrhagic, 143, 143*t*, 144–145
    ischemic, 143, 143*t*
    management goals for patients, 145
    prior risk factors, 141–142
    warning signs, 142
Stroke volume, 216
Subarachnoid hemorrhage (SAH), 143
    signs/symptoms, 144–145
Subcutaneous skin layer, 45, 45*f*
Subcutaneous tissue, 233, 234*f*
"Sucking chest wound," 254

Suction catheters, 102
Suctioning techniques, 99, 101
Suction units, 101, 101–102f
Sudden infant death syndrome
     emergency management, 303
     signs/symptoms, 302
Suicidal ideation, warning signs
     of, 193–194
Suicide, 190, 193–194
Suicidology, defined, 193
Superfund Amendments and
     Reauthorizations Act
     (SARA), 358
Superior, anatomical term, 36
Supine, anatomical term, 36
Sympathetic nervous system, 242
Syncope
     causes of, 150
     emergency management, 150
     in geriatric patients, 315
System medical director, 9
System pressures, 217
Systolic blood pressure, 44, 131

T
TBIs. See Traumatic brain
     injuries (TBIs)
Technical Assistance Program
     Standards for EMS
     (NHTSA), 7
Technical hazards, 356, 357f
Tegretol, 148
Television, exposure to, toddlers
     and, 52
Temperament, infants, 50
Temperature, regulation of. See
     Environmental emergencies;
     Hyperthermia; Hypothermia
Tension pneumothorax, 255–256
Terminal drop hypothesis, 57
Terminally ill patients, 329–330
Terrorism. See also Weapons of mass
     destruction (WMD)
     defined, 372
     threat, 372–373
     World Trade Center, 373f
Testes, 182f, 183–184
Testicular torsion, 173, 198
Thorax, 36
Thorazine, 191
Threshold limit value (TLV), 363
Thyroid gland, 182, 182f
Tissue hypoxia, 39
Tissue perfusion, 218
TLV. See Threshold limit value (TLV)

TOA. See Tuboovarian abscess (TOA)
Toddlers, 50–52
     cardiovascular system, 50
     dental system, 51
     elimination patterns, 51
     immune system, 51
     musculoskeletal system, 51
     nervous system, 51
     psychosocial development, 51–52
     pulmonary system, 51
     renal system, 51
     weight of, 50
Tonic-clonic seizure, 146
     stages of, 147–148
Topamax, 148
Torso, anatomical term, 35
Tourniquet, to control bleeding, 221
Toxic injection poisoning, 159
Toxic shock syndrome (TSS), 210
Toxins, 376
Tracheotomy tube, and special needs
     pediatric patients, 305
Traction splinting, 264–265
Trade/brand name, medications, 61
Training, EMT
     formal origins of, 4
     specialty, 176
Transient ischemic attack, in geriatric
     patients, 314
Transportation
     patient refusal to, 28–29
     and semidecontaminated patient,
     371–372
Tranxene, 149
Trauma
     assessment of, 79–83, 80t
     blast injuries, 231
     blunt, 227–230
     falls, 231
     and geriatric patient, 315–316
     head. See Traumatic brain injuries
     (TBIs)
     kinematics, 226–227
     patient assessment, 231–232
     in pediatric patients, 303
     penetrating, 231
Trauma patients. See also Injury
     assessment; Mechanism of
     injury (MOI)
     geriatric, 311
     guidelines for assessment, 82t
     high-risk, 81–83
Traumatic brain injuries (TBIs), 238,
     327–328
     signs/symptoms, 240

Trendelenburg, anatomical term, 36
Triage
     benefits of, 358
     purpose of, 358
     secondary, 360–361
     START, 358–361, 360f
Trileptal, 148
TSS. See Toxic shock
     syndrome (TSS)
Tuboovarian abscess (TOA), 210

U
Umbilical cord, 281
Universal precautions, 175–177
Unresponsive patient
     assessment for spinal injury, 244
     medical, 84
Upper airway, 95
Upper extremities, 37
Upper GI hemorrhage, 170–171
Ureterolithiasis, 198
Urinary calculi, 198. See also Kidney
     stones
Urinary incontinence. See
     Incontinence
Urinary tract infections (UTIs),
     172, 197
     causes, 198
     classifications, 198
Uterine rupture, 285
Uterus, 281
UTIs. See Urinary tract
     infections (UTIs)

V
Vagina, 281
Vaginitis, 210
Valium, 149
Vapor density (VD), 363
Vapor pressure, 363
VD. See Vapor density (VD)
Vectors, 378
Veins, 43, 130
Venae cavae, 43, 130
Ventilators, home, and special needs
     pediatric patients, 305
Ventolin, 64–65
Ventral, anatomical term, 36
Ventricle, 40
Ventricular fibrillation, recurrent,
     135, 135f
Ventricular tachycardia, 134, 134f
Venule, 43, 130
Verbal communication, 18
Vicks VapoRub, 165

Violence
   assessment in behavioral
      emergencies, 195
   victim of, crime scene
      and, 179
Viruses, 376
Visual acuity, toddlers, 51
Visual impairments, 319
Voice production disorders, 320
Voluntary (skeletal)
   muscles, 44

W
Warm zone, hazardous materials, 359,
   362f, 363
Wasps sting, 274, 276
Water solubility, 363

Weapons of mass destruction
   (WMD), 372
   biological agents, 375–376
   chemical agents, 374–375
   dissemination devices,
      377–378
   ease of creating, 373–374
   indicators of attack, 374
   levels of protection
      against, 379
   limitations, 374
   outcomes of attack, 374
   personal protection against,
      378–379
   radiological/nuclear weapons,
      376–377
Wedsworth-Townsend Act, 5

Weight
   of infants, 47
   of toddlers, 50
Westley score, for croup severity, 299t
West syndrome, 147
White blood cells, 43, 130
Wind Chill chart, 268f
WMD. *See* Weapons of mass destruc-
   tion (WMD)
World Trade Center, 373f

Z
Zarontin, 148
Zonegran, 149
Zones, hazardous materials, 359,
   362–363, 362f. *See also*
   specific zones